Multidisciplinary Spine Tumor Management

Yoshiya Yamada • Mark H. Bilsky • Eric Lis
Editors

Multidisciplinary Spine Tumor Management

A Modern Approach

Springer

Editors
Yoshiya Yamada
Department of Radiation Oncology
Memorial Sloan Kettering Cancer Center
New York, NY, USA

Mark H. Bilsky
Department of Neurosurgery
Memorial Sloan Kettering Cancer Center
New York, NY, USA

Eric Lis
Department of Radiology
Memorial Sloan Kettering Cancer Center
New York, NY, USA

ISBN 978-3-032-07518-5 ISBN 978-3-032-07519-2 (eBook)
https://doi.org/10.1007/978-3-032-07519-2

This Springer imprint is published by the registered company Springer Nature Switzerland AG
The registered company address is: Gewerbestrasse 11, 6330 Cham, Switzerland

Contents

1 **Introduction** 1
Yoshiya Yamada, Eric Lis, and Mark H. Bilsky

2 **NOMS: Roadmap to Multidisciplinary Metastatic Spine Tumor Management** 3
Mark H. Bilsky, Alexandra Giantini-Larsen, Natasha Kharas, W. Christopher Newman, and Yoshiya Yamada

3 **The Role of Vertebral Cement Augmentation** 17
Eric Lis

4 **The Role of Surgery in the Modern Management of Primary Tumors of the Mobile Spine** 39
Mark H. Bilsky, Natasha Kharas, Alexandra Giantini-Larsen, W. Christopher Newman, and Yoshiya Yamada

5 **Separation Surgery for Spinal Metastatic Cancer** 51
W. Christopher Newman

6 **Minimally Invasive Surgery in Spine Oncology** 63
Rabih Bou Nassif, W. Christopher Newman, Mark H. Bilsky, and Ori Barzilai

7 **The Multidisciplinary Management of Sacral Tumors** 75
Max Vaynrub

8 **Radiotherapy for Primary Tumors of the Spine** 89
Daniel Higginson

9 **Stereotactic Radiotherapy for Spine Metastases** 123
Christopher Jackson, E. Christopher Dee, and Yoshiya Yamada

10 **Treatment Planning for Spine SBRT** 141
Masoud Zarepisheh, Lei Zhang, and Linda Hong

11 **Spine Radiation Toxicity and Management** 167
Boris Mueller

12 **Toxicities of Overlapping Spine Radiotherapy and Systemic Therapy** 183
Justin Haseltine

13 **Genomic Biomarkers to Guide the Management of Spine Metastases** 197
Gustav Cederquist and Adam Schmitt

14 **Pain Management of Spine Tumors** 213
Ingharan Siddarthan and Amitabh Gulati

15 **Rehabilitation of the Spine Tumor Patient** 235
Kristen de Vries and Lisa Marie Ruppert

16 **How a Multidisciplinary Spine Oncology Service Functions** 255
Mark H. Bilsky and Yoshiya Yamada

Index 263

Contributors

Ori Barzilai Department of Neurosurgery, Memorial Sloan-Kettering Cancer Center, New York, NY, USA

Mark H. Bilsky Department of Neurosurgery, Memorial Sloan Kettering Cancer Center, New York, NY, USA

Gustav Cederquist Department of Radiation Oncology, Memorial Sloan Kettering Cancer Center, New York, NY, USA

Kristen de Vries Rehabilitation Medicine Service, Department of Neurology, Memorial Sloan Kettering Cancer Center, New York, NY, USA

Department of Rehabilitation Medicine, Weill Cornell Medical Center, New York, NY, USA

E. Christopher Dee Department of Radiation Oncology, Memorial Sloan Kettering Cancer Center, New York, NY, USA

Alexandra Giantini-Larsen Department of Neurological Surgery, Memorial Sloan-Kettering Cancer Center, New York, NY, USA

Amitabh Gulati Department of Anesthesiology and Critical Care Medicine, Memorial Sloan Kettering Cancer Center, New York, NY, USA

Justin Haseltine Memorial Sloan Kettering Cancer Center, Department of Radiation Oncology, New York, NY, USA

Daniel Higginson Department of Radiation Oncology, Memorial Sloan Kettering Cancer Center, New York, NY, USA

Linda Hong Department of Medical Physics, Memorial Sloan Kettering Cancer Center, New York, NY, USA

Christopher Jackson Department of Radiation Oncology, Memorial Sloan Kettering Cancer Center, New York, NY, USA

Natasha Kharas Department of Neurological Surgery, Memorial Sloan-Kettering Cancer Center, New York, NY, USA

Eric Lis Department of Radiology, Memorial Sloan Kettering Cancer Center, New York, NY, USA

Boris Mueller MSKCC, Radiation Oncology, New York, NY, USA

Rabih Bou Nassif Department of Neurosurgery, Memorial Sloan-Kettering Cancer Center, New York, NY, USA

W. Christopher Newman Department of Neurological Surgery, Memorial Sloan-Kettering Cancer Center, New York, NY, USA

Lisa Marie Ruppert Rehabilitation Medicine Service, Department of Neurology, Memorial Sloan Kettering Cancer Center, New York, NY, USA

Department of Rehabilitation Medicine, Weill Cornell Medical Center, New York, NY, USA

Adam Schmitt Department of Radiation Oncology, Memorial Sloan Kettering Cancer Center, New York, NY, USA

Ingharan Siddarthan Department of Anesthesiology, Weill Cornell Medical College, New York, NY, USA

Department of Anesthesiology and Critical Care Medicine, Memorial Sloan Kettering Cancer Center, New York, NY, USA

Max Vaynrub Department of Surgery, Orthopaedic Service, Memorial Sloan Kettering Cancer Center, New York, NY, USA

Yoshiya Yamada Department of Neurological Surgery, Memorial Sloan-Kettering Cancer Center, New York, NY, USA

Spinal Oncology Service, Department of Radiation Oncology, Memorial Sloan Kettering Cancer Center, New York, NY, USA

Masoud Zarepisheh Department of Medical Physics, Memorial Sloan Kettering Cancer Center, New York, NY, USA

Lei Zhang Department of Medical Physics, Memorial Sloan Kettering Cancer Center, New York, NY, USA

Chapter 1
Introduction

Yoshiya Yamada, Eric Lis, and Mark H. Bilsky

Best practice care for spine tumor patients is important. Optimal treatment paradigms for spine malignancies are a rapidly evolving landscape as new diagnostic and treatment tools arrive at an ever-increasing pace. Advances in systemic therapy, molecular diagnostics, surgical techniques, interventional procedures, diagnostic imaging, and radiation therapy treatment tools and technologies have exponentially improved outcomes for spine tumors. In addition, new pain management approaches and the skills of rehabilitative medicine need to be incorporated into the treatment plans for the care of these often complex and vexing clinical conditions. In the twenty-first century, the optimal management of spine tumor patients is sufficiently complex that the best results can only be achieved as a multidisciplinary team. One of the goals of this book is to provide a summary of the individual components of multidisciplinary spine tumor care. This book emphasizes the importance of a multidisciplinary team approach focused on coordinating a diverse group of specialists whose collective skills and expertise can be exercised on behalf of the patient in need.

At Memorial Sloan Kettering Cancer Center, we have been practicing this model of multidisciplinary spine oncology care for nearly a quarter of a century. As a group, we have published over 250 peer-reviewed articles on various aspects of spine tumor management, which have been cited over 20,000 times in the medical literature. This book represents our collective experience in advancing spine tumor

Y. Yamada (✉)
Department of Radiation Oncology, Memorial Sloan Kettering Cancer Center, New York, NY, USA
e-mail: yamadaj@mskcc.org

E. Lis
Department of Radiology, Memorial Sloan Kettering Cancer Center, New York, NY, USA

M. H. Bilsky
Department of Neurosurgery, Memorial Sloan Kettering Cancer Center, New York, NY, USA

Y. Yamada et al. (eds.), *Multidisciplinary Spine Tumor Management*, https://doi.org/10.1007/978-3-032-07519-2_1

treatment. We hope that it will be of some benefit to those seeking to provide the best level of care for their patients.

Importantly, we gratefully acknowledge the critical contributions of the members of the spine oncology service at MSKCC, represented by neurosurgeons, radiation oncologists, orthopedic surgeons, interventional radiologists, physiatrists, pain specialists, as well as the dedicated nurses and allied providers, without whom none of this would have been possible.

Chapter 2
NOMS: Roadmap to Multidisciplinary Metastatic Spine Tumor Management

Mark H. Bilsky, Alexandra Giantini-Larsen, Natasha Kharas, W. Christopher Newman, and Yoshiya Yamada

Metastatic spine tumors are a major source of morbidity and mortality in the cancer population. The principal goals of treatment for metastatic tumors are to provide effective and durable palliation in terms of improving or maintaining neurologic function, providing mechanical stability, pain relief and quality of life. Over the past several decades, the treatment of metastatic tumors has transitioned significantly with the development of advanced surgical and radiation techniques, necessitating updates to treatment algorithms. Prior to the 1990s, conventional external beam radiation (cEBRT), e.g., 30 Gy in 10 fractions, had become the standard treatment as it was associated with equivalent outcomes and less morbidity compared to laminectomy without instrumentation [1]. Laminectomy was a poor approach to spine tumors as it was associated with neurologic decline, iatrogenic instability, progressive deformity, and pain. By the 1990s, revolutionary surgical advances included the development of segmental spine instrumentation, aggressive surgical approaches such as anterior transcavitary and *en bloc* resection [2–7], and embolization for hypervascular tumors [8]. In 2005, Patchell et al provided Class 1 evidence in a landmark prospective randomized trial demonstrating the significant benefits of surgery compared to cEBRT in treating myelopathy from solid tumor malignancies [9]. Based on these advances, the pendulum swung from radiation to surgery reflected in the proliferation of surgically based decision-making algorithms, such as the Tomita and Tokuhashi scores [2, 10]. Spine stereotactic radiosurgery (sSRS) represented the next revolutionary treatment of metastatic spine tumors, as it provided histology-independent durable responses by overcoming the radioresistance seen with cEBRT in solid tumor malignancies. The development, integration, and

M. H. Bilsky (✉) · A. Giantini-Larsen · N. Kharas · W. C. Newman · Y. Yamada
Department of Neurological Surgery, Memorial Sloan-Kettering Cancer Center, New York, NY, USA
e-mail: bilskym@mskcc.org

Y. Yamada et al. (eds.), *Multidisciplinary Spine Tumor Management*,
https://doi.org/10.1007/978-3-032-07519-2_2

evolution of sSRS ushered in the modern era of multidisciplinary decision making for spine metastases represented in the NOMS decision framework [11–17].

The NOMS decision framework was initially proposed at Memorial Sloan Kettering Cancer Center (MSKCC) in 2004 to simplify and codify complex multidisciplinary assessments of metastatic spine tumors that frequently require urgent or emergent treatment. The treatment of metastatic spine tumors requires multidisciplinary care and is predicated on the consensus opinions of physicians, including radiation oncologists, spine surgeons, medical oncologists, interventional radiologists, interventional pain specialists, and physiatrists. NOMS provides a comprehensive analysis of the fundamental issues that need to be considered by the multitude of physicians who often have siloed expertise. For instance, when NOMS was developed 20 years ago, radiation oncologists possessed a nuanced understanding of differential histology-dependent tumoral responses to conventional external beam radiation (cEBRT) but had very little concept of fracture-related instability. Irradiating multiple myeloma with an unstable burst fracture at the thoracolumbar junction has a high probability of achieving tumor control but has no impact on addressing the severe mechanical pain. Conversely, spine surgeons understood the concept of instability but had no sense of how exquisitely sensitive multiple myeloma is to radiation. This disconnect led to innumerable patients undergoing complicated multi-level surgery for tumor control while incurring substantial morbidity that could have been avoided with conventional external beam radiation (cEBRT) alone. Ultimately, effective palliation can only be achieved by understanding and addressing critical issues in spine-tumor management.

At MSKCC, NOMS is the cornerstone of our multidisciplinary effort, as it provides a framework for making consistent, timely, and individualized decisions on this complicated patient population to meet the goals of palliation in the context of overall cancer care. The four sentinel decision points in NOMS are Neurologic, Oncologic, Mechanical (stability) and Systemic disease (Fig. 2.1). The Neurologic assessment considers both clinical and radiographic parameters, including the presence of myelopathy, functional radiculopathy and the degree of epidural spinal cord compression (ESCC). The Oncologic consideration reflects the most effective strategy for achieving local tumor control, which is principally based on the expected response to radiation therapy and systemic treatment. Mechanical stability considers whether a pathologic fracture creates significant movement-related pain that requires an interventional procedure or external orthosis. The final consideration is the extent of systemic disease and medical comorbidities, which traditionally have been an assessment of a patient's ability to tolerate a proposed procedure based on NOM and the predicted survival; however, the recent additional NOMS systemic considerations are whether local treatment for spine metastases impacts overall survival and decreases the propensity for distant metastases.

Whereas the four sentinel decision points of NOMS have remained the same since its inception in 2004, the treatment decisions based on these assessments have changed dramatically over the past 20 years, with the integration of evidence-based medicine and new technologies significantly impacting every domain of spine tumor care. NOMS remains a decision framework, but new updated algorithms are

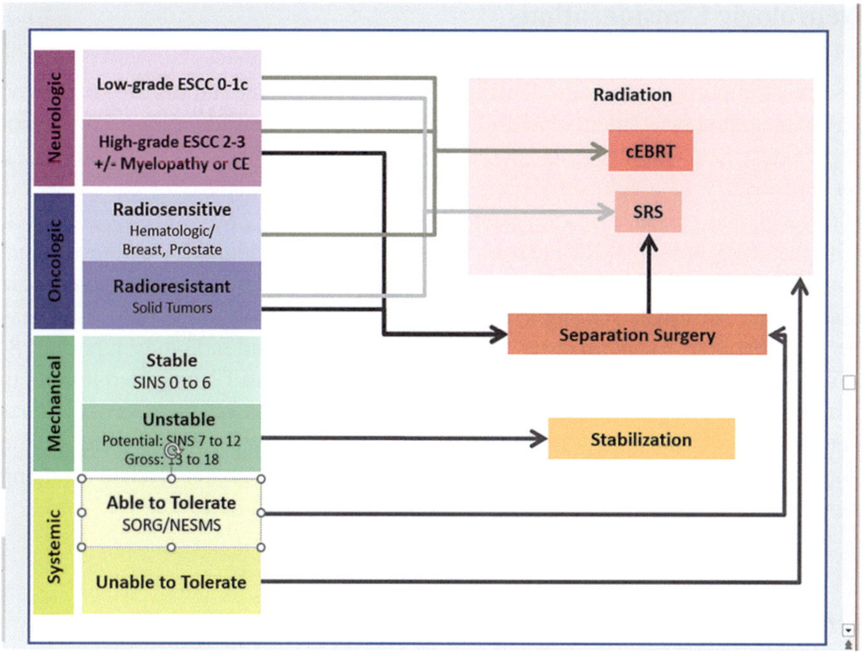

Fig. 2.1 NOMS figures

created and published approximately every 5 years based on the incorporation of these advances. The most disruptive technology impacting NOMS since its inception is the development and integration of spine stereotactic radiosurgery (sSRS). The ability of sSRS to deliver ablative radiation that is both histology and volume independent changed the indications for and type of surgery required. It has all but eliminated the need for *en bloc* or intralesional gross total resection in the metastatic population in lieu of definitive radiation or hybrid therapy, i.e., separation surgery followed by sSRS. In addition to proton beam and carbon ion radiation, sSRS has shown similarly great promise in the treatment of primary bone tumors such as chordoma, which will be covered in a separate chapter. Many centers do not have advanced technology integrated into the latest NOMS algorithm; however, NOMS can be modified based on the existing resources in any institution. The most critical issue is coordinating multidisciplinary care and finding a consensus agreement on each NOMS domain to facilitate timely care and optimize outcomes. The current iteration of the NOMS framework is presented along with new changes being integrated and several case examples.

Neurologic Considerations

The most important treatment decisions for metastatic spine tumors are predicated on an integrated assessment of neurologic and oncologic considerations. The neurologic assessment is both clinical and radiographic. The clinical assessment is based on the severity of myelopathy (i.e., ASIA score), completeness of cauda equina syndrome, and presence of a functional radiculopathy (i.e., MRC scale). However, with the integration of sSRS into treatment paradigms, radiographic epidural spinal cord compression (ESCC) also became a major determinant in the neurologic assessment. An ESCC scoring system, eponymously termed the Bilsky score, has been validated to standardize reporting in the literature and radiology reports [18] (Fig. 2.2). The ESCC score is a 6-point grade based on axial T2-weighted images in which 0 is bone only; 1a, 1b, and 1c are progressively increasing degrees of epidural deformation without spinal cord compression; 2 and 3 are spinal cord compression with or without CSF visualized, respectively. Traditionally, for decision-making purposes, ESCC grades 2 and 3 are considered to be high-grade.

Oncologic Considerations

The oncologic consideration assesses the optimal strategy to achieve local tumor control and is fundamentally dependent on the radiation and systemic therapy response. For spine tumors, cEBRT dose strategies include 30 Gy in 10 fractions,

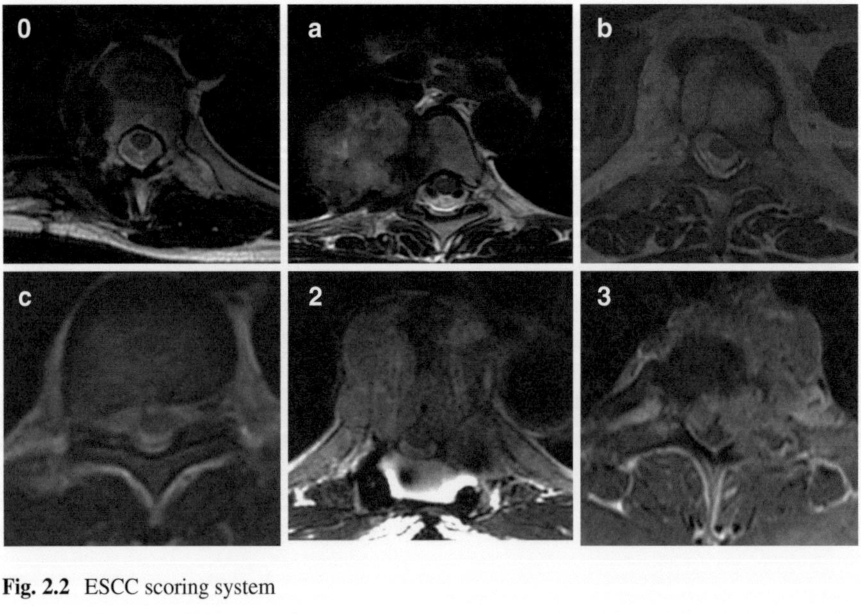

Fig. 2.2 ESCC scoring system

40 Gy in 20 fractions, and more recently 8 Gy single fraction. These doses were largely chosen because they were well within the tolerance of the spinal cord and other adjacent at-risk organs, but consequently were largely ineffective for ablating most spine metastases, resulting in early recurrences and local-tumor progression. cEBRT demonstrates a differential response based on tumor histology. The hematologic malignancies, such as lymphoma and multiple myeloma, are highly radiosensitive whereas the hormone-driven solid tumor malignancies, such as breast and prostate carcinoma, are moderately sensitive to cEBRT with durable response rates of greater than 80% at 2 years. However, the remainder of solid tumor malignancies are moderately to highly radioresistant to cEBRT and response rates in some series are reported to be as low as 30% at 3 months [19]. Thus, cEBRT is ineffective for treating very common spine metastases such as melanoma, sarcoma, colon, renal cell, and non-small cell lung carcinoma (NSCLC) in either the upfront or postoperative setting. Conversely, sSRS provides histology-independent responses, overcoming radioresistance using conformal high-dose hypofractionated radiation, typically given as 16–24 Gy single fraction or 24 to 30 Gy in 3 fractions [20–23]. However, sSRS cytotoxic tumoral doses are well above the tolerance of the spinal cord and other organs at risk such as the esophagus, bowel, and kidneys. Tight dose constraints on the spinal cord and cauda equina have been established such as a cord Dmax of 14 Gy for single fraction or 23.7 Gy for hypofractionated (e.g., 27 Gy in 3 fractions) treatment. The need to deliver an ablative tumoral dose tolerant of the spinal cord and cauda equina provides the rationale for surgery in patients with high-grade ESCC, even in the absence of myelopathy or cauda equina syndrome. However, the histology and volume independent responses to sSRS as a postoperative adjuvant have reduced the surgical goals from intralesional gross total resection or *en bloc* excision to simple separation surgery, i.e., posterolateral epidural decompression to reconstitute the thecal sac combined with posterior segmental fixation [14]. The combination of separation surgery followed by sSRS is commonly referred to as hybrid therapy.

Neurologic and Oncologic Decision-Making

Radiosensitive Tumors

ESCC 0 to 1c/2: cEBRT or SRS
ESCC 2/3 without myelopathy: cEBRT
ESCC 2/3 with myelopathy or cauda equina syndrome

Hematologic Malignancies cEBRT
Breast/Prostate Carcinoma: Hybrid Therapy

Radiosensitive tumors provide the widest range of treatment options, which continue to evolve. In principle, radiosensitive tumors can always be effectively treated with cEBRT regardless of the degree of ESCC in the absence of myelopathy or cauda equina syndrome. The hematologic malignancies in this setting are often treated with definitive systemic therapy rather than radiation. Many radiosensitive tumors are now receiving SRS, which is not only equally as effective as cEBRT but also decreases the number of fractions, thereby increasing the probability of compliance. SSRS also reduces the extent of soft tissue receiving radiation, which is particularly important if patients require subsequent spine surgery. Additionally, as noted in the subsequent systemic consideration's section, SRS portends a survival advantage compared to cEBRT for oligometastatic tumors [22, 23].

The quandary becomes the treatment of high-grade ESCC with myelopathy or cauda equina syndrome. Hematologic malignancies are exquisitely radiosensitive, demonstrating an apoptotic response with an expedient decompression of the spinal cord. Even though breast and prostate respond to cEBRT in the setting of high-grade ESCC, the cytoreductive effect takes weeks to months; thus, there is no effective immediate decompression. In our experience, neurologically symptomatic hormone-driven solid tumors are better treated with hybrid therapy rather than cEBRT only.

Radioresistant Tumor ESCC 0 to 1c: SSRS

Numerous studies have demonstrated the benefit of using sSRS in achieving durable local control rates greater than 85%, as definitive treatment for radioresistant solid tumor metastases presenting with ESCC 0 to 1c [20–23]. Yamada et al. demonstrated dose-dependent outcomes in 811 tumors treated in a cohort of 657 patients at MSK [20]. The prescription dose to the planning target volume ranged from 16 to 24 Gy for a single fraction. In this study, the low-dose cohort received a median dose of 16.4 Gy and the high-dose cohort received a median dose of 22.4 Gy. The local failure rate in the low-dose and high-dose cohorts was 5% vs. 0.41% at one year and 20% vs. 2.1% at 4 years, respectively. The only significant factor in the incidence of local failure was the dose of sSRS. As opposed to cEBRT, the tumor histology and size of the tumor did not impact tumor control rates for sSRS. SRS led to a change in the recommended treatment of solid tumor spine metastases presenting with ESCC 0 to 1c from *en bloc* resection to sSRS alone. This was reflected in a Cochrane review by Bilsky et al., who made a strong recommendation that patients with RCC in the absence of spinal cord compression (i.e., ESCC 0 to 1c) undergo stereotactic radiosurgery rather than en bloc resection [24]. This paper represented a major paradigm shift and helped sSRS become first-line therapy for radioresistant oligometastatic disease rather than en bloc resections. This paradigm shift was critical as en bloc resections were increasingly being applied to oligometastatic spine disease despite a paucity of published data demonstrating improved local-tumor control or survival, and most case reports uniformly failed to account for the significant surgical morbidity associated with the technique [3–5, 25, 26].

Radioresistant Tumor ESCC 2 Without Myelopathy: sSRS (Hypofractionated) or Hybrid Therapy

Traditionally, radioresistant tumors with ESCC 2 without neurologic symptoms are and continue to be treated with hybrid therapy. However, Rothrock et al. reviewed a series of 29 patients with ESCC 2 treated with hypofractionated sSRS using 24 to 30 Gy in 3 fractions [27]. All had contraindications to separation surgery. The 1-year and 2-year cumulative incidence of loco-regional failure was 10.4% and 22%, respectively, and those requiring same-level surgery at 2 years were 14.5%. Sophisticated radiation delivery system such as volumetric arc therapy, and further refinement of dose constraints, provides increasingly effective palliation using radiation alone. More recently Jackson, et.al., reported sSRS outcomes in 2702 lesions irradiated in 1838 patients using 3 dose strategies 24 Gy single fraction or 24 to 30 Gy in 3 fractions. In the cohort receiving hypofractionated sSRS, no difference was seen in the 2-yr local failure rates comparing ESCC 0 to 1c versus 2 to 3, 14% vs. 17% (p=0.3), respectively. Excluding breast and prostate carcinoma, solid tumor malignancies with ESCC 2 or 3 did seem to benefit from separation surgery plus sSRS compared to sSRS alone with 2-year LF rates of 7.9% vs. 20% (p=.051). However, this benefit may be less impactful in short-term survivors or high-risk surgical candidates [28].

Radioresistant Tumor ESCC 2–3 With or Without Myelopathy: Hybrid Therapy

Patchell et al. reported a landmark prospective randomized trial comparing cEBRT to surgery followed by cEBRT for patients presenting with high-grade spinal cord compression due to radioresistant solid-tumor malignancies [9]. Exquisitely radiosensitive hematologic malignancies and germ cell tumors were excluded. In every outcome variable, the surgical arm demonstrated improved outcomes compared to the cEBRT cohort, including maintenance or recovery of ambulation and bowel and bladder function, lower narcotic requirements, and improved survival. Based on the Patchell trial and numerous other studies demonstrating good surgical outcomes, Bilsky et al. reported a Cochrane review–based recommendation from the Spine Oncology Study Group (SOSG) that patients with high-grade spinal cord compression resulting from solid tumor malignancies should undergo surgery followed by radiation therapy [24].

Whereas the indications for surgery have remained unchanged since the publication of the Patchell study, the efficacy of postoperative sSRS has shifted surgical objectives [14, 29–31]. The improved local control of sSRS allowed for separation surgery, a surgical technique whereby the thecal sac is decompressed and reconstituted to create a 2mm margin between the tumor and the spinal cord for targeting constraints. Laufer et al. evaluated the strategy of separation surgery followed by sSRS (i.e., hybrid therapy) in 186 patients operated on for high-grade ESCC for predominantly radioresistant tumor histologies, with 50% of those patients having failed prior radiation therapy [14]. The three dose strategies used were high-dose single fraction (24 Gy), high-dose hypofractionated (24 to 30 Gy in 3 fractions) and low-dose hypofractionated (18 to 36 in 5 to 6 fractions). The 1-year cumulative recurrence rate was 16.4%, but patients undergoing high-dose single fraction or high-dose hypofractionated radiation had local recurrence rates of 9% and 4%, respectively. MSKCC subsequently examined histology-specific outcomes in patients undergoing hybrid therapy with a median postoperative adjuvant dose of 27 Gy in 3 fractions. Hussain et al. recently reported hybrid therapy for RCC in 90 patients using the same dose, demonstrating 1-year and 2-years cumulative incidence of recurrence were 4.6% and 8.2%, respectively [29]. Overall, 90% of patients remained ambulatory with an ECOG of 0 to 2 at one-year follow-up. Similarly, Chakravarthy et al. demonstrated similarly good outcomes in 103 patients undergoing hybrid therapy for non-small cell lung carcinoma, demonstrating 2-year local control rates of 94.6% (95% CI:89.8–99.3) [32]. Overall survival was impacted by initiating EGFR-targeted therapy in patients who harbored the mutation and were EGFR-inhibitor naïve. Similarly, Chakravarthy et al. examined outcomes in colorectal carcinoma, demonstrating LC in 86.7% at 2 years [33]. Of note, the adenomatous polyposis coli gene mutation conveyed a poor prognosis.

Unknown Tumor with Myelopathy: Hybrid Therapy

Tumors with an unknown histology often present as emergencies with high-grade ESCC and myelopathy or cauda equina syndrome. The default oncologic assessment in these patients is to assume the tumor is radioresistant and requires separation surgery as per the Patchell trial [9]. This is predicated on the fact that establishing a definitive histology in a timely manner is often very difficult and patients who are neurologically impaired frequently progress to paralysis in a relatively short period of time, even on high-dose steroids. Definitive surgical decompression ensures the best chance of neurologic recovery regardless of the ultimate tumor diagnosis. At surgery, if a presumptive radiosensitive diagnosis is made, our recommendation is to complete the spinal cord decompression rather than only biopsy in order to optimize the chance of neurologic recovery and provide time for wound healing prior to definitive radiation or chemotherapy. Surgeons have argued that emergency intralesional separation surgery of chordomas for spinal cord decompression jeopardizes cure, as these tumors have traditionally been treated with *en bloc* excision. However high-grade ESCC precludes *en bloc* spondylectomy to achieve the wide margins necessary to surgically cure chordoma. Additionally, chordoma is remarkably sensitive to sSRS as a postoperative adjuvant following intralesional resection with 90% 5-year local tumor control [34]. Regardless of histologic diagnosis or tumor radiosensitivity, prioritizing neurologic recovery with emergency separation surgery provides the best chance of effective palliation.

Mechanical Instability Decision-Making

Mechanical instability is a separate assessment from the neurologic and oncologic considerations as it is reflective of symptomatic spine fractures and will not respond to tumor-directed treatment such as radiation or chemotherapy therapy. Pathologic fractures often differ from traumatic fractures as they maintain the integrity of the interspinous ligaments and require a different means of assessment from commonly used trauma scores. The SINS criteria were developed to define instability in the neoplastic setting and provide guidance regarding the need for interventional procedures [35]. SINS has 6 criteria, which are weighted by their contribution to instability. The criteria include only one clinical assessment reflective of the presence of movement-related or axial load-pain in counter-distinction to biologic or tumor-related pain, which is present at night and morning, but improves with movement and walking. The remaining 5 assessments are all radiographic parameters with the highest point scores per category given to junctional spine levels, lytic bone destruction, presence of fracture subluxation, >50% vertebral body collapse, and bilateral posterior element destruction. SINS scores 0 to 6 are considered stable and often present as lytic vertebral compression fractures without significant movement-related pain. These commonly do not require brace application or a stabilization procedure and can be irradiated with no further surgical interventions. Scores of 7 to 12 are potentially unstable and management is largely left to the discretion and resources of the surgeon or interventional radiologist. Most painful burst or compression thoracic and lumbar fractures in this category can be effectively treated with percutaneous vertebral body cement augmentation, i.e., vertebra- or kyphoplasty, and/or an external orthosis. The CAFÉ study addresses pathologic fractures in this category and provides class 1 evidence that kyphoplasty is significantly better than medical management in terms of pain relief at 1-month and 1-year follow-up [36]. Scores >13 typically represent junctional vertebral body fractures with posterior element involvement and an additional subluxation. In our experience, these fractures require not only kypho- or vertebroplasty at the index level, but also a posterior tension band such as cement-augmented percutaneous pedicle screws 1-level above and below the index level or open surgery in the cervical spine. This scenario also occurs commonly in the atlanto-axial spine, which can be addressed posteriorly only with occipital-cervical fixation [37].

Systemic Decision-Making

The final critical assessment in NOMS is the impact of systemic disease and medical comorbidities on the patient's ability to tolerate treatment and whether it makes sense in the context of palliation to offer either surgery or even radiation therapy. In my practice, approximately 30% of the patients who have firm indications for surgery based on NOM are excluded based on the systemic assessment. This assessment is in many ways the most complicated of the NOMS framework as it is predicated not only on an urgent assessment of both a global health concerns related to cardiac, pulmonary, and hematologic issues as with any spine surgery, but also predicting survival based on cancer-related issues such as expected response to often third-line systemic agents or new targeted agents in clinical trials. It is perhaps the most difficult discussion a physician can have with a patient to recommend foregoing surgery, even with the inevitability that the patient will progress to paraplegia with loss of bowel and bladder function. However, in the context of palliation, it is very difficult to justify taking a patient to surgery who is predicted to have a very poor survival, has no realistic chance of returning to activities of daily living, or has a high probability of postoperative life-threatening medical complications. As healthcare providers, we put a priority on ambulation, but in the context of metastatic cancer care, there may well be other end-of-life priorities that are disrupted by spending time recovering from a futile surgery.

Expected survival is often used as a major determinant in the systemic assessment. The integration of biologics and checkpoints has extended survival for virtually every tumor histology and thus necessitates the development of new predictive models. Both the SORG nomogram and the New England Spinal Metastases Score were developed and validated in the era of these newer systemic therapies, making them significantly more impactful in decision-making than older models such as the Tomita, modified Tokuhashi, and Bauer scores [2, 10, 38–41]. Frailty indices are currently being developed and validated in this population to help with this assessment. These models can be used as general guides, but physician judgment, particularly from medical oncologists, still plays a big role in this assessment.

In addition to predictive models of survival based on cancer parameters, the additional assessments are based on existing medical comorbidities. The acute onset of myelopathy may preclude a full medical work-up, but there is often time to optimize medical issues such as medication adjustments for cardiac issues and pleural effusion drainage. Nadir counts can often be corrected with transfusions but also may respond within a couple of days to agents such as pegfilgrastim for neutropenia and romiplostim for thrombocytopenia. Deep venous thrombosis (DVT) is very commonly detected in non-ambulatory patients, occurring in 24% of spine-surgery patients on preoperative screening dopplers [42]. Patients may benefit from screening dopplers to identify occult DVTs. These can be managed with inferior vena cava filters, delaying full-dose anticoagulation for three weeks after surgery.

The quantum leap in the NOMS systemic assessment has occurred over the past 5 years in the domain of oligometastatic disease. Two sentinel prospective studies demonstrated the impact of SRS on not only local control but systemic disease control and survival. The SABR-COMET trial is a European phase 2 randomized trial comparing SBRT to cEBRT combined with best medical management [23]. In this study, the cohort undergoing SBRT had not only better local tumor control but also a significant improvement in overall survival. The PISA trial was a bone-only trial comparing two single-fraction SRS strategies, 16 Gy vs 24 Gy [22]. The 24-Gy cohort demonstrated improved local tumor control but, somewhat unexpectedly, a significant decrease in distant metastases. These studies have started to change radiation recommendations from only treating symptomatic or at-risk lesions to treating even small asymptomatic oligometastatic tumors.

Case Example (Fig. 2.3): A 78-year-old man with a history of metastatic Stage IV papillary thyroid carcinoma presented with progressive low back pain at night for 5 weeks. 5 days ago, his pain progressed to being severe axial load pain that worsened with lying flat, as well as a radiculopathy present with axial load. On neurological examination, the patient was full strength in the bilateral upper and lower extremities, had full sensation to light touch and pinprick in the upper and lower extremities, and had normal deep tendon reflexes. His MRI of the thoracic spine demonstrated a planum burst fracture at T5 with extension of tumor into the bilateral pedicles (Fig. 2.3a, b), with a CT scan (not shown) demonstrating lytic disease. Medically, the patient has a history of coronary artery disease with 4 stents, he takes aspirin daily, and he has chronic COPD without an oxygen requirement. His current systemic disease burden is limited to the left iliac bone, right posterior 8th rib, right humerus, and multiple subcentimeter pulmonary nodules.

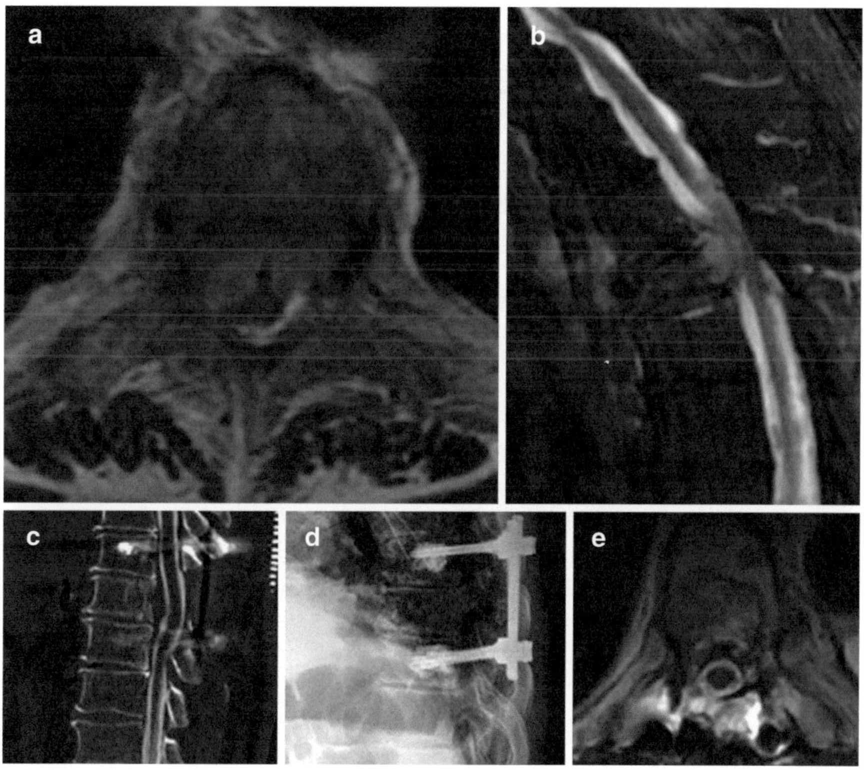

Fig. 2.3 Case example

NOMS Assessment

Neurologic: Patient was neurologically intact with ESCC Grade 3 based on the MRI.

Oncologic: Papillary thyroid cancer is a radioresistant histology.

Mechanical: The patient has evidence of mechanical instability and mechanical radiculopathy manifested by his worsening pain with standing upright, radiculopathy upon axial loading, and his difficulty with lying flat and pushing into his thoracic curvature. His SINS score is 14.

Systemic: The patient's systemic disease is progressive, but it is not overwhelming in terms of progression. The SORG nomogram predicts a 70% 1-year survival. Medically, his comorbidities are stable with no acute exacerbations. The medical evaluation described him as a moderate risk for postoperative cardiopulmonary complications.

The patient has mechanical instability with associated radiculopathy and a radioresistant tumor histology with high-grade epidural spinal cord compression (Grade 3). The mechanical instability represents its own surgical indication for palliation of the patient's pain with surgical fixation. Additionally, the radioresistant nature of the tumor with high-grade ESCC requires decompression of the spinal cord to create a radiation target that is amenable to SBRT to achieve durable local control. While the patient does have a moderate risk of post-surgical cardiopulmonary complications, without surgery to create an appropriate SBRT target, the patient's tumor will progress and lower extremity paralysis will occur. Therefore, the patient underwent separation surgery in the form of a T5 to T7 posterior segmental fixation with cement augmentation as well as T6 laminectomy and bilateral pediculectomy for the resection of the epidural tumor (Fig. 2.3c, d). The result was circumferential reconstitution of the thecal sac (Fig. 2.3e) and SBRT to the area in the form of 27 Gy delivered in 3 fractions.

Conclusion

This chapter presents an updated version of NOMS, which will continue to evolve with newer technologies and evidence-based medicine, but the cornerstone of metastatic spine tumor management continues to be reflected in the four sentinel decision points: Neurologic, Oncologic, Mechanical Instability and Systemic Disease. The NOMS decision framework provides a multidisciplinary framework that can be adopted by any institution to existing technology that allows radiation oncologists, spine surgeons, and interventional radiologists to make expeditious decisions regarding optimal patient management. Coordinated care will ultimately lead to better outcomes in terms of better tumor control with less morbidity in an ever-evolving cancer milieu in which patients need long-term solutions for metastatic tumors.

References

1. Gilbert RW, Kim JH, Posner JB. Epidural spinal cord compression from metastatic tumor: diagnosis and treatment. Ann Neurol. 1978;3(1):40–51.
2. Tomita K, Kawahara N, Kobayashi T, Yoshida A, Murakami H, Akamaru T. Surgical strategy for spinal metastases. Spine (Phila Pa 1976). 2001;26(3):298–306.
3. Walsh GL, Gokaslan ZL, McCutcheon IE, et al. Anterior approaches to the thoracic spine in patients with cancer: indications and results. Ann Thorac Surg. 1997;64(6):1611–8.
4. Klekamp J, Samii H. Surgical results for spinal metastases. Acta Neurochir (Wien). 1998;140(9):957–67.
5. Sundaresan N, DiGiacinto GV, Krol G, Hughes JE. Spondylectomy for malignant tumors of the spine. J Clin Oncol. 1989;7(10):1485–91.
6. Hall DJ, Webb JK. Anterior plate fixation in spine tumor surgery. Indications, technique, and results. Spine (Phila Pa 1976). 1991;16(3 Suppl):S80–3.
7. Hosono N, Yonenobu K, Fuji T, Ebara S, Yamashita K, Ono K. Vertebral body replacement with a ceramic prosthesis for metastatic spinal tumors. Spine (Phila Pa 1976). 1995;20(22):2454–62.
8. Sundaresan N, Scher H, DiGiacinto GV, Yagoda A, Whitmore W, Choi IS. Surgical treatment of spinal cord compression in kidney cancer. J Clin Oncol. 1986;4(12):1851–6.
9. Patchell RA, Tibbs PA, Regine WF, et al. Direct decompressive surgical resection in the treatment of spinal cord compression caused by metastatic cancer: a randomised trial. Lancet. 2005;366(9486):643–8.
10. Tokuhashi Y, Matsuzaki H, Oda H, Oshima M, Ryu J. A revised scoring system for preoperative evaluation of metastatic spine tumor prognosis. Spine (Phila Pa 1976). 2005;30(19):2186–91.
11. Barzilai O, Fisher CG, Bilsky MH. State of the art treatment of spinal metastatic disease. Neurosurgery. 2018;82(6):757–69.
12. Barzilai O, Laufer I, Yamada Y, et al. Integrating evidence-based medicine for treatment of spinal metastases into a decision framework: neurologic, oncologic, mechanicals stability, and systemic disease. J Clin Oncol. 2017;35(21):2419–27.
13. Laufer I, Bilsky MH. Advances in the treatment of metastatic spine tumors: the future is not what it used to be. J Neurosurg Spine. 2019;30(3):299–307.
14. Laufer I, Iorgulescu JB, Chapman T, et al. Local disease control for spinal metastases following "separation surgery" and adjuvant hypofractionated or high-dose single-fraction stereotactic radiosurgery: outcome analysis in 186 patients. J Neurosurg Spine. 2013;18(3):207–14.
15. Laufer I, Rubin DG, Lis E, et al. The NOMS framework: approach to the treatment of spinal metastatic tumors. Oncologist. 2013;18(6):744–51.
16. Liu JK, Laufer I, Bilsky MH. Update on management of vertebral column tumors. CNS Oncol. 2014;3(2):137–47.
17. Newman WC, Laufer I, Bilsky MH. Neurologic, oncologic, mechanical, and systemic and other decision frameworks for spinal disease. Neurosurg Clin N Am. 2020;31(2):151–66.
18. Bilsky MH, Laufer I, Fourney DR, et al. Reliability analysis of the epidural spinal cord compression scale. J Neurosurg Spine. 2010;13(3):324–8.
19. Gerszten PC, Mendel E, Yamada Y. Radiotherapy and radiosurgery for metastatic spine disease: what are the options, indications, and outcomes? Spine (Phila Pa 1976). 2009;34(22 Suppl):S78–92.
20. Yamada Y, Katsoulakis E, Laufer I, et al. The impact of histology and delivered dose on local control of spinal metastases treated with stereotactic radiosurgery. Neurosurg Focus. 2017;42(1):E6.
21. Sahgal A, Myrehaug SD, Siva S, et al. Stereotactic body radiotherapy versus conventional external beam radiotherapy in patients with painful spinal metastases: an open-label, multicentre, randomised, controlled, phase 2/3 trial. Lancet Oncol. 2021;22(7):1023–33.
22. Zelefsky MJ, Yamada Y, Greco C, et al. Phase 3 multi-center, prospective, randomized trial comparing single-dose 24 Gy radiation therapy to a 3-fraction SBRT regimen in the treatment of oligometastatic cancer. Int J Radiat Oncol Biol Phys. 2021;110(3):672–9.

23. Palma DA, Olson R, Harrow S, et al. Stereotactic ablative radiotherapy for the comprehensive treatment of oligometastatic cancers: long-term results of the SABR-COMET Phase II Randomized Trial. J Clin Oncol. 2020;38(25):2830–8.
24. Bilsky MH, Laufer I, Burch S. Shifting paradigms in the treatment of metastatic spine disease. Spine (Phila Pa 1976). 2009;34(22 Suppl):S101–7.
25. Gokaslan ZL, York JE, Walsh GL, et al. Transthoracic vertebrectomy for metastatic spinal tumors. J Neurosurg. 1998;89(4):599–609.
26. Molina C, Goodwin CR, Abu-Bonsrah N, Elder BD, De la Garza RR, Sciubba DM. Posterior approaches for symptomatic metastatic spinal cord compression. Neurosurg Focus. 2016;41(2):E11.
27. Rothrock RJ, Li Y, Lis E, et al. Hypofractionated spinal stereotactic body radiation therapy for high-grade epidural disease. J Neurosurg Spine. 2020:1–8.
28. Jackson CB, Boe LA, Zhang L, et. al. Histologic classifier of radiosensitivity to spine stereotactic body radiation therapy. Int J radiat oncolo biol phys 2025; 123(3):829–838. PMID 40516631
29. Hussain I, Goldberg JL, Carnevale JA, et al. Hybrid therapy (surgery and radiosurgery) for the treatment of renal cell carcinoma spinal metastases. Neurosurgery. 2022;90(2):199–206.
30. Newman WC, Amin AG, Villavieja J, Laufer I, Bilsky MH, Barzilai O. Short-segment cement-augmented fixation in open separation surgery of metastatic epidural spinal cord compression: initial experience. Neurosurg Focus. 2021;50(5):E11.
31. Amankulor NM, Xu R, Iorgulescu JB, et al. The incidence and patterns of hardware failure after separation surgery in patients with spinal metastatic tumors. Spine J. 2014;14(9):1850–9.
32. Chakravarthy VB, Schachner B, Amin AG, et al. The impact of targetable mutations on clinical outcomes of metastatic epidural spinal cord compression in patients with non-small-cell lung cancer treated with hybrid therapy (Surgery followed by stereotactic body radiation therapy). Neurosurgery. 2023;92(3):557–64.
33. Chakravarthy VB, Schachner B, Amin A, et al. Long-term clinical outcomes of patients with colorectal cancer with metastatic epidural spinal cord compression treated with hybrid therapy (Surgery followed by stereotactic body radiation therapy). World Neurosurg. 2023;169:e89–95.
34. Jin CJ, Berry-Candelario J, Reiner AS, et al. Long-term outcomes of high-dose single-fraction radiosurgery for chordomas of the spine and sacrum. J Neurosurg Spine. 2019:1–10.
35. Fourney DR, Frangou EM, Ryken TC, et al. Spinal instability neoplastic score: an analysis of reliability and validity from the spine oncology study group. J Clin Oncol. 2011;29(22):3072–7.
36. Berenson J, Pflugmacher R, Jarzem P, et al. Balloon kyphoplasty versus non-surgical fracture management for treatment of painful vertebral body compression fractures in patients with cancer: a multicentre, randomised controlled trial. Lancet Oncol. 2011;12(3):225–35.
37. Moulding HD, Elder JB, Lis E, et al. Local disease control after decompressive surgery and adjuvant high-dose single-fraction radiosurgery for spine metastases. J Neurosurg Spine. 2010;13(1):87–93.
38. Paulino Pereira NR, McLaughlin L, Janssen SJ, et al. The SORG nomogram accurately predicts 3- and 12-months survival for operable spine metastatic disease: external validation. J Surg Oncol. 2017;115(8):1019–27.
39. Schoenfeld AJ, Ferrone ML, Schwab JH, et al. Prospective validation of a clinical prediction score for survival in patients with spinal metastases: the New England Spinal Metastasis Score. Spine J. 2021;21(1):28–36.
40. Massaad E, Hadzipasic M, Alvarez-Breckenridge C, et al. Predicting tumor-specific survival in patients with spinal metastatic renal cell carcinoma: which scoring system is most accurate? J Neurosurg Spine. 2020:1–11.
41. Bauer H, Tomita K, Kawahara N, Abdel-Wanis ME, Murakami H. Surgical strategy for spinal metastases. Spine (Phila Pa 1976). 2002;27(10):1124–6.
42. Zacharia BE, Kahn S, Bander ED, et al. Incidence and risk factors for preoperative deep venous thrombosis in 314 consecutive patients undergoing surgery for spinal metastasis. J Neurosurg Spine. 2017;27(2):189–97.

Chapter 3
The Role of Vertebral Cement Augmentation

Eric Lis

Cancer patients are at risk of developing vertebral compression fractures (VCF). Often, this is a consequence of metastatic disease to the spine. The spine is the most common site for bone metastasis, with the metastatic disease often lytic in nature, resulting in structural weakening of the vertebral body and a pathologic compression fracture [1]. Solid tumors that are often associated with lytic metastatic disease include breast, lung, kidney, and thyroid cancer. The most common hematologic tumor resulting in lytic disease and VCF is multiple myeloma.

Cancer treatments also contribute to an increased risk of patients developing VCF. Steroids are commonly utilized in the treatment of many tumors or to minimize the side effects of chemotherapy, resulting in osteoporosis. Hormonal therapy, estrogen blockade and aromatase inhibitors in patients with breast cancer and anti-androgens in patients with prostate cancer can result in generalized demineralization/osteoporosis contributing to VCF. Radiation therapy, whether it is directed at metastatic disease within the spine or collaterally involves the spine, such as in the treatment of lung and pancreatic primaries, can also result in VCFs [2].

Regardless of the etiology of the VCF, pathologic/metastatic versus therapy-related or a combination of the two can result in significant back pain and morbidity for the cancer patient. Vertebral cement augmentation (VCA) is a general term for the percutaneous infusion of PMMA (polymethyl methacrylate) into a collapsed vertebral body. Percutaneous kyphoplasty (PKP) and percutaneous vertebroplasty (PVP) are the two most common minimally invasive procedures that can reduce the pain associated with pathologic VCFs [3, 4]. PVP is the percutaneous injection of PMMA into a pathologically collapsed vertebra. PKP is a modification of PVP that involves percutaneous placement of bone tamps (balloons) into the collapsed

E. Lis (✉)
Department of Radiology, Memorial Sloan Kettering Cancer Center, New York, NY, USA
e-mail: lise@mskcc.org

Y. Yamada et al. (eds.), *Multidisciplinary Spine Tumor Management*,
https://doi.org/10.1007/978-3-032-07519-2_3

vertebrae that are inflated and then deflated, creating a cavity within the vertebrae prior to the infusion of PMMA.

Multiple publications have documented the effectiveness of kyphoplasty in patients with metastatic disease and for pathologic compression fractures [5]. The "Cancer Patient Fracture Evaluation (CAFE) study" was a multicenter randomized controlled clinical trial that showed decreased pain and overall improvement in quality of life in cancer patients that underwent balloon kyphoplasty in the management of their painful vertebral body compression fractures versus conservative non-interventional management [6].

Though it is beyond the scope of this chapter to cover every scenario of a patient with a VCF, this chapter, through clinical examples, will focus on how the MSK multidisciplinary spine team incorporates kyphoplasty into the management of cancer patients with painful pathologic VCFs, focusing on imaging evaluation, pre-procedure strategies and technical modifications.

Patient Selection

Patients with pathologic compression fractures that are candidates for kyphoplasty typically have movement-related axial/mechanical back pain that is exacerbated with transitional movements such as getting up out of bed or up from a chair and which corresponds to the level of the VCF. The pain can be sharp or stabbing and often associated with muscle spasm. This pain typically improves with recumbency or with staying still. Movement-related back pain (fracture pain) is distinguished from the most common cause of back pain in patients with metastatic disease, which is biological pain. Biological pain is typically more constant throughout the day, not associated with movement and often is dull—achy or throbbing in character. It is also typically worsened at night secondary to the diurnal decrease in intrinsic steroids. This biological pain is often related to regional factors such as tumor cytokine release and periosteal irritation. Biological pain typically improves with steroids. Often biological pain and mechanical back pain coexist, though for patients that benefit from kyphoplasty, the mechanical pain dominates [7].

All patients to be considered for kyphoplasty require recent, cross-sectional imaging, preferably an MRI. Ideally, imaging should be within 30 days of the planned procedure. However, if there is a question of significant disease progression or development of new neurological symptoms, repeat imaging of the spine should be performed. The MRI should be of the entire spine, not only to characterize the symptomatic compression fracture but also to identify additional, though possibly less symptomatic, pathologic VCFs that could benefit from cement stabilization at the same time. In addition, the spinal canal will need to be assessed for epidural disease not only at the index VCF level but also throughout the remainder of the spine. The pain related to the compression fracture may mask relatively occult though significant epidural disease that may take priority over the compression fracture.

The vertebral fracture ideally will be limited to the vertebral body. Patients exhibiting extensive lytic destruction with little remaining intact vertebral body or fracture of the posterior elements or dominant radicular pain, or myelopathy are not candidates for kyphoplasty and need to be evaluated by neurosurgery, as often these patients require instrumented stabilization and possibly decompression [8]. MRI has the capability to assess disease involving the posterior elements but may underestimate a fracture extending into the posterior elements, pedicle or facet joints. If there is a question regarding a fracture through the posterior elements, then a CT scan through the level in question can provide additional information and ultimately help decide whether VCA can provide enough stability as a stand-alone procedure or if the patient needs neurosurgical instrumented fusion (Fig. 3.1)

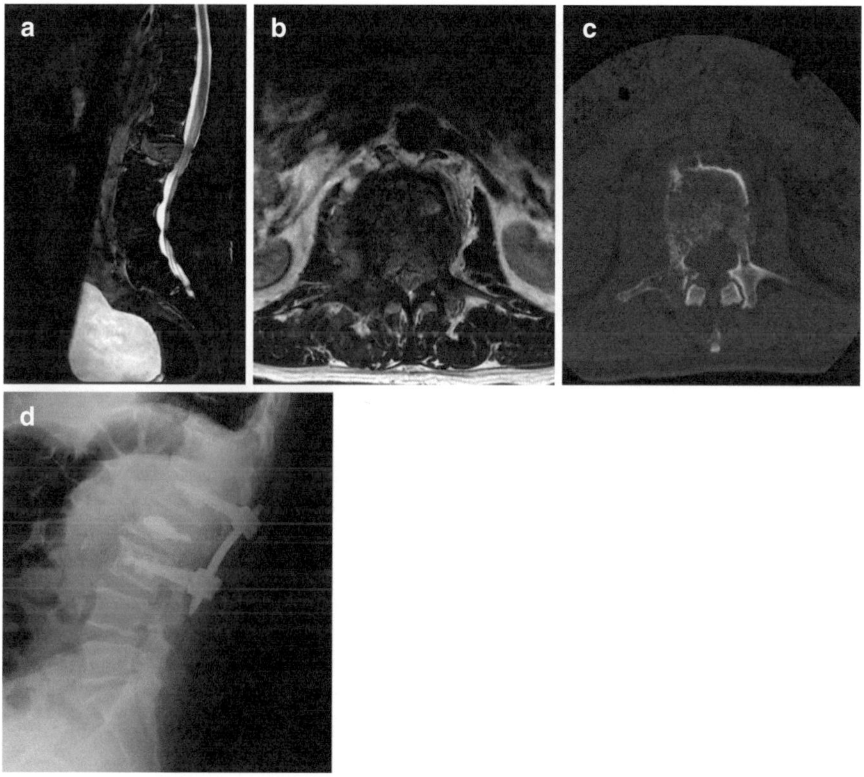

Fig. 3.1 (**a–d**) A 71-year-old male patient with lung cancer and biological and mechanical back pain without a radicular component referred to the neurointerventional service for kyphoplasty. Sagittal T2 STIR (**a**) and axial T1 (**b**) weighted images show metastatic involvement of L2 with a pathologic collapsed deformity and ventral epidural disease resulting in moderate canal compromise. Axial CT (**c**) shows mixed lytic permeative changes throughout the entire vertebral body with involvement of the posterior elements bilaterally, right greater than left, and with fractures involving the pedicles. Based on the imaging, epidural disease and involvement of the posterior elements with associated pedicle fractures, it was determined that kyphoplasty as a stand-alone procedure would not provide enough stabilization, necessitating neurosurgical evaluation. Benefited by the seamless multidisciplinary approach, the patient underwent L2 kyphoplasty (**d**) in conjunction with laminectomy/decompression and cemented short-segment instrumented fusion, followed by radiation therapy, resulting in near complete resolution of the presenting symptoms

Lastly, as with any procedure, the patient needs to be medically able to tolerate the procedure. They will need to be off anticoagulation and have a platelet count generally 50 K or greater and an INR 1.5 or less. The absolute neutrophil count (ANC) should be greater than 1. The patient should be without an underlying active infection or sepsis.

Goals and Expectations

The primary goal or indication of the VCA is to reduce the mechanical/movement-related back pain associated with a pathologic vertebral compression fracture. The second goal of the procedure is to limit fracture progression that can ultimately result in a worsening kyphosis, sagittal imbalance, which can contribute to long-term back pain and in more severe cases of fracture progression may require neurosurgical stabilization.

Reviewing realistic goals and expectations of VCA with the patient will lead to greater patient satisfaction. In our experience the pain relief provided by this procedure in the setting of a pathologic compression fracture is that the Visual Analogue Scale (VAS) pain score typically will decrease from a 7–10/10 level to about 3–4/10 level. Included in the discussion is that pain relief is not instantaneous, though typically our patients see improvement between day 3 and day 7 post kyphoplasty, with sometimes pain improvement taking upwards of 2 weeks. For the patients with painful VCFs that are undergoing kyphoplasty prior to radiation therapy, verbalizing to the patient the understanding that the kyphoplasty will reduce the mechanical movement-related back pain though the biological tumor-related pain will often persist and sometimes become more apparent. Kyphoplasty is often combined with radiation treatment or effective systemic therapy to provide durable local tumor control and ultimately allow further improvement in tumor-associated back pain. Another important aspect in the management of these patients treated with VCA is a referral to rehabilitative medicine to target core muscle weakness and general deconditioning that often accompanies pathologic compression fractures. Post VCA valuation for lightweight bracing can also be beneficial as a noninvasive way of improving pain associated with an increased kyphosis-sagittal imbalance.

Discussing with the patient beforehand that most patients that are determined to be candidates for VCA do well, there are a subset of patients that may not get significant relief from their mechanical back pain. Communicating that VCA is the least invasive procedure that can effectively reduce mechanical back pain, though if the procedure does not provide satisfactory reduction in their back pain, there are other options such as epidural steroid injections or erector spinae paraspinal injections that often can help. If dominant mechanical pain exists post VCA, further stabilization with percutaneous rods and screws will often work [9]. The patient having this knowledge that there are effective options if the procedure does not provide acceptable pain relief will also lead to their overall satisfaction.

Technical Aspects and Clinical Examples

Technical "hands-on" training in the performance of VCA, PKP/PVP is commonly available through various spine societies and vendor-sponsored training programs. This chapter is not meant to replace those training programs. This chapter will focus on how kyphoplasty is typically performed at our institution, highlighting some technical aspects that we have found helpful. The procedure is typically performed under fluoroscopy, with most patients receiving general anesthesia. In patients with significant pulmonary disease, the procedure is occasionally done under monitored anesthesia care. After the induction of general anesthesia, the patient is carefully rolled into a prone position onto the fluoroscopy/angio table. Careful padding and addressing pressure points is very important in this patient population as they often have disease in other bones, i.e., ribs or pelvis, that potentially could be fractured with patient positioning.

Technical aspects of the procedure are individualized to the patient and the type of fracture, though we will focus on the more common techniques and thought processes in addressing the needs of patients with symptomatic pathologic VCFs [10]. Walking through a successful case of kyphoplasty can highlight technical aspects that can be applied to most cases. Outlining this is an example of an 88-year-old male with a history of metastatic prostate cancer, treated with various forms of androgen deprivation therapy and who also received prior radiation therapy to metastatic disease to his thoracic spine. The patient acutely developed severe mid to lower thoracic back pain with a VAS of 9/10. He describes the pain as sharp and stabbing and worsened with transitional movements such as getting out of bed (mechanical) and with bending and coughing and sneezing. The pain was limited to the back and the immediate paraspinal regions. He felt most comfortable either lying flat in bed or semi-recumbent in a chair, with the pain also generally less intense once he was up and ambulating. The patient had an MRI of their spine through our urgent care center and subsequently was referred for kyphoplasty (Fig. 3.2). The MRI of the spine shows marrow edema within T10 consistent with an acute compression fracture. The posterior elements are intact and the collapsed deformity results in minimal spinal canal compromise. The absence of an epidural or paraspinal soft tissue component with relative preservation of the posterior elements favors that this compression fracture is likely on a nonmalignant basis, in an area that likely represents treated disease, previously irradiated. Based on the clinical findings, mechanical back pain referable to this part of the spine, no medical contraindications to a procedure and concordant imaging findings, the patient was determined to be a good candidate for VCA, percutaneous kyphoplasty.

Cross-sectional imaging, preferably an MRI, is crucial in planning the procedure. Analyzing the axial and sagittal images can help identify potential anatomic

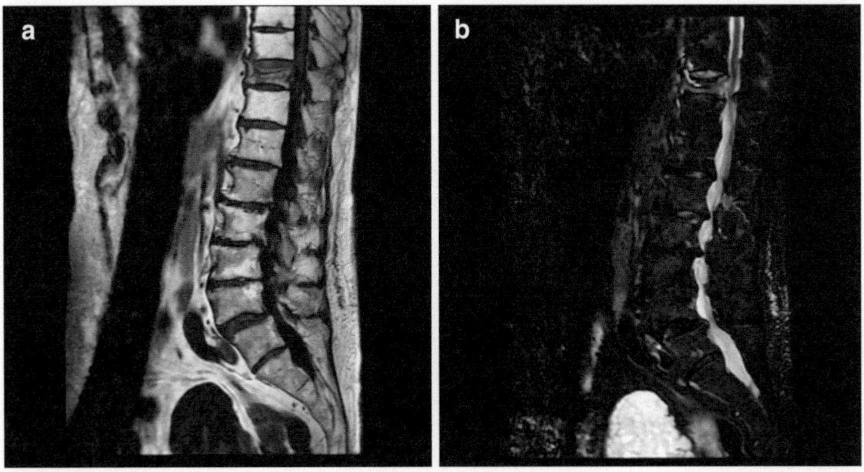

Fig. 3.2 (**a** and **b**) 88-year-old male with metastatic prostate cancer and prior palliative radiation therapy to the thoracic spine who presents with acute midthoracic back pain. Sagittal T1 (**a**) and sagittal T2 STIR (**b**) revealing a moderate collapsed deformity of the T10 vertebral body with a small fluid-filled cleft along the infracted superior endplate. Background vertebral radiation change is evident

abnormalities or variants that are important to be aware of during the procedure or that may modify the planned needle trajectory. Regional anatomy that can be visualized on the MRI is the location of the aorta, the adjacent lungs, and the overall size of the pedicles, to make sure that there are no significant perineural cysts that would need to be avoided. It also allows the opportunity to determine if there is any epidural disease or possible destruction of the posterior vertebral body cortex. Based on the axial images (Fig. 3.3) a potential needle trajectory can be planned. In this case a bilateral transpedicular approach is drawn on the axial image. The distance between the skin entry points as measured on the MRI is transferred to the patient's skin at the time of the procedure, in this case marked with a clamp and a scissor and is shown on AP X-ray (Fig. 3.4a). In the lateral projection the clamp and scissor are moved in a cephalad or caudad direction on the patient's skin, further determining the skin entry point and the trajectory of the kyphoplasty trocars. In this case the skin entry points were adjusted for a transpedicular approach and to accommodate the plane of the superior endplate infraction (Fig. 3.4b). An important point that cannot be overemphasized is to make sure that, under fluoroscopy, true AP and laterals are obtained. This way the spinal canal can be easily identified and unintentional trocar placement either into the spinal canal or neural foramina or adjacent structures can be avoided. Slowly advancing the needle imaging in both the AP and lateral projections allows the trocars to safely advance into the vertebral body, avoiding the spinal canal and the adjacent neural foramina (Fig. 3.5). After the kyphoplasty trocars were advanced into the posterior 3rd of the vertebral body, a biopsy was performed and then a manual intra-osseous drill was utilized to create a tract for the bone tamps. The bone tamps are slowly inflated within the vertebral

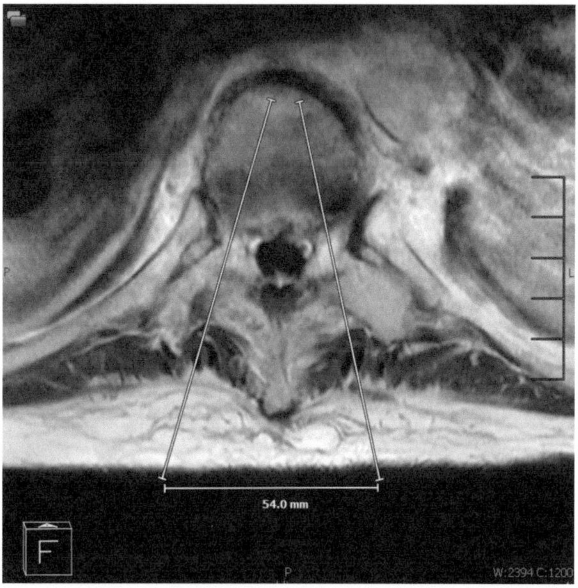

Fig. 3.3 Axial T1-weighted image through T10. Bilateral transpedicular needle trajectory is planned with the puncture sites approximately 5.4 cm apart

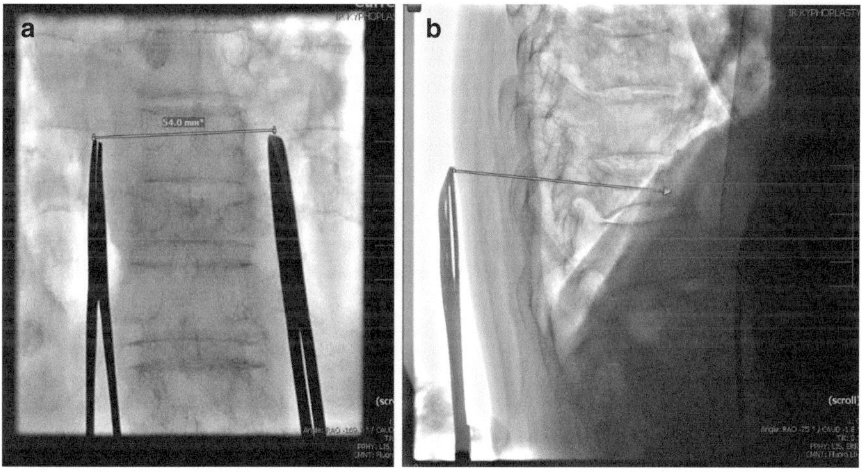

Fig. 3.4 AP and lateral fluoroscopic images of T10. True AP X-ray of T10 (**a**) showing equal distance between the spinous process and the medial margins of the pedicles. The clamp and scissor placed on the patient's skin, localizing potential entry points for a bilateral transpedicular approach. The distance between the clamp in the scissor is about 5.4 cm, approximating the measurement determined on the axial MRI (Fig. 3.3). True lateral X-ray of T10 (**b**) with a line showing the planned trajectory of the kyphoplasty trocars into the T10 vertebral body

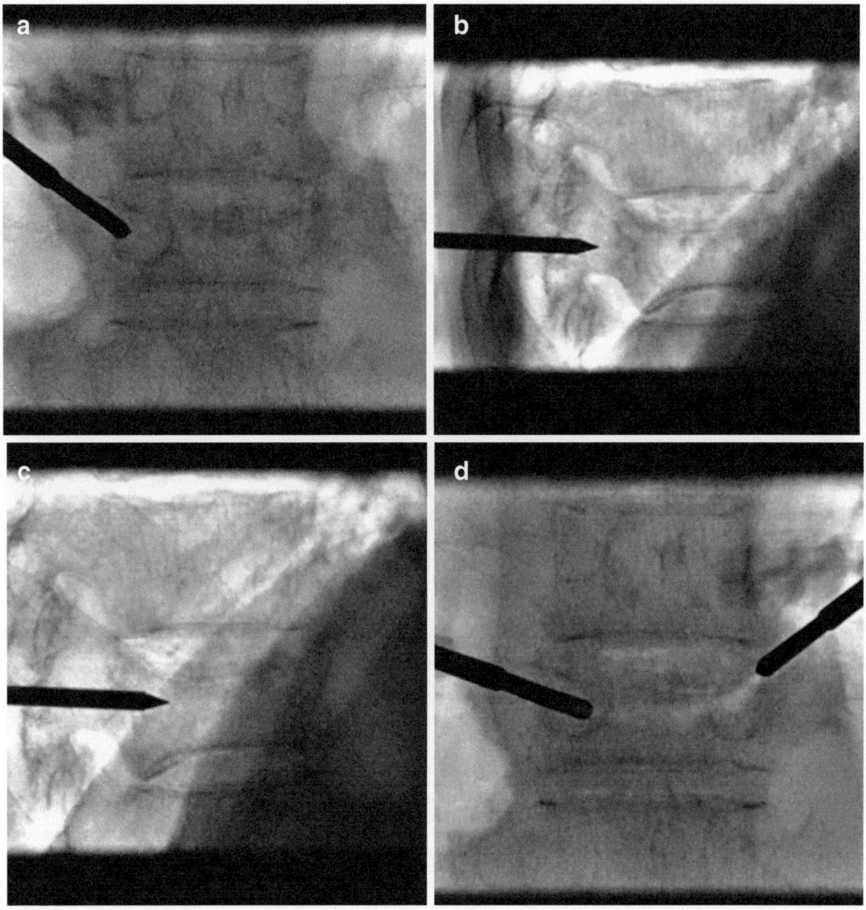

Fig. 3.5 Consecutive AP (**a** and **d**) and lateral X-rays (**b** and **c**) showing the kyphoplasty trocar being advanced into the T10 vertebral body via a transpedicular approach. Notice in Fig. 3.5d that an air-filled cleft is evident

body, again imaging in both the AP and lateral projections (Fig. 3.6). The bone tamps are then deflated and exchanged for "bone Fillers" that allow radiopaque PMMA to be injected into the cavities created by the bone tamps (Fig. 3.7). The consistency of the PMMA that is injected is equivalent to a thick toothpaste and as a rule a thicker consistency of the PMMA is better in limiting extra-vertebral extravasation. While infusing the PMMA into the vertebral body, fluoroscopic imaging is performed in the AP and lateral projections, making sure that there's no extravasation of the PMMA either into the spinal canal or the epidural venous plexus. Similarly, close fluoroscopic assessment of the paravertebral soft tissues is required to make sure that there is no paraspinal venous extravasation that can result in PMMA emboli. The amount of PMMA that is injected into the vertebral body, in part, depends on the volume that the bone tamps were inflated to. Typically, the

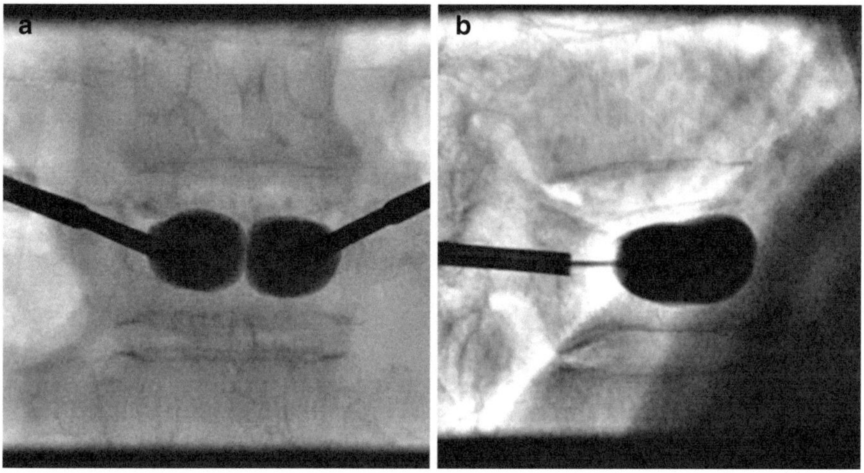

Fig. 3.6 AP (**a**) and lateral (**b**) X-rays showing the inflated bone tamps

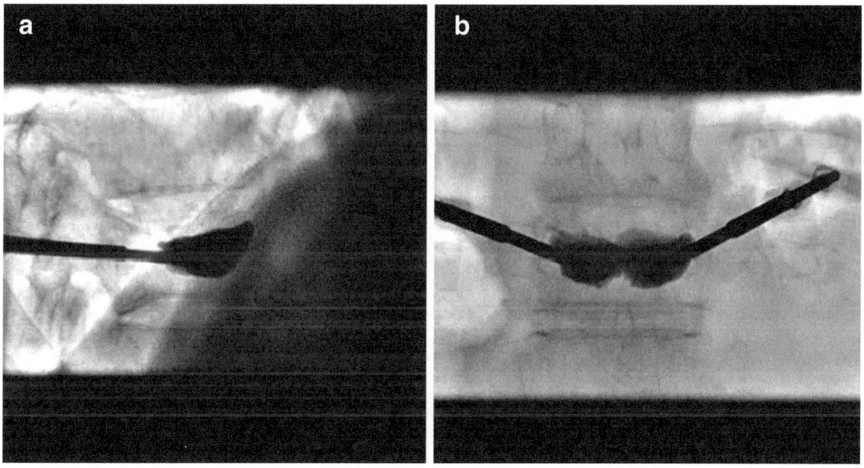

Fig. 3.7 Lateral (**a**) and AP (**b**) X-rays showing the radio-opaque PMMA filling the cavities created by the bone tamps. Intermittent fluoroscopy during the PMMA infusion in both the AP and lateral projections is evaluated for any extravasation either into the epidural space or paraspinal veins

PMMA infusion is stopped when the cavity created by the bone tamp is completely opacified and the PMMA interdigitates into the adjacent cancellous bone. The PMMA infusion is also stopped when the PMMA approaches the posterior vertebral body or neural foramina. The PMMA infusion is also terminated when there is extra vertebral venous extravasation, epidural or paraspinal venous. Ultimately, the total volume of cement that is infused into the vertebral body comes down to striking a balance between getting enough of the PMMA to provide structural support

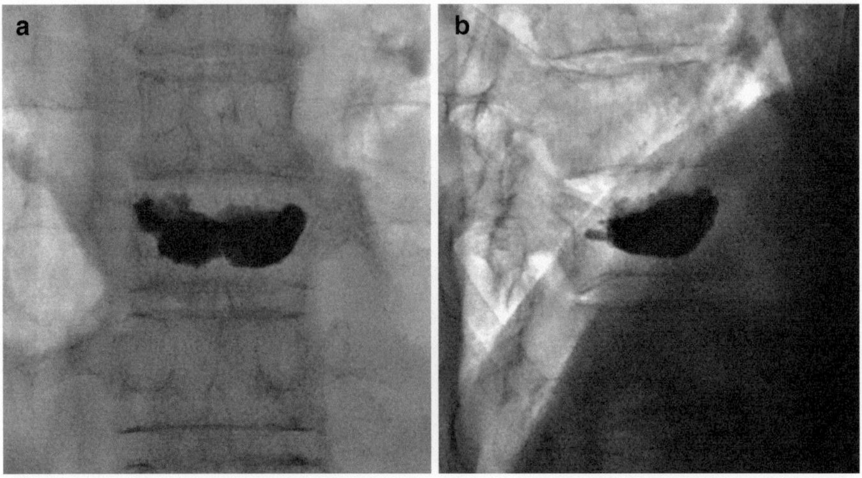

Fig. 3.8 Final AP (**a**) and lateral (**b**) X-rays

while avoiding extra vertebral extravasation or encroachment upon the neural elements. When the PMMA infusion is complete, the bone filler is removed and replaced with the kyphoplasty trocars. The trocars are then removed, and hemostasis is achieved with manual pressure and sterile dressings are applied. Final AP and lateral X-rays are taken (Fig. 3.8). The patient is then returned to the supine position and transferred to the recovery room for pain management and observation. The patient was discharged home after about 2 hour observation peroid in the recovery room, continuing basic spine precautions, avoiding any heavy lifting and no deep bending or twisting. The patient reported that his movement-related back pain had nearly completely resolved about 4 days after the procedure. The biopsy was negative for viable tumor, revealing a treatment change and osteonecrosis. A staging CT scan 3 weeks after the kyphoplasty shows good cement augmentation of T10 with minor asymptomatic fracture progression (Fig. 3.9).

Effects of Kyphoplasty upon the Spinal Canal

There is always potential for the kyphoplasty to result in increasing encroachment upon the spinal canal or neural foramina. This may be secondary to direct cement extravasation into these areas or extension into the epidural or foraminal venous plexus (Fig. 3.10). Scrutiny of the fluoroscopic images at the time of the PMMA fusion, especially as the PMMA approaches the posterior 3rd of the vertebral body, is of utmost importance. Kyphoplasty also has the potential to further displace preexisting epidural tumors posteriorly into the epidural space, resulting in increased spinal canal compromise [11]. This most often occurs when there is destruction of the posterior vertebral body cortex (Fig. 3.11). Soft tissue displacement is not

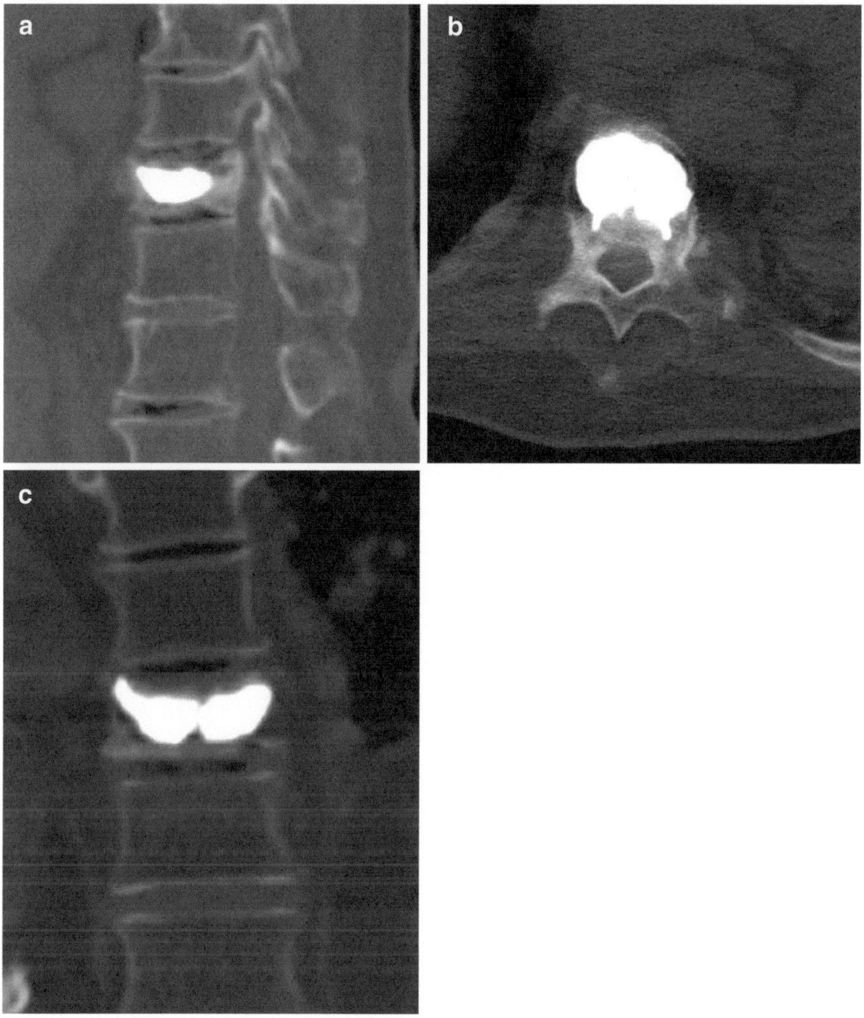

Fig. 3.9 Sagittal (**a**) and axial (**b**) and coronal (**c**) CT images 3 weeks post kyphoplasty showing good cement augmentation of T10. There has been slight asymptomatic fracture progression compared to the post-kyphoplasty X-rays (Fig. 3.8). The axial images show previously treated sclerotic metastatic disease involving the posterior aspect of the vertebral body and right posterior elements

fluoroscopically visualized, and a complete assessment of the pre-kyphoplasty cross-sectional imaging with regard to epidural disease, the degree of spinal canal compromise and the integrity of the posterior vertebral body cortex are important findings the operator should be aware of. The significance is that posterior displacement of the tumor has the potential to alter radiation treatment plans and possibly result in neurological complications requiring surgical decompression.

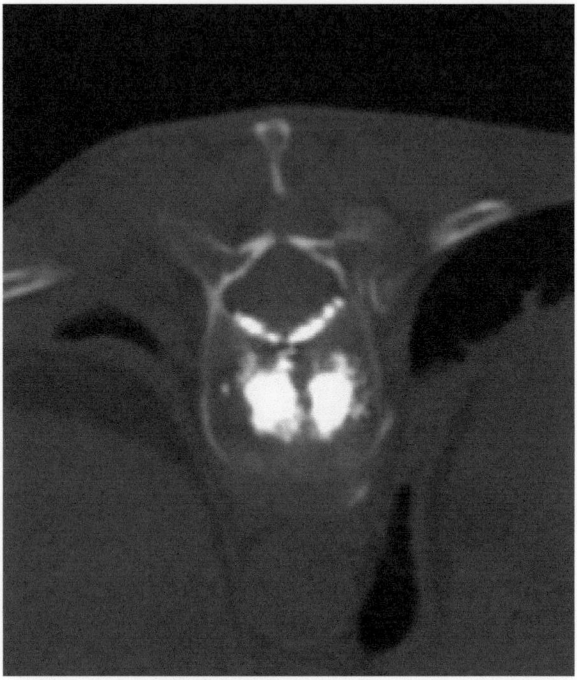

Fig. 3.10 Post-kyphoplasty CT showing PMMA extravasation into the ventral epidural venous plexus

Persistent or Recurrent Pain Post Kyphoplasty—Post-kyphoplasty Fracture Progression

When there is no significant pain relief following kyphoplasty or when the pain worsens after a period of improvement, there are several things that can be considered, some of which may require further intervention. This usually requires further imaging, preferably MRI. The first concern is recurrent or progressive metastatic disease at the treated or adjacent levels, accounting for the ongoing or recurrent back pain post kyphoplasty. If local tumor control cannot be achieved at the treated level, ultimately the kyphoplasty will fail secondary to further loss of vertebral structural integrity or involvement of neural elements. Adjacent level fractures are always a possibility, especially in a patient that has been previously radiated [12]. Post-radiation paraspinal myositis can result in recurrent pain or persistent back pain [13]. However, a commonly seen and a potential cause for recurrent back pain in a patient post VCA is fracture progression [14]. The treated vertebrae continue to collapse, usually down to the PMMA. Often this fracture progression is minor and asymptomatic, or the recurrent pain is limited and can be managed medically/conservatively. Fracture progression could result in a worsening kyphosis and the pain and morbidity associated with the sagittal imbalance. In more severe cases fracture progression can result in the patient requiring further stabilization, post-kyphoplasty instrumented fusion.

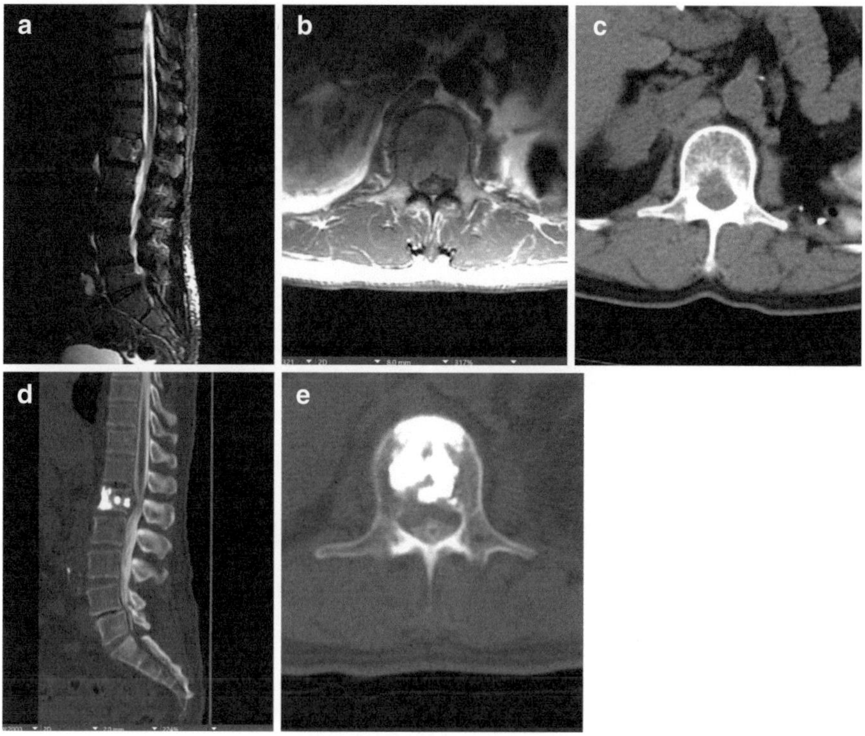

Fig. 3.11 73-year-old male with kidney cancer and L1 metastasis. Pre kyphoplasty sagittal T2 (**a**), axial T1 (**b**) and axial CT (**c**) showing the L1 metastasis with destruction of the vertebral body cortex and ventral epidural disease resulting in moderate spinal canal compromise. Post-kyphoplasty CT myelogram sagittal (**d**) and axial (**e**) showing increased ventral epidural disease and increased spinal canal compromise compared to the pre-kyphoplasty imaging

The reasons for fracture progression in patients with metastatic pathologic compression fractures are multifactorial [15]. The presence of lytic metastatic disease with the destruction of not only the cancellous bone but often of the vertebral cortical margins, especially the superior/inferior endplates, contributes to the fracture progression that is seen post kyphoplasty. While the underlying metastatic disease ultimately resulted in the pathologic compression fracture, the less affected bone of the treated vertebrae often fails at some point, resulting in fracture progression. This is typically from treatment-related factors that weaken this more normal bone that is already subjected to increased stress from re-distributed loads caused by the adjacent lytic disease. Radiation therapy can weaken this relatively more normal bone, making it susceptible to fracture progression, as will systemic therapy in combination with nutritional and metabolic abnormalities that are often present in patients with metastatic disease, leading to underlying general poor bone health, susceptible to fracture.

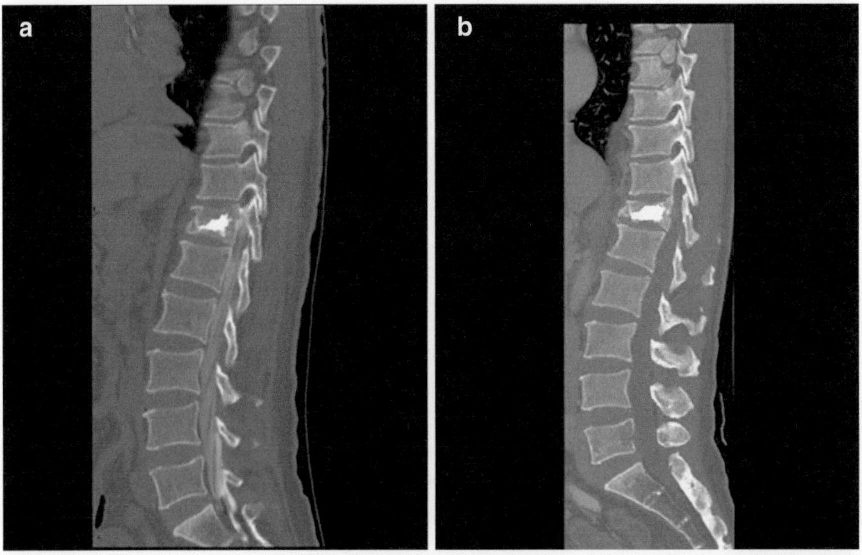

Fig. 3.12 48-year-old male with colon cancer and T12 metastasis. Sagittal CT images obtained immediately post T12 kyphoplasty (**a**) and 8 weeks later (**b**) showing fracture progression; fracturing down to the cement

As an example, the second patient presented in this chapter underwent T10 kyphoplasty with complete resolution of his back pain, though on follow-up imaging, he did have minor fracture progression, essentially fracturing down to the cement, but fortunately, he remained asymptomatic and no further intervention was required (Fig. 3.9). Factors that contributed to the fracture progression were prior high-dose radiation therapy in combination with years of androgen deprivation therapy.

Another example of fracture progression is in a 48-year-old male with metastatic colon cancer with a symptomatic T12 compression fracture treated with kyphoplasty followed by high-dose single-fraction radiation therapy. The patient initially had significant post-kyphoplasty pain relief though several weeks after the procedure the pain recurred, not as bad as what was experienced prior to the procedure, though significant enough to require further medical management. Post kyphoplasty Fig. 3.12a shows the absence of PMMA in the anterior and superior aspect of the T12 vertebral body. This region of the vertebral body is what ultimately failed, resulting in fracture progression (Fig. 3.12b). A more extreme example of fracture progression is illustrated in Fig. 3.13. The post-kyphoplasty sagittal CT scan shows cement augmentation just along the superior aspect of the T6 vertebral body with subjacent lytic disease that ultimately failed and with the patient acutely developing severe mechanical back pain requiring surgical stabilization.

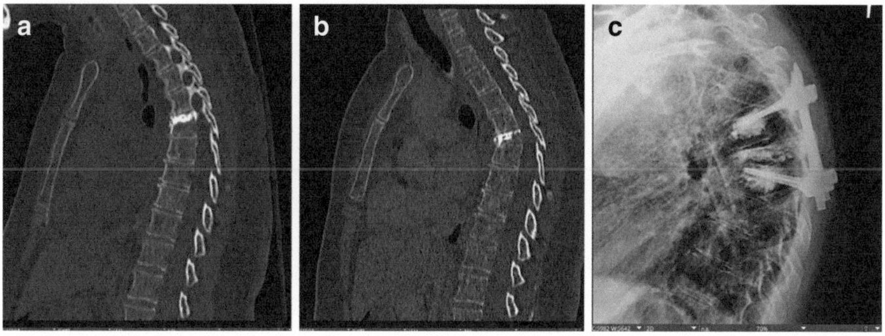

Fig. 3.13 53-year-old female with lung cancer and T6 metastasis. Sagittal CT images obtained post-kyphoplasty (**a**) and after the patient was admitted with acute severe back pain (**b**) showing marked fracture progression requiring surgical stabilization (**c**)

Limiting Fracture Progression-Achieving Adequate "Top to Bottom" Fill

Fracture progression can result in increased morbidity, possibly leading to further surgical intervention [14]. The goal is to safely incorporate more PMMA into the targeted vertebral body to limit fracture progression. It is not necessarily the total volume of PMMA that matters, but rather the targeted placement of the PMMA, resulting in an adequate "top to bottom" fill of the vertebral body to limit fracture progression. As previously illustrated and in many cases, the vertebral body will continue to collapse, eventually limited by the PMMA. In our experience the best way to address fracture progression starts prior to the procedure. Inspection of the pre-VCA imaging can determine strategies, particularly targeted needle placement, which may result in a better "top to bottom" fill. This is illustrated in this 47-year-old female patient with kidney cancer and mechanical back pain referable to a T12 metastasis who was referred from radiation oncology for VCA prior to radiation therapy. Figure 3.14 shows metastatic involvement of the T12 vertebral body, right greater than left, with underlying lytic destruction of almost 40% of the vertebral body and an early superior endplate infraction with mild vertebral body height loss. This patient with oligometastatic disease will be treated with high-dose radiation therapy with the expectation of durable local control and overall prolonged survival. This junctional zone metastasis with dominant lytic disease is at risk for fracture progression. The VCA should be capable of not only reducing the associated mechanical back pain but also providing a reasonable expectation of limiting fracture progression. Based on imaging, the pre-kyphoplasty plan is not only to address the right-sided lytic destruction, which has already started to fracture, but also to reinforce the more normal appearing bone on the left that is also at risk for fracture secondary to increased stress related to altered regional biomechanics and which will further weaken secondary to demineralization following high-dose radiation therapy. By achieving adequate "top to bottom" fill, cement augmentation of the

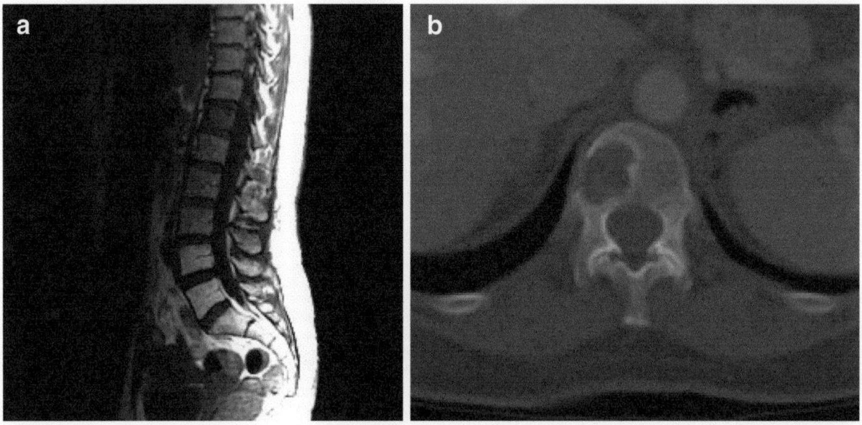

Fig. 3.14 47-year-old male with kidney cancer and a T12 metastasis. Sagittal T1 MRI (**a**) and the axial CT (**b**) showing the T12 metastasis with an early superior endplate infraction and with approximately 40% lytic destruction

dominant lytic component on the right (kyphoplasty) and cement reinforcement of the more normal appearing bone on the left (vertebroplasty) will give the patient the best chance of having adequate pain relief and just as important long-term structural stability to complement the durable local control that will be achieved by radiation therapy.

Figure 3.15a–i shows sequential intraprocedural fluoroscopic images taken during the T12 VCA-PKP. Initially the kyphoplasty trocars were directed inferiorly. On the right bone, the tamp easily expands into the area of lytic destruction, noting a low psi. On the left in the region of more normal appearing bone, the bone tamp is inflated to a much smaller volume with an observed higher psi. Inflating the bone tamp on the left just a little bit in the region of more normal appearing bone allows a greater surface area for PMMA permeation and an improved vertebroplasty effect. Care is taken not to overinflate the bone tamp on the left to the point that it may extend into the dominant lytic disease on the right. Under fluoroscopic visualization the PMMA is slowly infused into the cavity created on the right and allowed to infiltrate into more normal bone on the left. After the lower half of the vertebral body is augmented, the kyphoplasty trocars are withdrawn posteriorly and then, utilizing the trocars' bevel, directed superiorly, allowing for cement augmentation of the upper half of the T12 vertebral body. Figure 3.16 is a 6-month post-kyphoplasty/radiation therapy staging CT scan that shows little room for fracture progression. Figure 3.16a, b shows PMMA opacification, the dominant lytic disease on the right and the "stacking" of the PMMA as a result of the kyphoplasty trocar repositioning. Figure 3.16a, c shows PMMA infiltration of the left side of the vertebral body, the vertebroplasty effect, with left-sided trocar repositioning also contributing to inadequate "top to bottom" fill.

Another example is in a patient with colon cancer and a lytic T12 metastasis, the bone tamps are first inflated inferiorly and then repositioned superiorly, permitting

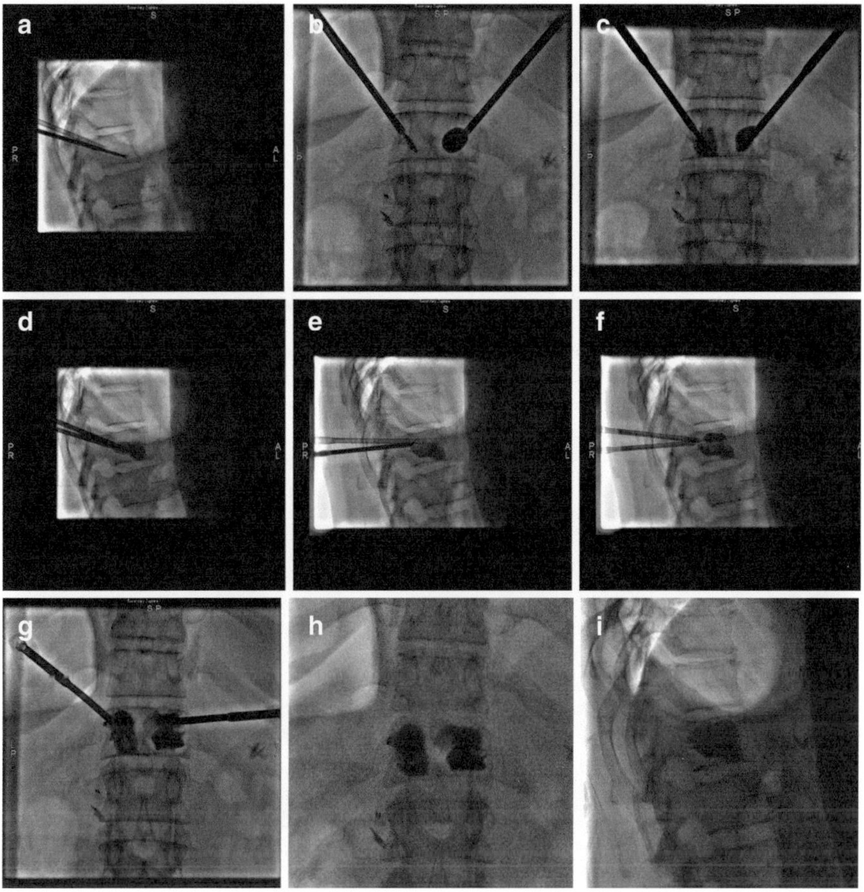

Fig. 3.15 Sequential intraoperative AP (**b**, **c**, **g**, and **h**) and lateral (**a**, **d**, **e**, **f**, and **I**) X-rays showing repositioning of the kyphoplasty working channels starting inferiorly and then angling superiorly to optimize "top to bottom" cement augmentation of the T12 vertebral body. Note that vertebroplasty was utilized on the left in the region of more normal appearing bone and cavity creation employed on the right in the region of lytic destruction

"top to bottom" PMMA augmentation. Figure 3.17. The previous two examples illustrate that repositioning of the kyphoplasty trocars can allow more complete opacification of the affected vertebral body and can limit significant fracture progression and, more importantly, potentially limit catastrophic fracture progression requiring further intervention, instrumented fusion. Repositioning does add additional time to the procedure, occasionally requiring a second PMMA mix. Repositioning of the kyphoplasty trocars can result in some increased pain in the immediate postoperative period. However, slightly increased procedure time and postprocedural pain that can be managed are outweighed by the potential long-term benefits of limiting fracture progression.

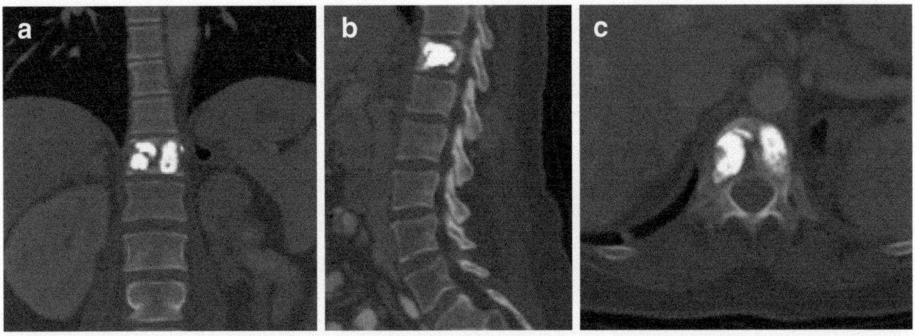

Fig. 3.16 Coronal (**a**), sagittal (**b**) and axial (**c**) CT images obtained 6 months post-T12 kyphoplasty and radiation therapy without significant fracture progression. The CT images show the "stacking" of the PMMA to allow better opacification of the dominant lytic disease on the right, with the vertebroplasty effect evident on the left

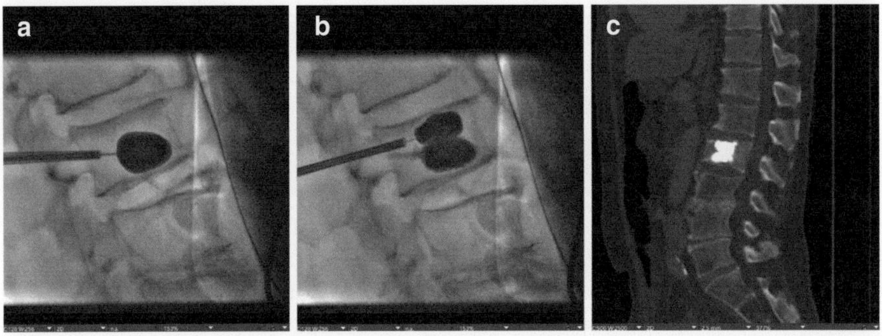

Fig. 3.17 L2 kyphoplasty in a patient with metastatic colon cancer. Lateral fluoroscopic image (**a**) with a bone tamp inflated. Repositioning of the kyphoplasty trocar cephalad allows redeployment of the bone tamp, creating a 2nd cavity (**b**). Six-month follow-up CT scan shows durable cement augmentation of L2 (c)

Beyond Fluoroscopy

The overwhelming majority of the kyphoplasty procedures are done with fluoroscopy. However, at times visualization of the collapsed vertebral body and, more importantly, the pedicles or attaining adequate true AP and lateral views of the fracture may be difficult with fluoroscopy alone. This may be due to a variety of reasons, often generalized osteopenia, fractures within the upper thoracic spine that could be obscured by the secondary to overlying structures such as the shoulders and paraspinal disease such as mediastinal adenopathy, pulmonary disease or even postsurgical changes following prior thoracotomy. CT, cone beam CT (CBCT), and image-based navigation systems can be employed in select cases where fluoroscopy alone can be challenging. The patient is a 47-year-old male with metastatic anaplastic thyroid cancer with a T4 metastasis previously treated with radiation therapy who now has increasing pain between the shoulder blades. CT-based navigation was

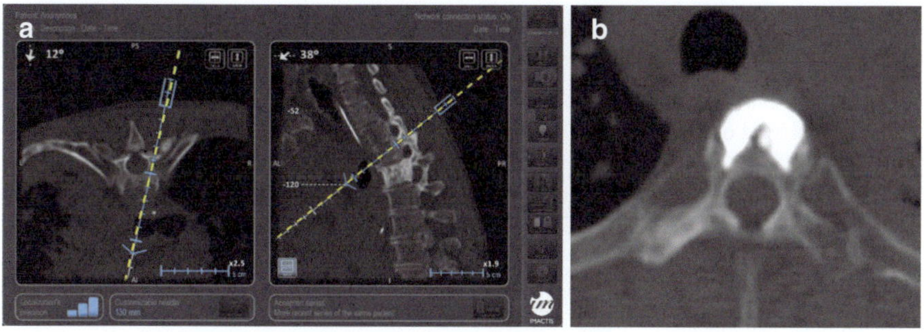

Fig. 3.18 47-year-old male with metastatic anaplastic thyroid cancer with a T4 pathologic compression fracture. Captured screen shot (**a**) from the CT base navigation system (IMACTIS, GE Medical) showing the planned trajectory. Post kyphoplasty axial CT scan (**b**) showing PMMA opacification of the dominant lytic components within the T4 vertebral body

used to place the kyphoplasty trocars with fluoroscopic and CT imaging confirming adequate trocar positioning, leading to successful VCA of T4 (Fig. 3.18).

Adding Ablation

Thermal ablation, most commonly RF ablation, can be implemented in the treatment of pathologic compression fractures prior to the infusion of PMMA [16, 17]. However, at MSK, vertebral ablation is used selectively. Ultimately it is the cement augmentation, PMMA restoring stability to the fractured vertebral body, which will reduce the patient's mechanical pain. Ablative therapy may address a component of the patient's pain, particularly the biological pain and pain derived from the basivertebral nerve, potentially offering quicker pain relief [17]. Most often RF ablation is usually reserved for the solitary pathologic compression fracture. In patients with oligometastatic disease and a pathologic compression fracture, almost always RF ablation is done, potentially and theoretically decreasing circulating tumor cells that can be released into circulation during the procedure [18]. For this reason, the two patients illustrated in Figures 3.14 and 3.17, both of which had oligometastatic disease, were treated with RF ablation prior to the infusion of the PMMA, and both were subsequently treated with high-dose radiation therapy to provide durable local control. The key points to remember are that while RF ablation can technically be added to the procedure of VCA, it is not a replacement for radiation therapy in providing local tumor control and RF ablation will not make up for less than optimal cement augmentation, because, as with radiation therapy, it does not address mechanical back pain.

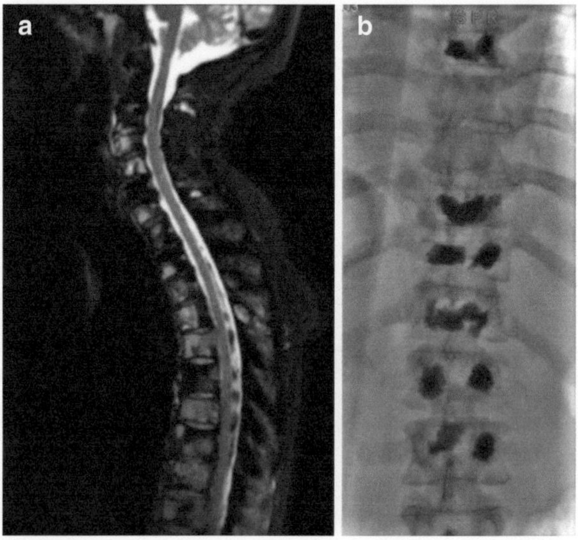

Fig. 3.19 61-year-old male with widely metastatic lung cancer admitted for a pain crisis with a sagittal MRI of the spine (**a**) revealing multiple osseous metastases and multiple pathologic collapsed deformities. The patient underwent multilevel thoracolumbar kyphoplasty (**b**) with a significant reduction in his mechanical back pain, with subsequent discharge 2 days later to hospice

End of Life

A subset of patients that greatly benefit from kyphoplasty are those patients with extensive metastatic disease, multiple pathologic compression fractures whose goals of care are supportive in nature [19]. Multilevel kyphoplasty can often quickly and safely be incorporated into the patient's end-of-life care plan, effectively reducing the patient's mechanical back pain and improving simple functional tasks such as getting out of bed with less assistance. In patients with limited life expectancy, pain palliation is the primary goal, with the technique often modified to treat multiple VCFs in one setting, sometimes with a unilateral approach and with less procedure time committed for maximum vertebral body filling (Fig. 3.19).

Conclusion

Vertebral cement augmentation is a minimally invasive procedure that can be easily incorporated into the patient's care plan to effectively reduce mechanical back pain associated with pathologic compression fractures. In patients with symptomatic pathological fractures, image analysis, technique modification and multidisciplinary evaluation when needed result in the best patient outcomes.

References

1. Bilsky MH, et al. The diagnosis and treatment of metastatic spinal tumor. Oncologist. 1999;4(6):459–69.
2. Rose PS, et al. Risk of fracture after single fraction image-guided intensity-modulated radiation therapy to spinal metastases. J Clin Oncol. 2009,27(30):5075–9.
3. Burton AW, Rhines LD, Mendel E. Vertebroplasty and kyphoplasty: a comprehensive review. Neurosurg Focus. 2005;18(3):e1.
4. Burton AW, Mendel E. Vertebroplasty and kyphoplasty. Pain Physician. 2003;6(3):335–41.
5. Vertebral augmentation involving vertebroplasty or kyphoplasty for cancer-related vertebral compression fractures: a systematic review. Ont Health Technol Assess Ser. 2016;16(11):1–202.
6. Berenson J, et al. Balloon kyphoplasty versus non-surgical fracture management for treatment of painful vertebral body compression fractures in patients with cancer: a multicentre, randomised controlled trial. Lancet Oncol. 2011;12(3):225–35.
7. Laufer I, et al. The NOMS framework: approach to the treatment of spinal metastatic tumors. Oncologist. 2013;18(6):744–51.
8. Barzilai O, et al. Minimal access surgery for spinal metastases: prospective evaluation of a treatment algorithm using patient-reported outcomes. World Neurosurg. 2018;120:e889–901.
9. Barzilai O, et al. Utility of cement augmentation via percutaneous fenestrated pedicle screws for stabilization of cancer-related spinal instability. Oper Neurosurg (Hagerstown). 2019;16(5):593–9.
10. Fourney DR, et al. Percutaneous vertebroplasty and kyphoplasty for painful vertebral body fractures in cancer patients. J Neurosurg. 2003;98(1 Suppl):21–30.
11. Lis E, et al. Change in the cross-sectional area of the thecal sac following balloon kyphoplasty for pathological vertebral compression fractures prior to spine stereotactic radiosurgery. J Neurosurg Spine. 2019;30(1):111–8.
12. Lockney DT, et al. Adjacent level fracture incidence in single fraction high dose spinal radiosurgery. Ann Transl Med. 2019;7(10):211.
13. Lockney DT, et al. Myositis following spine radiosurgery for metastatic disease: a case series. J Neurosurg Spine. 2018;28(4):416–21.
14. Dargelos-Descoubez M, et al. Progression toward vertebral collapse of vertebral metastases treated with percutaneous vertebroplasty: rate and risk factors. J Vasc Interv Radiol. 2024;35(1):59–68.
15. Virk MS, et al. Frequency of symptomatic vertebral body compression fractures requiring intervention following single-fraction stereotactic radiosurgery for spinal metastases. Neurosurg Focus. 2017;42(1):E8.
16. Chen AL, et al. Combination radiofrequency ablation and vertebral cement augmentation for spinal metastatic tumors: a systematic review and meta-analysis of safety and treatment outcomes. N Am Spine Soc J. 2024;17:100317.
17. Jain S, Kinch L, Rana M, Anitescu M. Comparison of post-operative pain scores and opioid use between kyphoplasty and radiofrequency ablation (RFA) systems combined with cement augmentation. Skeletal Radiol. 2020;49(11):1789–94.
18. Mohme M, et al. Circulating tumour cell release after cement augmentation of vertebral metastases. Sci Rep. 2017;7(1):7196.
19. Lee SK, Weiss B, Yanamadala V, Brook A. Percutaneous interventional management of spinal metastasis. Semin Intervent Radiol. 2019;36(3):249–54.

Chapter 4
The Role of Surgery in the Modern Management of Primary Tumors of the Mobile Spine

Mark H. Bilsky, Natasha Kharas, Alexandra Giantini-Larsen, W. Christopher Newman, and Yoshiya Yamada

Introduction

For the past 30 years, *en bloc* surgical excision has been the mainstay of treatment for aggressive benign and malignant primary spine tumors; however, the integration of ablative conformal radiation and the development of biologics is impacting the need for aggressive tumor resection in lieu of multi-modality therapy. Whereas primary spine neoplasms, such as giant cell tumor and chondrosarcoma, are most commonly seen in the appendicular skeleton and pelvis, conventional chordoma is uniquely found in the axial skeleton of the clivus, mobile spine and sacrum. Despite the rarity of chordoma—occurring in less than 1 case in one million population—it remains the most commonly encountered adult primary spine tumor and thus remains a major focus of attention for spine surgeons.

Limitations to *En Bloc* Resection

The current surgical treatment of chordoma is predicated on the principles espoused in the Enneking classification developed in 1980 for musculoskeletal tumors of the appendicular skeleton [1]. The Enneking classification proposed surgical recommendations wherein benign bone tumors are candidates for curettage, intralesional excision, but low-and high-grade malignancies require *en bloc excisions* to achieve marginal, wide, or radical margins. In the 1990s, the WBB classification adapted the surgical principles of the Enneking classification, thereby providing a roadmap for

M. H. Bilsky (✉) · N. Kharas · A. Giantini-Larsen · W. C. Newman · Y. Yamada
Department of Neurological Surgery, Memorial Sloan-Kettering Cancer Center, New York, NY, USA
e-mail: bilskym@mskcc.org

Y. Yamada et al. (eds.), *Multidisciplinary Spine Tumor Management*,
https://doi.org/10.1007/978-3-032-07519-2_4

en bloc excision of primary spine tumors [2]. The ensuing decades witnessed an explosion of case reports demonstrating increasingly aggressive *en bloc* excisions, which were extraordinary technical feats, but often did not meet the goals of wide excision. More importantly, these case reports failed to report long-term local tumor control or associated surgical morbidity.

In the Enneking classification, chordoma should be classified as a high-grade malignancy based on the propensity to present with satellite lesions and develop distant metastases. For a high-grade malignancy, the surgical approach recommendation is *en bloc* spondylectomy to achieve wide surgical margins defined as a cuff of normal tissue around the gross tumor. One must appreciate that the term "*en bloc*" is a surgical term simply denoting that the tumor was resected in a single piece as opposed to piecemeal or curettage resection. However, the critical issue in terms of local recurrence and overall survival is whether the *en bloc* excision achieved wide negative margins. With rare exceptions such as small intercompartmental tumors, en *bloc* wide excision in the mobile spine is rarely achievable due to significant anatomic constraints such as the dura, spinal cord, encased bilateral vertebral arteries or other adjacent critical structures such as the esophagus. Additionally, at the time of surgery, it is nearly impossible to account for skip and satellite lesions that often have been found to track several centimeters away from the gross tumor, especially in large, extracompartmental lesions that infiltrate adjacent soft tissues. Due to anatomic constraints and the increased morbidity associated with achieving wide margins, many surgeons perform *en bloc* marginal, marginal with intentional transgression, or intralesional resections typically employed for low-grade malignancies or aggressive benign tumors; however, marginal and intralesional marginal resections often leave viable microscopic tumor on the dura or other critical structures and do not account for soft tissue skip lesions. This residual microscopic disease largely explains early recurrences after extensive *en bloc* surgery.

What has been lost in the application of the WBB classification is the original concept expressed by Enneking in which he recognized that local control must be balanced against poor functional and neurologic outcomes and that effective adjuvant therapy may redefine the need for *en bloc* excision. At the time WBB was conceived, no study demonstrated a significant benefit to adjuvant therapy (e.g., low-dose photon beam therapy), rendering *en bloc* excision a reasonable approach despite the inherent morbidity of these procedures. However, over the past two decades, advances in radiation techniques and promising developments in biologic agents and immunotherapy have changed the role of *en bloc* excision in achieving local tumor control and improving overall survival for chordoma [3]. The truly revolutionary advances have been in the radiation domain as photon-based stereotactic body radiotherapy (SBRT), proton beam, and carbon ion radiation can all deliver a cytotoxic ablative radiation dose and have been used effectively as neoadjuvant, postoperative, and even definitive treatment. This chapter will focus on how the integration of advanced radiation has fundamentally changed treatment paradigms for chordoma.

En Bloc Resection: What's the Data?

Much of the recent justification for *en bloc* resection as definitive therapy for mobile spine chordoma is predicated on the study by Gokaslan, et al. who reported the AO spine forum multi-institutional retrospective registry comparing EA versus EI resection in 166 patients [4]. Enneking appropriate (EA) was defined as *en bloc* resection that achieved wide or marginal margins and EI was en bloc or curettage intralesional resection [4]. The mean age was 59 years with a male predominance. Notably, 30% of patients were undergoing surgery for recurrent tumors. Overall, EI versus EA resections were achieved in 59% and 41%, respectively. Adjuvant therapy was delivered in 51% and local recurrences were demonstrated in 35%. In univariate analysis, local recurrence was significantly higher in EI vs. EA resections, 46% vs.14% ($p < .001$), respectively. Additionally, those who underwent RT had a significantly higher recurrence rate, 38% vs. 27% ($p < .006$), respectively. This study has been used to support EA resection of chordoma compared to EI, which would be a reasonable conclusion if there was equivalency between the cohorts. However, the lack of parity in the EA and EI groups, as well as radiation being associated with worse outcomes, makes this study considerably less impactful. Known risk factors for local recurrence following surgery were not examined in this study, including intra- vs. extracompartmental location, primary surgery versus recurrence, and failure to use central pathology review to definitively differentiate chordoma from notochordal rests. Additionally, there is a high likelihood that recurrences were underestimated in both cohorts as the median follow-up of 2 years is short compared to the median time to local recurrence of 5.3 years. Moreover, in this retrospective review, the timing and strategy of surveillance imaging for recurrence is not known.

Additionally, reported surgical complications in the literature are upwards of 70% using *en bloc* techniques in the mobile spine but were not assessed or discussed [5]. The absence of this discussion limits the ability to apply this paper to preoperative patient counseling or to justify aggressive approaches from which many patients do not have a reasonable possibility of returning to activities of normal daily living [5]. Perhaps the most significant shortcoming of this paper is its implication that radiation treatment is a negative prognostic factor, a finding that has led surgeons to continue to believe chordomas are radioresistant and that radiation has no role in the treatment of chordomas. As contemporary studies have shown, the radiation dose and delivery strategy are fundamentally important to chordoma tumor control, but unfortunately, these details were not reported in this paper and severely limit the reader's ability to draw meaningful conclusions regarding the impact of radiation on tumor control.

Advanced Radiation: Game Changer

Chordomas have traditionally been considered radioresistant in large part because initial strategies employed conventionally fractionated low-dose radiation (i.e., <65 Gy in 1.8– 2.0 Gy/fraction), demonstrating overall survival (OS) and local control (LC) rates no better than surgery alone. Dose escalation required techniques that could deliver an ablative dose to the tumor within the constraints of normal tissue tolerance, most importantly, the spinal cord and cauda equina. Proton-beam and carbon ion radiation techniques take advantage of charged particles to deliver energy at a distance from the source based on the Bragg peak effect. The advantage of these techniques is the limited dose delivered to tissues distal to the target, significantly reducing the probability of radiation toxicity to visceral organs and the esophagus; however, there can be significant skin toxicity. Photon-based stereotactic radiosurgery uses techniques such as image-guided intensity modulated radiation therapy and volumetric arc therapy to deliver a cytotoxic tumoral dose remaining within tight dose constraints to critical organs based on inverse treatment planning. Chordoma studies using proton beam typically have employed doses >70 Gy relative biological effectiveness (RBE) in 1.8 to 2.0 Gy/fraction with a biologic equivalent dose of 76 Gy RBE. Carbon ion studies have used a hypofractionated dose of 70 Gy in 4 to 5 Gy RBE to reach a biologic equivalent dose of 85 to 105 Gy RBE. The single study from Memorial Sloan Kettering Cancer Center used SBRT to deliver a median dose of 24 Gy in a single fraction, which constituted a BED of 156 Gy RBE [3]. Establishing chordoma as a radiosensitive tumor to these advanced radiation techniques allows for the integration of radiation into treatment paradigms and study designs as a neoadjuvant, postoperative adjuvant, or even definitive therapy. Although the results of carbon ions for chordoma treatment have been impressive, they have almost exclusively been applied to sacral chordoma, and their availability currently is limited to Japan and Europe, so they will not be discussed further in this paper.

Proton beam radiation has been used since the early 1990s for chordoma, but its use was largely limited to postoperative treatment for residual disease or recurrence [6]. The past decade has witnessed a proliferation of less expensive proton facilities with advanced conformal pencil beam technology that have created a resurgent interest in the treatment of chordoma, including at our own institution. Many of the studies and parameters for treatment were developed and reported by Tom Delaney's efforts at Massachusetts General Hospital (MGH). From this group, Rotondo et al. reported a series of 126 sacrococcygeal, thoracic, and lumbar chordomas treated at a mean total dose of 72.4 Gy RBE using mixed proton and photon beam radiation [7]. Patients received neoadjuvant radiation to a maximal dose of 50.4Gy RBE to a clinical target volume, followed by surgical resection and a postoperative proton boost. In those patients in whom this represented the primary treatment, 5-year local control (LC) was 89% in those receiving surgery and RT vs. 56% in those undergoing resection alone. In terms of resection technique, the 5-year LC in the *en bloc* versus the intralesional cohort was 72% and 55%, respectively. In multivariate analysis, *en bloc* excision was the only significant intervention impacting local control ($p < .04$). However, the 28 patients with primary chordomas who completed neoadjuvant and postoperative radiation combined with *en bloc* resection demonstrated no local recurrences in this series.

A second series from MGH further demonstrated the true impact of proton beam radiation on tumor control. Banfield et al. reviewed a series of 67 patients who received definitive radiation for unresectable chordomas of the mobile spine and sacrum in which the surgical morbidity was deemed to be prohibitively high either due to medical comorbidities or unacceptable expected neurologic deficits [8, 9]. The median tumoral dose was 77.4 Gy RBE (range 77.4 Gy RBE to 85.9 Gy RBE in 1.8 to 2.0 GY fractions). With a median follow-up of 56.2 months, 5- and 8-year local progression-free survival was 81.8% and 63.6%, respectively. Overall, distant control was 72.5% at 8 years. The most common complications were sacral insufficiency fracture (22.4%), followed by sacral neuropathy (7.5%), but no patient developed a spinal cord injury. At a minimum, this series shows that a proton beam can deliver an ablative dose to chordoma, providing long-term control without incurring the additional burden of surgical morbidity.

At MSKCC, much of the effort to integrate radiation into the treatment of chordoma has been led by the Multidisciplinary Spine Tumor Service with a focus on integrating high-dose photon-based stereotactic radiosurgery. This interest was partly predicated on long-term data in our metastatic population in which we demonstrated 98% 4-years LC in a cohort receiving 24-Gy single fraction as definitive therapy to radioresistant solid tumor malignancies [10]. Additionally in patients undergoing SBRT as a postoperative adjuvant following separation surgery, 2-years LC for markedly radioresistant tumors, such as renal cell carcinoma and non-small cell lung carcinoma, was greater than 92% at a median dose of 27 Gy in 3 fractions [10, 11]. The second piece of evidence that we could deliver an ablative radiation dose to chordoma came at a time when we were still fairly wedded to *en bloc* resection for these tumors. At this time, we encountered an 80-year-old, extremely frail patient with an intracompartmental chordoma whose significant comorbidities precluded an L3 *en bloc* spondylectomy [12]. The patient was irradiated with 24 Gy in a single fraction and at 2 months post SRS developed a fracture for which he underwent kyphoplasty and biopsy. The biopsy demonstrated a viable tumor. At 4 months, the patient demonstrated radiographic changes thought to be consistent with tumor progression and thus underwent curettage, intralesional gross total resection. Pathology demonstrated the tumor was 99.9% necrosis. The combination of the results from this case and our extensive experience successfully treating radioresistant spine metastases led us to explore the integration of SRS into our chordoma treatment paradigm in an effort to provide more effective tumor control with less associated treatment morbidity.

Subsequent to this experience, Jin et al. reviewed the MSKCC series of 35 patients treated for primary chordomas of the mobile spine in 17 patients (49%) and sacrum in 18 patients (51%) who received single-fraction SRS with a median dose to the planning target of 24 Gy (range 18 to 24 Gy) [13]. SRS was delivered as definitive treatment in 12 patients (34%), neoadjuvant in 12 (34%) and as a postoperative adjuvant in 11 (35%). Definitive radiation was given in 7 sacral and 5 mobile spine chordomas. Of the 11 (61%) sacral tumors that underwent surgical resection, all had an *en bloc* excision of which 8 achieved wide margins and 2 achieved marginal resections. The mobile spine tumors that underwent surgery were principally operated on for high-grade epidural spinal cord compression (i.e., Bilsky Epidural Spinal Cord Compression grade 2 or 3) or other anatomic constraints that precluded achieving *en bloc* wide margin resections [14]. Mobile spine tumors were resected via curettage, intralesional gross total resection in 6 patients or simple separation surgery in 7 (Figs. 4.1 and 4.2). Overall, the 3- and 5-year local recurrence-free survival (LRFS) were 86.2% and 80.5%, respectively. However, in the 32

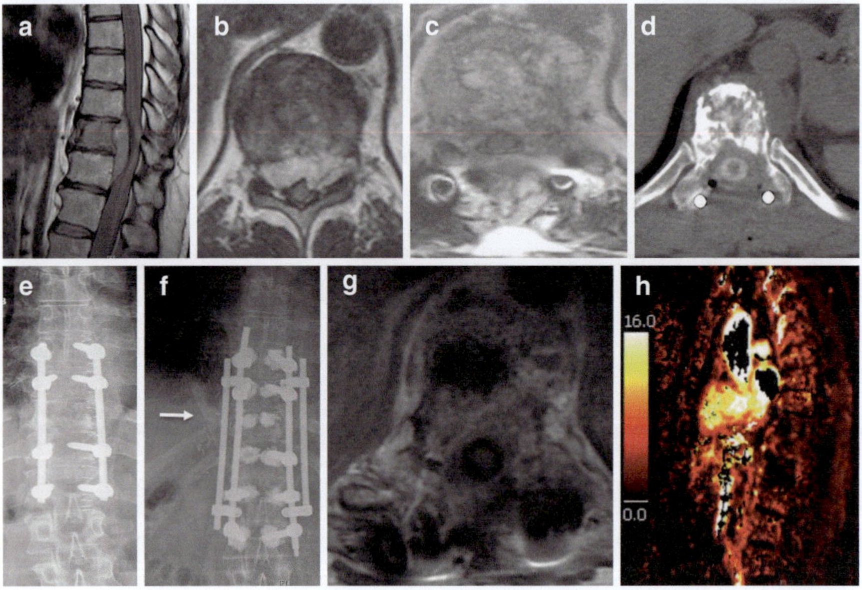

Fig. 4.1 53-year-old healthy, athletic male presented emergently to an outside emergency room with progressive myelopathy resulting in lower extremity weakness and numbness requiring ambulation with a walker. (**a** and **b**) MR sagittal (**a**) T1-weighted image and axial (**b**) T2-weighted image demonstrated T10-T11 high-grade epidural spinal cord compression (Bilsky grade 3) with infiltrative bone marrow involvement but without fracture. The patient underwent emergent separation surgery, resulting in recovery of neurologic function by 6 weeks. (**c**) Postoperative axial T2-weighted image demonstrated reconstitution of the thecal sac (Bilsky grade 1c). (**d**) Despite excellent recovery of neurologic function, the patient underwent a second separation surgery with reconstitution of the thecal sac seen on CT myelogram axial to create a target for 24 Gy single fraction within spinal cord constraints. The patient received 24 Gy single fraction 15 days postoperatively. (**e**) Plain AP X-rays demonstrate the original construct, which was good for short-term stability but was concerning for long-term failure. (**f**) Plain AP X-rays demonstrate re-instrumentation for a PMMA-augmented pedicle screw placement with a dual rod construct and kyphoplasty at the T10 index level with a right rib graft harvested on the segmental vascular pedicle and placed as a posterolateral graft (arrow). An additional autologous iliac crest graft was placed. (**g**) 2-year post hybrid therapy axial T1-postcontrast shows no evidence of recurrence both on axial T1-post-contrast imaging or (**h**) sagittal perfusion plasma volume (Pv) imaging (arrow)

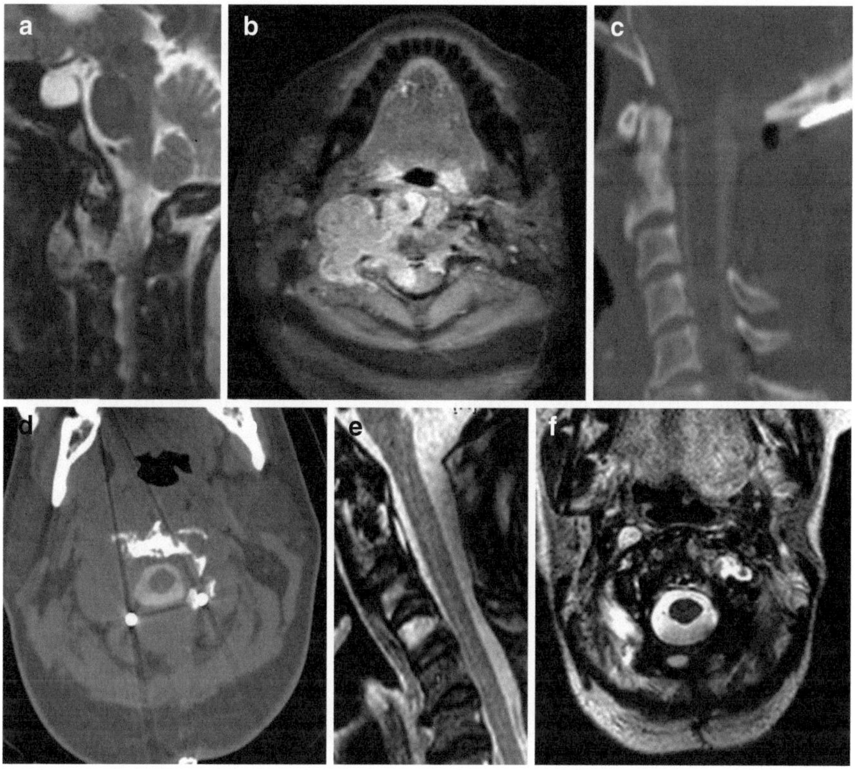

Fig. 4.2 54-year-old female presented with high-cervical myelopathy resulting in clumsy hand syndrome. Needle biopsy was consistent with chordoma. (**a** and **b**) Sagittal and axial T2-weighted imaging demonstrates high grade spinal cord compression (ESCC 3), bilateral vertebral artery encasement and the large paraspinal mass abutting the pharynx. The patient underwent separation surgery with occipital cervical fixation with recovery of neurologic function. (**c** and **d**) Sagittal and axial CT myelogram demonstrated spinal cord decompression following separation surgery. The patient underwent 24-Gy single fraction SRS. (**e** and **f**) Follow-up sagittal and axial T2-weighted MR images demonstrate no evidence of residual or recurrent tumor

patients receiving 24-Gy single fraction, the 3- and 5-year LRFS were 96.3% and 89.9% respectively. The 3- and 5-year overall survival rates were 90.0% and 84.3%, respectively. The only significant factor that impacted LRFS was the SBRT dose of 24 Gy single fraction. When using SBRT as definitive therapy, the extent or type of surgery did not impact LRFS, OS, or symptom relief. Complications in this series were assessed using Common Terminology Criteria for Adverse Events (version 5.0). *En bloc* resection was associated with a significantly higher surgical complication rate compared to intralesional gross total or separation surgery. Grade 2 or greater radiation-related toxicity was experienced in 31% of patients, including tissue necrosis, laryngeal nerve palsy, transient myelopathy, vertebral body fracture and a secondary malignancy.

The Jin et al. paper provides solid data that SBRT delivered as a 24 Gy single fraction is ablative for chordoma [13]. The impact of high-dose SBRT can be seen clearly as the MSKCC data compares very favorably to the AO spine EA cohort, despite only 31% of the tumors undergoing an EA resection in our series. However, 24 Gy single fraction remains well within acceptable tissue tolerances for adjacent organs. Whereas our initial approach for mobile spine high-grade ESCC in chordoma was intralesional gross total resection, we have largely transitioned to separation surgery with the goal of decompressing the spinal cord to reconstitute the thecal sac and allow for full dose delivery to the planning target volume within the spinal cord constraints (i.e., cord Dmax of 14 Gy for single fraction) (Figs. 4.1 and 4.2). For other organs at risk, organ displacement techniques are being used to improve target delineation and dose delivery. Saline can be infused into the retroperitoneum to displace the bowel and kidneys from the tumor [15]. Esophageal displacement at the cervicothoracic junction is accomplished via a thoracoscopic placement of hydrogel, which can provide a 2 cm margin from the tumor [16]. Additionally, omental slings can be created laparoscopically to create safe margins on critical organs. These techniques enable the treatment of large paraspinal masses often encountered in chordoma by improving the probability of delivering definitive ablative therapy within the dose constraints of adjacent organs at risk.

Systemic Options

Primary bone tumors have been largely resistant to systemic therapy; however, there are major exceptions, such as osteogenic sarcoma, giant cell tumor, and aneurysmal bone cysts where the integration of chemotherapy or biologics has redefined cure rates and significantly reduced surgical morbidity. Whereas the integration of advanced radiation techniques has been extremely meaningful in improving chordoma outcomes, ultimately, the development of effective systemic therapy is still critical for the upfront treatment of chordomas, locally recurrent tumors, or metastases. A number of clinical trials have been conducted using biologics to target molecular pathways such as platelet-derived growth factor receptor (PEGFR), vascular endothelial growth factor receptor (VEGFR), epidermal growth factor receptor (EGFR), mammalian target of rapamycin (mTOR), and SMARCB1, which uniquely targets an epigenetic driver [17]. Although these targets continue to hold potential promise, responses to current biologics targeting them have been modest at best. In a similar vein, immunotherapy is a second avenue of active investigation, both in terms of vaccines and checkpoint inhibitors. While studies are conflicting, chordomas have been shown to express PD-L1 in the tumor microenvironment [18, 19]. Both Pembrolizumab and Nivolumab are currently being used in clinical trials to assess the impact of checkpoint inhibitors in combination with SBRT to improve local tumor control and possibly induce an abscopal response for metastases.

Current MSKCC Algorithm for Mobile Spine Chordoma

At MSKCC, the current treatment algorithm for mobile spine chordoma largely mirrors the paradigm that has evolved for spine metastases and is predicated on the integration of SBRT and proton beam therapy, which has transformed the definition of this tumor from extremely radioresistant to exquisitely radiosensitive to these advanced radiation techniques. This new paradigm remains a work in evolution; however, the current data demonstrates equipoise in terms of LC and OS between *en bloc* resection and SBRT as definitive, neoadjuvant, or adjuvant therapy. In our experience, patients typically will elect to incorporate SBRT into their chordoma therapy to preserve function and limit disability while maintaining equivalent if not improved tumor control and survival. A thoroughly informed consent discussion is critically important, including expectations of long-term outcomes and treatment-related morbidity for both *en bloc* excision and radiation. Currently at MSKCC, our formal recommendation for mobile spine chordomas is as follows:

1. *Patients who are candidates for en bloc wide margin resection that can be achieved with limited functional morbidity are offered an en bloc surgery or definitive SBRT, 24 Gy single fraction.* Medical comorbidities and age are both factored into this recommendation.
2. *Patients who are not candidates for a wide margin en bloc excision based on anatomic constraints or medical comorbidities with ESCC 1b or less are offered definitive SBRT 24Gy single fraction.* Organ displacement is used to improve the delivery of ablative doses within the constraints of organs at risk such as the bowel, esophagus, and kidneys.
3. *Patients with tumors creating ESCC 1c or greater with or without myelopathy or cauda equina syndrome are recommended for hybrid therapy (i.e., separation surgery followed by 24-Gy single fraction as a postoperative adjuvant).* Separation surgery reconstitutes the thecal, ensuring delivery of an ablative dose to the entire planning target volume, including the dural margin within spinal cord constraints. Resection of the vertebral body and paraspinal masses is typically not resected as there is no benefit regarding the delivery of ablative radiation. This strategy prevents surgical injuries to paraspinal organs and vascular structures such as the vertebral arteries. In our experience, marginal seeding from intralesional resection is rare although it can be seen with percutaneous biopsies that were not performed with a coaxial needle.
4. *Patients with local recurrence can be re-treated with an ablative dose of SBRT or proton beam radiation without or without separation surgery, depending on the degree of ESCC.* Patients who meet criteria may be offered a Phase I/II protocol combining Nivolumab with SBRT.

Conclusion

Multidisciplinary input is critical for optimal management of primary spinal tumors. The treatment of mobile spine chordoma will continue to evolve in all domains but is currently being redefined and substantially impacted by the integration of ablative radiation using photon-based SBRT and proton beam radiation used as definitive radiation or in the neo- or postoperative setting. The era of aggressive *en bloc* spondylectomy with its incumbent morbidity and relatively poor cure rates has largely ended, having undergone a major transformation with the integration of advanced radiation techniques. As with metastatic tumors, the current treatment of chordoma requires a multidisciplinary approach that truly addresses the anatomic constraints and biology of this uniquely neuroaxis tumor. Ultimately, we will have additional systemic agents that will be equally as impactful, particularly in the metastatic setting, but may also improve local control in combination with radiation therapy.

References

1. Enneking WF, Spanier SS, Goodman MA. A system for the surgical staging of musculoskeletal sarcoma. Clin Orthop Relat Res. 1980;153:106–20.
2. Boriani S, Weinstein JN, Biagini R. Primary bone tumors of the spine. Terminology and surgical staging. Spine (Phila Pa 1976). 1997;22(9):1036–44.
3. Konieczkowski DJ, DeLaney TF, Yamada YJ. Radiation strategies for spine chordoma: proton beam, carbon ions, and stereotactic body radiation therapy. Neurosurg Clin N Am. 2020;31(2):263–88.
4. Gokaslan ZL, Zadnik PL, Sciubba DM, et al. Mobile spine chordoma: results of 166 patients from the AOSpine Knowledge Forum Tumor database. J Neurosurg Spine. 2016;24(4):644–51.
5. Molina CA, Ames CP, Chou D, et al. Outcomes following attempted en bloc resection of cervical chordomas in the C-1 and C-2 region versus the subaxial region: a multiinstitutional experience. J Neurosurg Spine. 2014;21(3):348–56.
6. Hug EB, Fitzek MM, Liebsch NJ, Munzenrider JE. Locally challenging osteo- and chondrogenic tumors of the axial skeleton: results of combined proton and photon radiation therapy using three-dimensional treatment planning. Int J Radiat Oncol Biol Phys. 1995;31(3):467–76.
7. Rotondo RL, Folkert W, Liebsch NJ, et al. High-dose proton-based radiation therapy in the management of spine chordomas: outcomes and clinicopathological prognostic factors. J Neurosurg Spine. 2015;23(6):788–97.
8. Banfield W, Ioakeim-Ioannidou M, Goldberg S, et al. Definitive high-dose, proton-based radiation for unresected mobile spine and sacral chordomas. Radiother Oncol. 2022;171:139–45.
9. Kabolizadeh P, Chen YL, Liebsch N, et al. Updated outcome and analysis of tumor response in mobile spine and sacral chordoma treated with definitive high-dose photon/proton radiation therapy. Int J Radiat Oncol Biol Phys. 2017;97(2):254–62.
10. Yamada Y, Katsoulakis E, Laufer I, et al. The impact of histology and delivered dose on local control of spinal metastases treated with stereotactic radiosurgery. Neurosurg Focus. 2017;42(1):E6.
11. Hussain I, Goldberg JL, Carnevale JA, et al. Hybrid therapy (Surgery and radiosurgery) for the treatment of renal cell carcinoma spinal metastases. Neurosurgery. 2022;90(2):199–206.

12. Wu AJ, Bilsky MH, Edgar MA, Yamada Y. Near-complete pathological response of chordoma to high-dose single-fraction radiotherapy: case report. Neurosurgery. 2009;64(2):E389–90. discussion E390
13. Jin CJ, Berry-Candelario J, Reiner AS, et al. Long-term outcomes of high-dose single-fraction radiosurgery for chordomas of the spine and sacrum. J Neurosurg Spine. 2019:1–10.
14. Bilsky MH, Laufer I, Fourney DR, et al. Reliability analysis of the epidural spinal cord compression scale. J Neurosurg Spine. 2010;13(3):324–8.
15. Katsoulakis E, Solomon SB, Maybody M, et al. Temporary organ displacement coupled with image-guided, intensity-modulated radiotherapy for paraspinal tumors. Radiat Oncol. 2013;8:150.
16. Boerner T, Jin CJ, Harrington C, Bilsky MH, Yamada YJ, Molena D. Efficacy of an esophageal spacer for spine radiosurgery: first experience. Pract Radiat Oncol. 2022;12(4):e312–6.
17. Ozair MZ, Shah PP, Mathios D, Lim M, Moss NS. New prospects for molecular targets for chordomas. Neurosurg Clin N Am. 2020;31(2):289–300.
18. Mathios D, Ruzevick J, Jackson CM, et al. PD-1, PD-L1, PD-L2 expression in the chordoma microenvironment. J Neurooncol. 2015;121(2):251–9.
19. Feng Y, Shen J, Gao Y, et al. Expression of programmed cell death ligand 1 (PD-L1) and prevalence of tumor-infiltrating lymphocytes (TILs) in chordoma. Oncotarget. 2015;6(13):11139–49.

Chapter 5
Separation Surgery for Spinal Metastatic Cancer

W. Christopher Newman

Introduction

Spine metastases are increasingly common, impacting an estimated 20% of cancer patients, and are a significant source of morbidity in the oncology population [1, 2]. Despite significant advances in systemic therapy for the management of metastatic disease, the treatment of spine and epidural metastases has remained largely palliative, focused on pain relief, neurologic preservation or recovery, and long-term local tumor control. Historically, the goal of surgical intervention for spinal metastatic disease was often *en bloc* or gross total resection. Modern advances in radiation techniques have allowed for a shift in this goal away from complete resection toward the current modality of separation surgery.

The term "separation surgery" is attributed to Dr. Edward Benzel and Dr. Lilyana Angelov. It describes a surgical approach focused on the removal of tumor from the epidural space in order to separate or create space between the spinal cord and the tumor-involved structures [3]. The goal of this approach is both to decompress the neural elements and to create space between the radiation target—the tumor—and the critical structures at risk of radiation toxicity—the spinal cord and nerve roots. The resultant tumor volume can then be targeted more effectively with a higher ablative dose of radiation, thereby achieving high rates of local tumor control with minimal rates of radiation-related side effects.

W. C. Newman (✉)
Department of Neurological Surgery, Memorial Sloan-Kettering Cancer Center, New York, NY, USA
e-mail: newmanw@mskcc.org

Y. Yamada et al. (eds.), *Multidisciplinary Spine Tumor Management*,
https://doi.org/10.1007/978-3-032-07519-2_5

Historical Evolution of Separation Surgery

The surgical philosophy underlying the management of metastatic epidural disease underwent a foundational paradigm shift with the 2005 publication of the Patchell trial, a prospective, randomized trial of conventional external beam radiation therapy (cEBRT) versus surgical decompression followed by cEBRT [4]. Prior to this study, the management of metastatic epidural disease largely consisted of decompressive laminectomies without instrumentation, which were associated with postoperative neurological decline and poor outcomes due to iatrogenic instability [5]. In the 1990s, segmental instrumentation was introduced in spinal reconstruction for metastatic disease with concomitant improvements in patient outcomes [6–8]. However, it was not until the 2005 Patchell et al. study that the management pendulum swung more firmly in the direction of surgical decompression for metastatic epidural spinal cord compression (MESCC). This study showed the benefits of surgery combined with cEBRT compared to cEBRT alone, with patients in the surgical arm demonstrating higher rates of maintenance or recovery of ambulation, longer post-treatment ability to ambulate, and longer overall survival [4].

The surgical success of the Patchell trial ushered in a new era of aggressive surgical interventions in the management of spinal metastatic disease. Corpectomies, spondylectomies, multi-segment fusions, transthoracic approaches, and other surgical approaches with substantial associated morbidity became more commonplace in order to achieve extensive reductions in index-level tumor volume prior to the patient undergoing cEBRT [7–9]. Aggressive tumor resection was pursued in an attempt to use cytoreduction to provide durable tumor control given the poor outcomes using cEBRT as a postoperative adjuvant. However, these approaches were associated with significant morbidity that, in some cases, proved to be prohibitively high.

It was not until the advent of spine stereotactic radiosurgery (sSRS) and its ability to deliver highly conformal, ablative doses of radiation that the relative radioresistance of solid tumor malignancies could be overcome [10–12]. This allowed for histology-independent local control rates that have exceeded 86% across studied solid tumor histologies [11–13]. As a result of improved radiation techniques, the goals of surgery shifted from maximal tumor resection to targeted partial resection to create space between the tumor and neural structures such that an ablative dose of radiation could be delivered without exceeding the toxicity thresholds of the spinal cord and nerve roots. The need for this space is the basis upon which separation

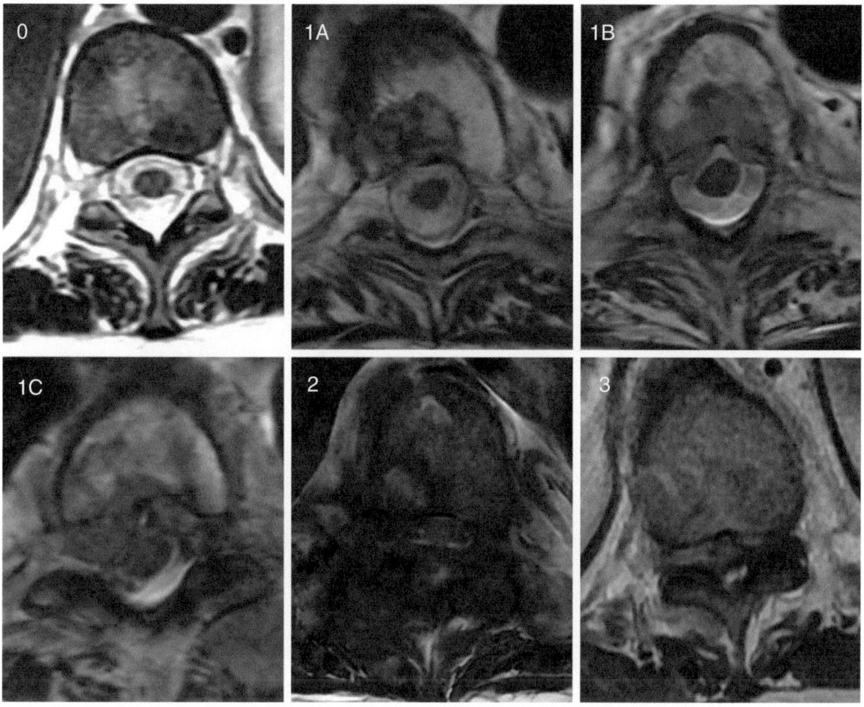

Fig. 5.1 Imaging of various degrees of metastatic epidural spinal cord compression (MESCC) as described by Bilsky M, et al. Grades are displayed in the upper left corner of the image. Grade 0 MESCC describes bone-only disease with no encroachment into the epidural space. Grades 1a to 1c describe increasing degrees of violation of tumor into the epidural space, with Grade 1a being epidural impingement without compression of the thecal sac, 1b being deformation of the thecal sac without abutment of the spinal cord, and 1c being deformation of the thecal sac with abutment of the spinal cord. Grade 2 MESCC describes spinal cord compression with CSF still visible, whereas Grade 3 describes spinal cord compression with no CSF visible around the cord. Grades 2 and 3 MESCC are considered high-grade

surgery is predicated, and when separation surgery is combined with postoperative sSRS, it is termed hybrid therapy [13, 14]. Practically speaking, in patients with radioresistant histologies with Bilsky grade 0–1c MESCC, sSRS can be pursued without the need for separation surgery. However, in those with Bilsky grade 2 and 3 MESCC (i.e., high-grade MESCC), separation surgery is a critical technique for creating an appropriate radiation target within the dose constraints of the spinal cord [12–15] (Figs. 5.1 and 5.2).

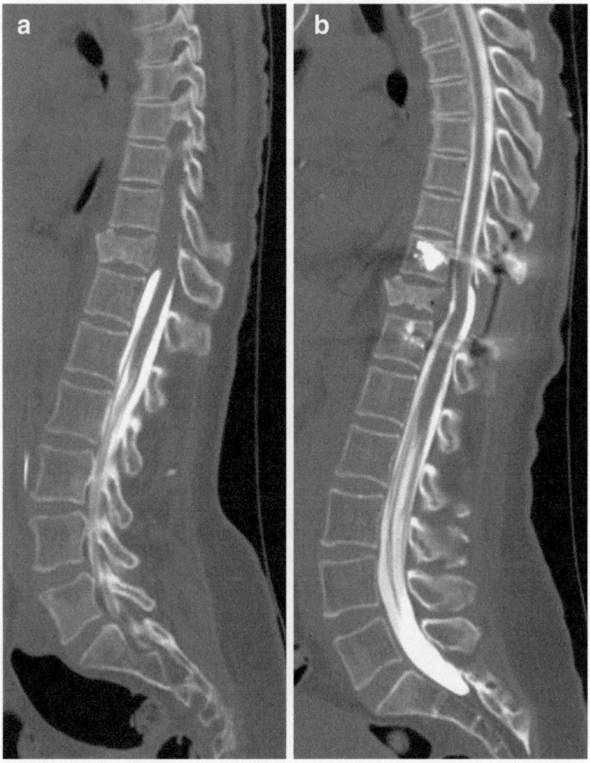

Fig. 5.2 Sagittal CT myelogram demonstrating (**a**) preoperative complete myelographic block at the level of T11 consistent with ESCC Grade 3 and (**b**) postoperative CT myelogram after decompression and stabilization. Reconstitution of the epidural space is visualized by the presence of intrathecal contrast at the level of T11 and above

Surgical Technique

As a technique, separation surgery focuses on the reconstitution of the thecal sac through the circumferential resection of epidural tumor and bony fragments that compress the thecal sac and spinal cord. Most patients who undergo separation surgery will require spinal instrumentation to restore spinal stability that may have been compromised due to tumor involvement of the vertebral body and posterior elements or the need for surgical pedicle resection to access the ventral epidural space safely [14].

Separation surgery typically utilizes a standard posterior midline exposure. After the exposure, spinal instrumentation is placed 1 to 2 levels above and below the index level, depending on adjacent segment anatomy and the extent of tumor involvement. This is followed by a laminectomy and resection of the dorsal epidural tumor. Lateral exposure is then obtained by performing a facetectomy and using the high-speed drill to remove the pedicle down to the level of the vertebral body.

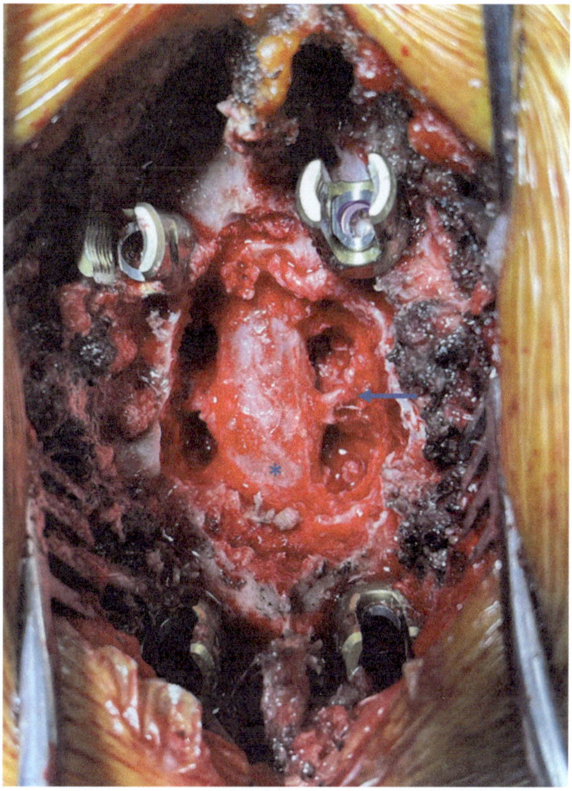

Fig. 5.3 Intraoperative photograph showing separation surgery with circumferential decompression of the thecal sac (asterisk). Tumor has been resected from the dorsal epidural space and the index level pedicles have been resected bilaterally, leaving the exiting nerve roots (arrow) exposed. The spaces cephalad and caudal to the nerve roots allow for access to the ventral epidural space and resection of tumor in this compartment. Pedicle screws can be seen at the levels above and below the decompression and will be used at the end of the case for placement of the rod

Drilling the bilateral pedicles allows for access to the ventral epidural space and the vertebral body. The posterior longitudinal ligament is then cut using tenotomy scissors, and the tumor is resected away from the ventral dura. Further decompression is achieved by depressing the epidural tumor ventrally away from the dura and into the vertebral body using a Woodson dissector or curettes (Fig. 5.3). Once the decompression is completed, confirmation of the adequacy of the decompression is done using an intraoperative ultrasound (Fig. 5.4). Adequate spinal cord decompression is essential to allow for the safe delivery of sufficient postoperative radiation to the osseous and residual epidural metastatic disease within spinal cord dose constraints. The creation of space between the radiation target and the neural structures is critical for achieving long-term local tumor control and optimizing the outcomes of hybrid therapy (Fig. 5.5).

Initially, separation surgery relied on large, multi-segmental constructs in order to overcome the intrinsic limitations of bone quality in patients with osseous metastatic disease as well as the issue of adjacent segment tumor involvement [16]. These longer constructs were associated with longer operating times, increased blood loss, and longer incisions. The advent of fenestrated screws that allowed for the extrusion of polymethyl methacrylate (PMMA) through the pedicle screws and into the vertebral body overcame the limitations of poor bone quality. The

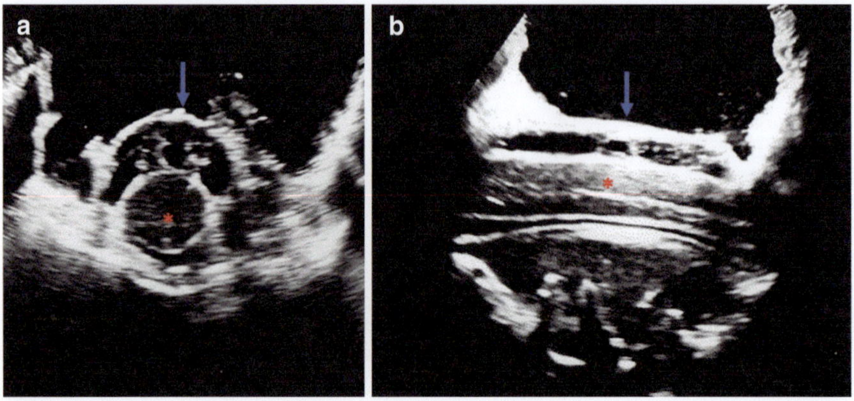

Fig. 5.4 Axial (**a**) and sagittal (**b**) views of the spinal cord and thecal sac utilizing intraoperative ultrasound to demonstrate the extent of spinal cord decompression. Arrows delineate the dorsal aspect of the thecal sac in both views and the red asterisks indicate the spinal cord. Note how in both views, CSF can be seen circumferentially around the spinal cord, confirming the adequacy of the decompression

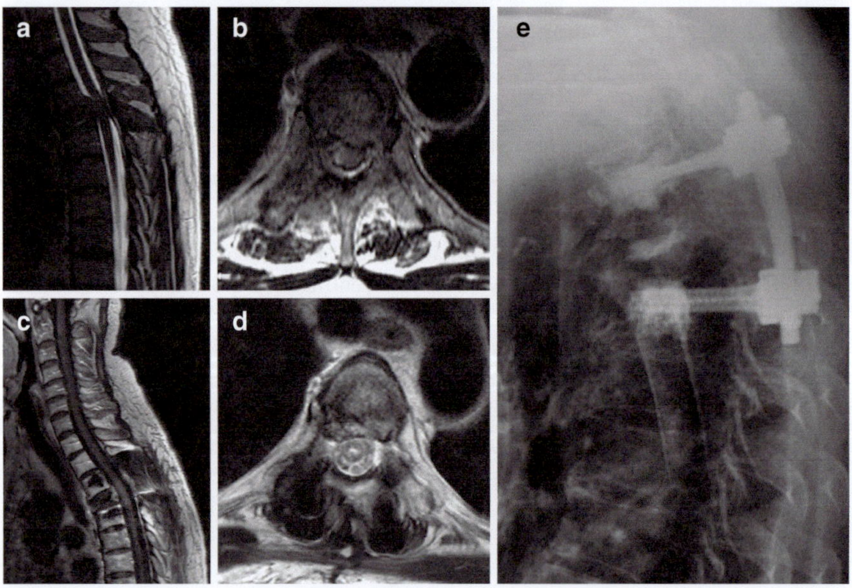

Fig. 5.5 Preoperative T2-sagittal (**a**) and axial (**b**) images demonstrating Grade 3 thoracic metastatic epidural spinal cord compression with signs of spinal cord signal change. After completion of a separation surgery followed by adjuvant stereotactic radiosurgery, 6-month follow-up MRI T1-sagittal (**c**) and T2-axial (**d**) demonstrate complete reconstitution of the thecal sac with no signs of disease recurrence at the index level. (**e**) Lateral X-ray demonstrating the short-segment construct with cement augmentation and index-level kyphoplasty used for stabilization

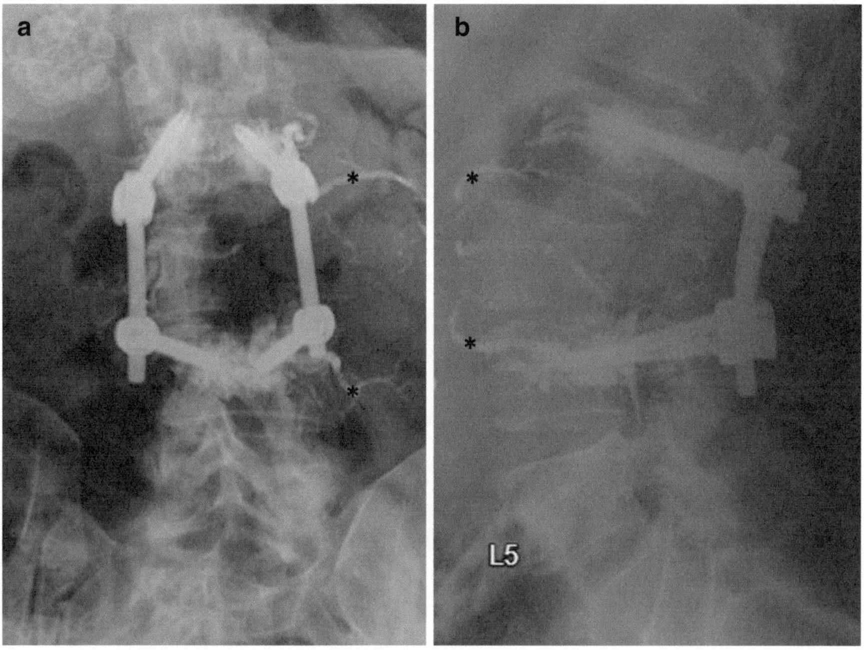

Fig. 5.6 AP (**a**) and lateral (**b**) X-ray images showing the appearance of fenestrated screws with cement augmentation used in spinal reconstruction during separation surgery for renal cell carcinoma metastasis involving the left two-thirds of the L4 vertebral body and extending into the psoas musculature. Embolic material (asterisks) related to the preoperative tumor embolization is also visualized

combination of fenestrated screws with PMMA is known as cement augmentation. PMMA augmentation improves screw pullout strength by allowing the cement extruded through the screw to interdigitate with the cancellous architecture of the vertebral body, thereby linking the two [17–19] (Fig. 5.6). Additionally, when sufficient cement is extruded into the vertebral body, this can also serve to support the vertebral body architecture, similar to a vertebroplasty. Like vertebroplasty and kyphoplasty, during the extrusion of PMMA into the vertebral body via fenestrated pedicle screws, attention must be paid to watch for any signs that the cement is extending beyond the cortical boundaries of the vertebral body as this may denote entry of the cement into the vasculature anteriorly or the epidural space posteriorly. Each of these complications can have devastating effects if they occur in sufficient volume (e.g., cement pulmonary embolus and cement-related epidural spinal cord compression, respectively).

Outcomes of Separation Surgery and Hybrid Therapy

Hybrid therapy has been associated with histology-independent local tumor control, with data demonstrating similar levels of control between traditionally radioresistant tumor histologies. For example, in multiple series by Chakravarthy et al. and Hussain et al., they demonstrated 2-year local control rates as high as 91.8% for renal cell carcinoma and 86.7% for colorectal carcinoma spine metastases undergoing hybrid therapy [13, 20]. Even more impressive, in patients with targetable mutations in non-small cell lung cancer with spine metastases undergoing hybrid therapy, Chakravarthy et al. were able to demonstrate a 95% local tumor control at 2 years [12]. These rates of local tumor control are far superior to the historical control rates reported with cEBRT.

While hybrid therapy represents a significant advance in the management of MESCC, it is not without its limitations. With respect to cement-augmented constructs for spinal reconstruction, a review of early fenestrated screw experience by Newman et al. demonstrated a failure rate of 2.8% for long-segment constructs and 2.2% for short-segment constructs, rates similar to traditional longer-segment fusions [19]. While the failure rates were similar to traditional constructs, the failure patterns were different—rather than the screw pullout frequently seen with long-segment fusions, the authors noted more instances of fracture at the screw-tulip interface. Similar to traditional constructs, both cement-augmented and traditional constructs can experience rod fractures.

With respect to separation surgery itself, studies demonstrate postoperative complication rates as high as 18% when measuring all surgical complications (e.g., urinary tract infection, pneumonia, etc.). Regarding surgical complications requiring a return to the operating room (e.g., wound infection or hardware failure), these rates are lower than those seen for larger, more aggressive surgical interventions and are approximately 12% or less, depending on the series [12, 14, 19, 21]. This demonstrates that while hybrid therapy may limit patient morbidity through the need for less aggressive surgical approaches, it is not a panacea without limitations.

Minimally Invasive Trends in Separation Surgery

Separation surgery in its earliest iterations involved long constructs often spanning three or more segments above and below the index level. However, as much of spine surgery for degenerative pathologies has trended toward minimally invasive approaches, so too has spine surgery for metastatic pathologies. This trend toward minimally invasive surgery for MESCC and the stabilization of pathologic fractures makes use of fenestrated screws with cement augmentation, percutaneous fixation, and tubular decompression to achieve the same goals of surgery with a more minimal surgical footprint.

Fenestrated screws with cement augmentation have allowed for the utilization of shorter constructs by overcoming bone quality limitations through increasing screw pullout strength and enabling shorter constructs with similar durability compared to historical longer segment constructs. The subsequent combination of cement augmentation with percutaneous rod-screw systems was another major advance in the trend toward more minimally invasive approaches to spine oncology. Percutaneous instrumentation allowed for the stabilization of pathological fractures without the need for long midline incisions to place the pedicle screws and rod as percutaneous screw and rod placement only requires multiple 1–2 cm paraspinal incisions. This decreased incision size allowed for shorter operative times, less blood loss, and smaller incisions that were easier to heal.

Combining percutaneous instrumentation with the ability to perform paramedian tubular or midline mini-open posterior approaches for surgical decompression of the spinal cord allowed for separation surgery to be performed while still utilizing a smaller incision than traditional approaches. The next step in the evolution of spinal cord decompression came in the application of tubular technologies to the treatment of MESCC, with tubular retractors allowing for the use of the same paraspinal incisions to access the ventral epidural space and achieve epidural tumor resection and spinal cord decompression. This transition to shorter constructs and more minimally invasive approaches has been associated with shorter operative times, less blood loss, and lower rates of wound complications compared to longer segment surgeries.

In total, this series of advances toward minimally invasive approaches to spine oncology has allowed for shorter surgeries, reduced blood loss, and smaller incisions with a reduced surgical footprint without compromising on outcomes in appropriately selected patients. As surgical technology continues to advance and as spine surgeons adapt technologies from other disciplines, the impact of minimally invasive techniques on spine oncology patients should continue to improve.

Conclusions

Separation surgery and its combination with postoperative radiation have fundamentally changed outcomes in patients with MESCC. Multiple studies have demonstrated that the ability to deliver ablative doses of radiation results in histology-independent local tumor control, firmly establishing the effectiveness of hybrid therapy. Subsequently, there has been a trend away from larger, more aggressive surgical interventions and toward more minimally invasive approaches with associated improvements in patient outcomes and recovery times. As technology, radiation, and systemic therapy options continue to evolve, so too will the role of separation surgery in the management of MESCC.

References

1. Loblaw DA, Laperriere NJ, Mackillop WJ. A population-based study of malignant spinal cord compression in Ontario. Clin Oncol (R Coll Radiol). 2003;15(4):211–7. https://doi.org/10.1016/s0936-6555(02)00400-4.
2. Mundy GR. Metastasis to bone: causes, consequences and therapeutic opportunities. Nat Rev Cancer. 2002;2(8):584–93. https://doi.org/10.1038/nrc867.
3. Spratt DE, Beeler WH, de Moraes FY, et al. An integrated multidisciplinary algorithm for the management of spinal metastases: an international spine oncology consortium report. Lancet Oncol. 2017;18(12):e720–30. https://doi.org/10.1016/S1470-2045(17)30612-5.
4. Patchell RA, Tibbs PA, Regine WF, et al. Direct decompressive surgical resection in the treatment of spinal cord compression caused by metastatic cancer: a randomised trial. Lancet. 2005;366(9486):643–8. https://doi.org/10.1016/S0140-6736(05)66954-1.
5. Gilbert RW, Kim JH, Posner JB. Epidural spinal cord compression from metastatic tumor: diagnosis and treatment. Ann Neurol. 1978;3(1):40–51. https://doi.org/10.1002/ana.410030107.
6. Sundaresan N, DiGiacinto GV, Krol G, Hughes JE. Spondylectomy for malignant tumors of the spine. J Clin Oncol. 1989;7(10):1485–91. https://doi.org/10.1200/JCO.1989.7.10.1485.
7. Walsh GL, Gokaslan ZL, McCutcheon IE, et al. Anterior approaches to the thoracic spine in patients with cancer: indications and results. Ann Thorac Surg. 1997;64(6):1611–8. https://doi.org/10.1016/s0003-4975(97)01034-5.
8. Gokaslan ZL, York JE, Walsh GL, et al. Transthoracic vertebrectomy for metastatic spinal tumors. J Neurosurg. 1998;89(4):599–609. https://doi.org/10.3171/jns.1998.89.4.0599.
9. Nazzaro JM, Arbit E, Burt M. "Trap door" exposure of the cervicothoracic junction. Technical note. J Neurosurg. 1994;80(2):338–41. https://doi.org/10.3171/jns.1994.80.2.0338.
10. Yamada Y, Bilsky MH, Lovelock DM, et al. High-dose, single-fraction image-guided intensity-modulated radiotherapy for metastatic spinal lesions. Int J Radiat Oncol Biol Phys. 2008;71(2):484–90. https://doi.org/10.1016/j.ijrobp.2007.11.046.
11. Yamada Y, Katsoulakis E, Laufer I, et al. The impact of histology and delivered dose on local control of spinal metastases treated with stereotactic radiosurgery. Neurosurg Focus. 2017;42(1):E6. https://doi.org/10.3171/2016.9.FOCUS16369.
12. Chakravarthy VB, Schachner B, Amin AG, et al. The impact of targetable mutations on clinical outcomes of metastatic epidural spinal cord compression in patients with non-small-cell lung cancer treated with hybrid therapy (surgery followed by stereotactic body radiation therapy). Neurosurgery. 2023;92(3):557–64. https://doi.org/10.1227/neu.0000000000002247.
13. Hussain I, Goldberg JL, Carnevale JA, et al. Hybrid therapy (surgery and radiosurgery) for the treatment of renal cell carcinoma spinal metastases. Neurosurgery. 2022;90(2):199–206. https://doi.org/10.1227/NEU.0000000000001780.
14. Barzilai O, Laufer I, Robin A, Xu R, Yamada Y, Bilsky MH. Hybrid therapy for metastatic epidural spinal cord compression: technique for separation surgery and spine radiosurgery. Oper Neurosurg (Hagerstown). 2019;16(3):310–8. https://doi.org/10.1093/ons/opy137.
15. Laufer I, Iorgulescu JB, Chapman T, et al. Local disease control for spinal metastases following "separation surgery" and adjuvant hypofractionated or high-dose single-fraction stereotactic radiosurgery: outcome analysis in 186 patients. J Neurosurg Spine. 2013;18(3):207–14. https://doi.org/10.3171/2012.11.SPINE12111.
16. Amankulor NM, Xu R, Iorgulescu JB, et al. The incidence and patterns of hardware failure after separation surgery in patients with spinal metastatic tumors. Spine J. 2014;14(9):1850–9. https://doi.org/10.1016/j.spinee.2013.10.028.

17. Choma TJ, Pfeiffer FM, Swope RW, Hirner JP. Pedicle screw design and cement augmentation in osteoporotic vertebrae: effects of fenestrations and cement viscosity on fixation and extraction. Spine (Phila Pa 1976). 2012;37(26):E1628–32. https://doi.org/10.1097/BRS.0b013e3182740e56.
18. Moussazadeh N, Rubin DG, McLaughlin L, Lis E, Bilsky MH, Laufer I. Short-segment percutaneous pedicle screw fixation with cement augmentation for tumor-induced spinal instability. Spine J. 2015;15(7):1609–17. https://doi.org/10.1016/j.spinee.2015.03.037.
19. Newman WC, Amin AG, Villavieja J, Laufer I, Bilsky MH, Barzilai O. Short-segment cement-augmented fixation in open separation surgery of metastatic epidural spinal cord compression: initial experience. Neurosurg Focus. 2021;50(5):E11. https://doi.org/10.3171/2021.2.FOCUS217.
20. Chakravarthy VB, Schachner B, Amin A, et al. Long-term clinical outcomes of patients with colorectal cancer with metastatic epidural spinal cord compression treated with hybrid therapy (surgery followed by stereotactic body radiation therapy). World Neurosurg. 2023;169:e89–95. https://doi.org/10.1016/j.wneu.2022.10.053.
21. Echt M, Stock A, De la Garza Ramos R, et al. Separation surgery for metastatic epidural spinal cord compression: comparison of a minimally invasive versus open approach. Neurosurg Focus. 2021;50(5):E10. https://doi.org/10.3171/2021.2.FOCUS201124.

Chapter 6
Minimally Invasive Surgery in Spine Oncology

Rabih Bou Nassif, W. Christopher Newman, Mark H. Bilsky, and Ori Barzilai

Introduction

In recent years, the field of oncology has witnessed remarkable advancements in the diagnosis and treatment of various types of cancer. Among the many challenges posed by cancer, the presence of spinal tumors stands out as a significant concern, impacting patients' quality of life and overall prognosis. Spinal tumors can arise as primary neoplasms originating within the spine or as secondary metastatic lesions spreading from distant cancer sites. Regardless of their origin, these tumors often lead to neurologic deficits, intractable pain and spinal instability, necessitating prompt and effective treatment [1].

Minimally invasive spine surgery (MISS) has emerged as a transformative approach in the management of spinal disorders, including tumors. As opposed to traditional open surgical methods, which require extensive tissue dissection and disruption of anatomical structures, MISS offers a less invasive alternative. By utilizing advanced surgical techniques and cutting-edge technology, MISS aims to achieve comparable surgical goals with reduced tissue trauma, minimized blood loss, and shorter hospital stays [2–4]. Such advantages not only translate to improved patient comfort but also contribute to faster postoperative recovery and rehabilitation. This is of utmost importance when the patient needs adjuvant therapy as soon as possible after the surgical intervention, leading to accelerated oncological treatment [5].

This research was funded in part through the NIH/NCI Cancer Center Support Grant P30 CA008748.

R. B. Nassif · W. C. Newman · M. H. Bilsky · O. Barzilai (✉)
Department of Neurosurgery, Memorial Sloan-Kettering Cancer Center, New York, NY, USA
e-mail: barzilao@mskcc.org

Y. Yamada et al. (eds.), *Multidisciplinary Spine Tumor Management*,
https://doi.org/10.1007/978-3-032-07519-2_6

As a result, it is vital for healthcare professionals, including spine surgeons, oncologists, and allied specialists, to be well-versed in the principles and applications of MISS in this specific context. This chapter aims to provide a comprehensive overview of minimally invasive spine surgery in the management of spinal tumors, helping foster informed decision-making and promoting optimal patient-centered care.

Traditional "Open" Versus Minimally Invasive Spine Surgery

Traditional open spine surgery has been the conventional approach for treating spinal tumors for many years. It involves making a midline incision over the affected area of the spine, which provides the surgeon with direct access to the tumor and surrounding structures. The surgical team then performs tissue dissection, necessitating the retraction and dissection of muscles and ligaments to gain visibility and access to the spine and subsequently to the tumor. The decompression of neural structures, resection of the tumor and subsequent spinal reconstruction are carried out through this open approach.

Open spine surgery offers several advantages. One of the key benefits is the excellent visualization it provides to surgeons. The direct and unobstructed view of the surgical field enables precise tumor resection and spinal reconstruction, enhancing surgical outcomes. Additionally, the versatility of the open approach stands out, as it can be adapted to various tumor locations and complexities. This adaptability makes it a reliable choice for addressing different challenging cases. Moreover, the familiarity that many surgeons have with traditional open techniques and anatomy adds to its appeal, making it a preferred option for cases that require a high level of expertise.

Despite its advantages, traditional open spine surgery comes with notable limitations. One significant drawback is the potential for tissue trauma. The dissection and retraction of tissues during the procedure can lead to significant muscle damage, which in turn may contribute to muscle necrosis, postoperative pain and a lengthy recovery process. Another drawback is the increased blood loss associated with larger incisions and the disruption of blood vessels, posing a concern during surgery. Particularly in the aging population, increased operative blood loss may increase postoperative complication rates and decrease survival [6]. Additionally, when compared to MISS techniques, this leads to prolonged hospital stays and extended recovery periods, which can be burdensome for patients. Moreover, wounds created in this approach increase the risk of infections [7, 8], heightening the overall risk of complications for patients undergoing open spine surgery, particularly in the oncology population, where wound-related issues such as infection and wound dehiscence are higher than in the general population, given poor nutritional status, systemic treatment including targeted and chemotherapy and local radiation [9–11].

MISS represents a revolutionary shift in spinal tumor management. It employs advanced surgical techniques and specialized instruments to achieve surgical goals with minimal disruption to surrounding tissues. The MISS strategies involve smaller incisions, often guided by real-time imaging such as fluoroscopy or intraoperative navigation systems. Through these small access points, surgical instruments are inserted, allowing for tumor resection, nerve decompression and spinal stabilization.

MISS presents several compelling advantages [12, 13]. One of the foremost benefits is the reduced tissue trauma associated with this approach. Smaller incisions and muscle-sparing techniques minimize disruption to tissues, resulting in diminished postoperative pain and accelerated recovery times for patients. Moreover, smaller incisions result in less blood loss during surgery, with reduced infection rates and shortened hospital stay [5].

Treatment Approach

The NOMS framework was established to standardize the treatment algorithm of spinal tumors and can be applied to both open and MISS procedures. The 4 components of the NOMS framework are the Neurologic, the Oncologic, the Mechanical and the Systemic status [14]. The Neurologic refers to the presence of a clinical radiculopathy or a myelopathy, as well as the radiological epidural spinal cord compression (ESCC) [15]. Oncologic status refers mainly to the tumor's potential response to current treatments. Mechanical stability serves as a separate surgical indication and assessment is aided using the Spinal Instability Neoplastic Score (SINS) [16]. The last component of NOMS is the Systemic status, which refers to the burden of disease and the capacity of the patient to tolerate the suggested treatment.

Currently, the main application of MISS techniques is in metastatic disease, where, for surgical decompression, the goals of surgery have shifted with the introduction of stereotactic body radiation therapy (SBRT). Rather than gross total resection and cytoreductive surgery, the goal transitioned to a simple posterolateral spinal cord decompression and stabilization (i.e., "separation surgery") [17, 18]. Separation surgery consists of creating a safe margin around the neural structures for adequate high-dose radiation treatment, which is a necessary second step in treatment (i.e., "hybrid therapy") [19–21]. This opened the door for more patients to benefit from MISS approaches before receiving adjuvant SBRT and resuming their oncologic treatment sooner than with traditional open surgery.

When stabilization of the spine is indicated, MISS also plays an important role, limiting the surgical footprint while providing durable stabilizing constructs. MISS stabilization can also be combined with MISS decompression whenever the patient could also benefit from a decompression for symptomatic relief and oncologic treatment. We have previously published our treatment algorithm for MISS applications in thoracolumbar spinal metastases (Fig. 6.1)

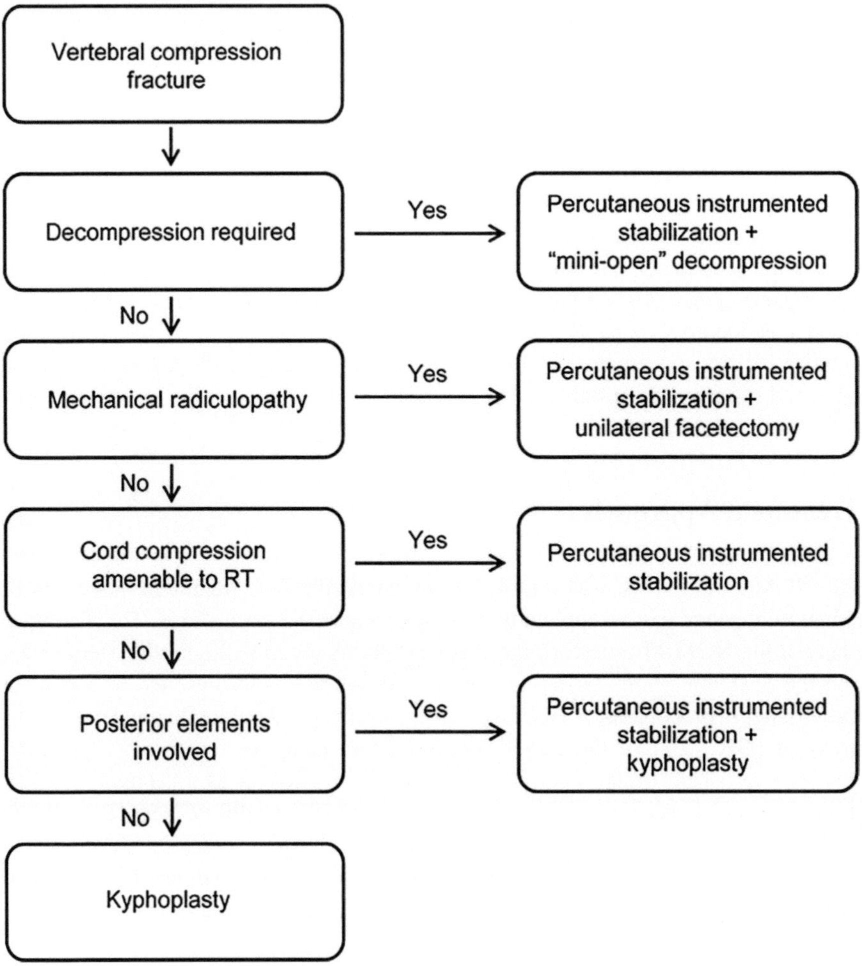

Fig. 6.1 MISS treatment algorithm for metastatic thoracolumbar compression fractures. Adapted from Barzilai et al. [22].

MISS Techniques in Spine Oncology

The field of MISS offers a spectrum of techniques, each with its own strengths and limitations. From cement augmentation to percutaneous pedicle screw instrumentation and tumor resection via minimally invasive means, the approach is far from one-size-fits-all. Instead, the art lies in combining these techniques in a synergistic manner, creating a tailored approach that aligns with the patient's specific condition.

Surgical Stabilization

Percutaneous Pedicle Screw Instrumentation and Vertebral Cement Augmentation

Vertebral cement augmentation has emerged as a versatile and innovative approach in the realm of spinal interventions, serving a dual purpose in pain relief and enhancing stability. This technique finds its application in both kyphoplasty and vertebroplasty, as well as in conjunction with fenestrated screws within percutaneous pedicle screw instrumentation (PPSI).

Kyphoplasty and vertebroplasty both provide reliable pain relief to individuals suffering from simple compression fractures that lack extensive cortical destruction or extension into the posterior elements of the spine. In both kyphoplasty and vertebroplasty, vertebral cement augmentation plays a pivotal role. A percutaneously placed needle allows for the injection of cement directly into the vertebral body. In vertebroplasty, the cement is introduced into the cancellous bone, while kyphoplasty involves creating a cavity using an inflatable balloon before cement injection. This process effectively stabilizes the fractured vertebral body, relieving pain and restoring function. However, caution is advised in cases involving epidural tumor extension, as cement injection might inadvertently push the tumor further into the spinal canal.

PPSI has revolutionized spinal stabilization, offering a minimally invasive alternative to conventional open posterior instrumentation. This technique is particularly beneficial for pathological fractures that do not lend themselves to standalone percutaneous cement augmentation as it stabilizes across the fractured segment, providing a posterior tension band. The Spine Instability Neoplastic Score (SINS) serves as a useful tool for the assessment and quantification of mechanical instability [23]. High instability usually requires surgical consultation, where the surgeons can assess and potentially recommend percutaneous stabilization to restore the mechanical stability of the spine [24].

PPSI minimizes disruption to surrounding soft tissues, avoiding complications like muscle necrosis, devascularization, and denervation, and also reduces blood loss [25]. It plays a major role in stabilization of the spine whenever the pathologic fracture is unstable and can be associated to decompression and tumor resection whenever warranted, either for pathologic diagnosis or decompression of nerve roots or the spinal cord [26, 27].

Carbon-fiber reinforced polyetheretherketone (CFRP) pedicle screw use has proven to provide some advantages in postoperative imaging, reducing artefact on postoperative MRI scans and providing better images for recurrence or progression of disease follow-up [28]. Additionally, even though focal MRIs and myelo-CT have been demonstrated to be sufficient for accurate radiation planning [29], CFRP screws could provide better images depending on the radiation oncology team's preferences [28]. CFRP screws can be placed using MIS techniques similar to titanium screws [30], but provide notably less haptic feedback during placement and the smallest diameter of 5.5 mm limits placement in small pedicles [31].

Polymethylmethacrylate (PMMA) bone cement augmentation through fenestrated screws offers additional screw pull-out strength, which is of high importance in patients with decreased bone density, a common issue in oncology. This opens the way for shorter segmental fusions, even for multilevel fractures. Cement injection is usually performed under live fluoroscopy monitoring to avoid spillage in the canal or anteriorly to the spine, as well as the distal embolus.

MIS Spinal Cord or Nerve Root Decompression with Tumor Resection

Spinal cord decompression constitutes one of the major neurosurgical emergencies. Even with the advances of SBRT, high-grade spinal cord compression (ESCC 2 or 3) from metastasis of a radioresistant tumor requires surgical decompression to establish an adequate radiation target enabling the delivery of an ablative radiation dose [32, 33]. In the lumbar spine, the main indication for surgical decompression is treatment-resistant radiculopathy.

Tubular MISS has become a very popular technique in degenerative spine surgery [34]. It provides access to the surgical target via tubular retractors when dilating, without harming muscular structures and limiting ligamentous and osseous disruption. Its popularity and the familiarity of surgeons with this technique made it gain traction in spinal tumor surgery. In select cases, tubular decompression allows resection of the tumor, posterior elements for nerve root decompression, ventral spinal cord decompression and even corpectomy with anterior column reconstruction [35–38]. It has been shown to be a safe and effective alternative to open approaches and would be mostly suitable for patients with hypo-vascular tumors [39].

Technological Innovation in MISS

Navigation and Robotics

Navigation in oncologic MISS constitutes an important pillar for accurate targeting and for percutaneous screw placement [40]. In addition to safely placing screws and accurately targeting decompression sites, spinal navigation helps by reducing the surgical staff and patient's radiation exposure [41]. Whether fluoroscopy or intraoperative computed tomography-based, these systems have become standard tools in spinal oncology surgery. Both have proven to be safe systems and help with highly accurate screw placement [42]. Navigation also has a role to play in endoscopy, where the surgical view can be limited. Navigating the endoscope helps confirm the trajectory and anatomical landmarks. Nevertheless, navigation should always be confirmed by other means as it can easily be uncalibrated by minimal movements of the patient or the navigation reference [43].

Robotics is another area that is transitioning into spine oncology surgery, after slowly gaining traction in general spine surgery. Multiple robotic systems have been in use in spine surgery, mainly for planning and execution of pedicle screw placement [44]. The use of robots has been shown to be safe and efficient in pedicle screw placement during spine tumor surgery [45]. Robotic-assisted spine surgery improves precision and patient outcomes, reducing blood loss, radiation exposure, and complications. However, only short-term research is available, and benefits regarding surgical duration and hospital stay are not yet conclusively proven [42].

Endoscopy

Endoscopic spine surgery is one of the most recent technical advances in spine surgery. It has been gaining popularity in degenerative spine surgery due to its ultra-minimal invasive nature. Endoscopy in tumor surgery is still in its debut stage, but it holds an important place and serves as a good tool in specific clinical situations [46]. Whether for pathologic diagnosis, tumor debulking or neural decompression, endoscopic spine surgery provides an even less invasive approach than other MISS techniques, helping speed up recovery in patients with multiple comorbidities, and can even be performed in situations where the patient wouldn't have been a surgical candidate due to the severity of the disease or to current treatments contraindicating more invasive surgeries. Initial reports have demonstrated endoscopic spine surgery's utility as a viable option for managing select spinal metastases and intradural-extramedullary tumors of the spinal column, yet more experience is necessary in order to evaluate its true potential to impact surgery for spinal tumors [47].

Laser Interstitial Thermotherapy

Image-guided laser interstitial thermal therapy (LITT) offers tumor ablation by thermal energy under real-time guidance by magnetic resonance imaging (MRI), initially described for intracranial tumors and later adopted for spine oncology [48–50]. LITT can also be combined with SBRT to provide tumor volume reduction with satisfactory pain control. This technique has nevertheless had limited adoption, likely due to significant technological requirements.

Current Limitations

MISS is not without its limitations. One significant challenge is the learning curve associated with performing MISS [51]. Surgeons require specialized training and expertise, and the transition from traditional open techniques to MISS can be steep, potentially affecting surgical outcomes during the early stages of adoption. Furthermore, the application of MISS is limited by factors such as tumor size, location, and patient anatomy [26]. Not all spinal tumors and complex cases are suitable for this approach, necessitating careful case selection. Additionally, the utilization of advanced surgical equipment and real-time imaging in MISS procedures can raise the overall cost of treatment, potentially impacting accessibility for some patients.

The comparison between traditional open spine surgery and minimally invasive spine surgery reveals the distinct advantages and limitations of each approach in the management of oncologic spinal tumors. While traditional open surgery has been the gold standard for many years and remains suitable for certain cases, the evolution of MISS has demonstrated compelling benefits in terms of reduced tissue trauma, faster recovery, and improved patient outcomes. However, it is essential for surgeons to carefully assess individual cases and choose the most appropriate surgical approach based on the tumor's characteristics, patient factors, and the surgeon's expertise in both techniques.

Conclusion

MISS has gained traction in spine oncology, particularly for treating spinal instability and metastatic epidural spinal cord compression. These techniques significantly reduce surgical blood loss and shorten hospital stays. MISS expands treatment options, offering surgical solutions to patients previously deemed ineligible for traditional open procedures. Crucially, minimally invasive approaches facilitate a quicker return to systemic treatments and radiation therapy, which is vital for improving oncologic prognosis. The reduced tissue trauma and faster recovery associated with MISS allow patients to resume critical cancer therapies sooner, potentially enhancing overall treatment efficacy. Technological advances in navigation and robotics have further enhanced the safety and precision of minimally invasive procedures. These innovations pave the way for exciting developments in endoscopic techniques, virtual reality-assisted surgery, and augmented reality guidance systems. Such advancements promise to revolutionize spine oncology by offering even less invasive, more accurate, and highly personalized surgical interventions. Moreover, the integration of artificial intelligence and machine learning algorithms with MISS techniques may enable real-time decision support, optimizing surgical outcomes and further reducing complications. As these technologies continue to evolve, they are likely to expand the scope and effectiveness of MISS in oncology, ultimately improving patient care and quality of life.

References

1. Choi D, Bilsky M, Fehlings M, Fisher C, Gokaslan Z. Spine oncology-metastatic spine tumors. Neurosurgery. 2017;80(3S):S131–7. https://doi.org/10.1093/NEUROS/NYW084.
2. Kumar N, Malhotra R, Maharajan K, et al. Metastatic spine tumor surgery: a comparative study of minimally invasive approach using percutaneous pedicle screws fixation versus open approach. Clin Spine Surg. 2017;30(8):E1015–21. https://doi.org/10.1097/BSD.0000000000000400.
3. Rao PJ, Thayaparan GK, Fairhall JM, Mobbs RJ. Minimally invasive percutaneous fixation techniques for metastatic spinal disease. Orthop Surg. 2014;6(3):187–95. https://doi.org/10.1111/OS.12114.
4. Hikata T, Isogai N, Shiono Y, et al. A Retrospective Cohort Study comparing the safety and efficacy of minimally invasive versus open surgical techniques in the treatment of spinal metastases. Clin Spine Surg. 2017;30(8):E1082–7. https://doi.org/10.1097/BSD.0000000000000460.
5. Uei H, Tokuhashi Y, Maseda M, et al. Clinical results of multidisciplinary therapy including palliative posterior spinal stabilization surgery and postoperative adjuvant therapy for metastatic spinal tumor. J Orthop Surg Res. 2018;13(1) https://doi.org/10.1186/S13018-018-0735-Z.
6. Hussain I, Hartley BR, McLaughlin L, et al. Surgery for metastatic spinal disease in octogenarians and above: analysis of 78 patients. Global Spine J. 2023;13(6):1481–9. https://doi.org/10.1177/21925682211037936.
7. Mueller K, Zhao D, Johnson O, Sandhu FA, Voyadzis JM. The difference in surgical site infection rates between open and minimally invasive spine surgery for degenerative lumbar pathology: a retrospective single center experience of 1442 cases. Oper Neurosurg (Hagerstown). 2019;16(6):750–5. https://doi.org/10.1093/ONS/OPY221.
8. Parker SL, Adogwa O, Witham TF, Aaronson OS, Cheng J, McGirt MJ. Post-operative infection after minimally invasive versus open transforaminal lumbar interbody fusion (TLIF): literature review and cost analysis. Minim Invasive Neurosurg. 2011;54(1):33–7. https://doi.org/10.1055/S-0030-1269904.
9. Kumar S, van Popta D, Rodrigues-Pinto R, et al. Risk factors for wound infection in surgery for spinal metastasis. Eur Spine J. 2015;24(3):528–32. https://doi.org/10.1007/S00586-013-3127-4.
10. Carl HM, Karim Ahmed A, Abu-Bonsrah N, et al. Risk factors for wound-related reoperations in patients with metastatic spine tumor. J Neurosurg Spine. 2018;28(6):663–8. https://doi.org/10.3171/2017.10.SPINE1765.
11. Demura S, Kawahara N, Murakami H, et al. Surgical site infection in spinal metastasis: risk factors and countermeasures. Spine (Phila Pa 1976). 2009;34(6):635–9. https://doi.org/10.1097/BRS.0B013E31819712CA.
12. Helal A, Yolcu YU, Kamath A, Wahood W, Bydon M. Minimally invasive versus open surgery for patients undergoing intradural extramedullary spinal cord tumor resection: a systematic review and meta-analysis. Clin Neurol Neurosurg. 2022:214. https://doi.org/10.1016/J.CLINEURO.2022.107176.
13. Raygor KP, Than KD, Chou D, Mummaneni PV. Comparison of minimally invasive transspinous and open approaches for thoracolumbar intradural-extramedullary spinal tumors. Neurosurg Focus. 2015;39(2):E12. https://doi.org/10.3171/2015.5.FOCUS15187.
14. Laufer I, Rubin DG, Lis E, et al. The NOMS Framework: approach to the treatment of spinal metastatic tumors. Oncologist. 2013;18(6):744. https://doi.org/10.1634/THEONCOLOGIST.2012-0293.

15. Bilsky MH, Laufer I, Fourney DR, et al. Reliability analysis of the epidural spinal cord compression scale: clinical article. J Neurosurg Spine. 2010;13(3):324–8. https://doi.org/10.3171/2010.3.SPINE09459.
16. Fisher CG, Schouten R, Versteeg AL, et al. Reliability of the Spinal Instability Neoplastic Score (SINS) among radiation oncologists: an assessment of instability secondary to spinal metastases. Radiat Oncol. 2014;9(1) https://doi.org/10.1186/1748-717X-9-69.
17. Laufer I, Iorgulescu JB, Chapman T, et al. Local disease control for spinal metastases following "separation surgery" and adjuvant hypofractionated or high-dose single-fraction stereotactic radiosurgery: outcome analysis in 186 patients. J Neurosurg Spine. 2013;18(3):207–14. https://doi.org/10.3171/2012.11.SPINE12111.
18. Moussazadeh N, Laufer I, Yamada Y, Bilsky MH. Separation surgery for spinal metastases: effect of spinal radiosurgery on surgical treatment goals. Cancer Control. 2014;21(2):168–74. https://doi.org/10.1177/107327481402100210.
19. Joaquim AF, Powers A, Laufer I, Bilsky MH. An update in the management of spinal metastases. Arq Neuropsiquiatr. 2015;73(9):795–802. https://doi.org/10.1590/0004-282X20150099.
20. Barzilai O, Laufer I, Robin A, Xu R, Yamada Y, Bilsky MH. Hybrid therapy for metastatic epidural spinal cord compression: technique for separation surgery and spine radiosurgery. Oper Neurosurg (Hagerstown). 2019;16(3):310–8. https://doi.org/10.1093/ONS/OPY137.
21. Rothrock R, Pennington Z, Ehresman J, et al. Hybrid therapy for spinal metastases. Neurosurg Clin N Am. 2020;31(2):191–200. https://doi.org/10.1016/J.NEC.2019.11.001.
22. Barzilai O, McLaughlin L, Amato MK, et al. Minimal access surgery for spinal metastases: prospective evaluation of a treatment algorithm using patient-reported outcomes. World Neurosurg. 2018;120:e889–901. https://doi.org/10.1016/j.wneu.2018.08.182.
23. Fisher CG, Dipaola CP, Ryken TC, et al. A novel classification system for spinal instability in neoplastic disease: an evidence-based approach and expert consensus from the Spine Oncology Study Group. Spine (Phila Pa 1976). 2010;35(22) https://doi.org/10.1097/BRS.0B013E3181E16AE2.
24. Mahakul DJ, Visen A, Agarwal J. The truly intermediate subgroup within the SINS "potentially unstable" category: the Matryoshka doll phenomenon. World Neurosurg; 2024. https://doi.org/10.1016/J.WNEU.2024.06.159.
25. Schupper AJ, Patel S, Steinberger JM, Germano IM. The role of minimally invasive surgery within a multidisciplinary approach for patients with metastatic spine disease over a decade: a systematic review. Neuro Oncol. 2024;26(3):417–28. https://doi.org/10.1093/NEUONC/NOAD206.
26. Barzilai O, Bilsky MH, Laufer I. The role of minimal access surgery in the treatment of spinal metastatic tumors. Global Spine J. 2020;10(2 Suppl):79S–87S. https://doi.org/10.1177/2192568219895265.
27. Kim CH, Chung CK, Sohn S, Lee S, Park SB. Less invasive palliative surgery for spinal metastases. J Surg Oncol. 2013;108(7):499–503. https://doi.org/10.1002/JSO.23418.
28. Ho D, Corde S, Chen C, Saade G, Betteridge C, Mobbs R. The use of carbon fiber/polyetheretherketone (CF/PEEK) in pedicle screw fixation for spinal neoplasms – potential advantages in postoperative imaging and radiotherapy planning. J Spine Surg. 2024;10(1):8–21. https://doi.org/10.21037/JSS-23-93/COIF).
29. Uhl M, Sterzing F, Habl G, et al. CT-myelography for high-dose irradiation of spinal and paraspinal tumors with helical tomotherapy: revival of an old tool. Strahlenther Onkol. 2011;187(7):416–20. https://doi.org/10.1007/S00066-011-2219-5.
30. de Paulo Martins Coelho Junior V, Dhaliwal JS, Chakravarthy VB. MIS technique for separation surgery in lumbar spine metastatic disease. Neurosurg Focus Video. 2024;10(2):2024. https://doi.org/10.3171/2024.1.FOCVID23222.
31. Alvarez-Breckenridge C, de Almeida R, Haider A, et al. Carbon fiber-reinforced polyetheretherketone spinal implants for treatment of spinal tumors: perceived advantages and limitations. Neurospine. 2023;20(1):317. https://doi.org/10.14245/NS.2244920.460.

32. Yamada Y, Katsoulakis E, Laufer I, et al. The impact of histology and delivered dose on local control of spinal metastases treated with stereotactic radiosurgery. Neurosurg Focus. 2017;42(1) https://doi.org/10.3171/2016.9.FOCUS16369.
33. Gerszten PC, Burton SA, Ozhasoglu C, Welch WC. Radiosurgery for spinal metastases: clinical experience in 500 cases from a single institution. Spine (Phila Pa 1976). 2007;32(2):193–9. https://doi.org/10.1097/01.BRS.0000251863.76595.A2.
34. Hernandez RN, Wipplinger C, Navarro-Ramirez R, et al. Ten-step minimally invasive cervical decompression via unilateral tubular laminotomy: technical note and early clinical experience. Oper Neurosurg (Hagerstown). 2020;18(3):284–94. https://doi.org/10.1093/ONS/OPZ156.
35. Saigal R, Wadhwa R, Mummaneni PV, Chou D. Minimally invasive extracavitary transpedicular corpectomy for the management of spinal tumors. Neurosurg Clin N Am. 2014;25(2):305–15. https://doi.org/10.1016/J.NEC.2013.12.008.
36. Laratta JL, Weegens R, Malone KT, Chou D, Smith WD. Minimally invasive lateral approaches for the treatment of spinal tumors: single-position surgery without the "flip". J Spine Surg. 2020;6(1):62–71. https://doi.org/10.21037/JSS.2019.12.12.
37. Lau D, Chou D. Posterior thoracic corpectomy with cage reconstruction for metastatic spinal tumors: comparing the mini-open approach to the open approach. J Neurosurg Spine. 2015;23(2):217–27. https://doi.org/10.3171/2014.12.SPINE14543.
38. Chou D, Lu DC. Mini-open transpedicular corpectomies with expandable cage reconstruction. Technical note. J Neurosurg Spine. 2011;14(1):71–7. https://doi.org/10.3171/2010.10.SPINE091009.
39. Cui Y, Mi C, Wang B, Pan Y, Lin Y, Shi X. Mini-open compared with the trans-tubular approach in patients with spinal metastases underwent decompression surgery – a retrospective cohort study. BMC Cancer. 2023;23(1) https://doi.org/10.1186/S12885-023-11730-4.
40. Helm PA, Teichman R, Hartmann SL, Simon D. Spinal navigation and imaging: history, trends, and future. IEEE Trans Med Imaging. 2015;34(8):1738–46. https://doi.org/10.1109/TMI.2015.2391200.
41. Jeys L, Matharu GS, Nandra RS, Grimer RJ. Can computer navigation-assisted surgery reduce the risk of an intralesional margin and reduce the rate of local recurrence in patients with a tumour of the pelvis or sacrum? Bone Joint J. 2013;95-B(10):1417–24. https://doi.org/10.1302/0301-620X.95B10.31734.
42. Zawar A, Chhabra HS, Mundra A, Sharma S, Kalidindi KKV. Robotics and navigation in spine surgery: a narrative review. J Orthop. 2023;44:36–46. https://doi.org/10.1016/J.JOR.2023.08.007.
43. Schmidt BT, Chen KT, Kim JS, Brooks NP. Applications of navigation in full-endoscopic spine surgery. Eur Spine J. 2024;33(2):429–37. https://doi.org/10.1007/S00586-023-07918-8/FIGURES/5.
44. Overley SC, Cho SK, Mehta AI, Arnold PM. Navigation and robotics in spinal surgery: where are we now? Neurosurgery. 2017;80(3S):S86–99. https://doi.org/10.1093/NEUROS/NYW077.
45. Menta AK, Weber-Levine C, Jiang K, et al. Robotic assisted surgery for the treatment of spinal metastases: a case series. Clin Neurol Neurosurg. 2024;243:108393. https://doi.org/10.1016/J.CLINEURO.2024.108393.
46. Ali R, Hagan MJ, Shaaya E, et al. Endoscopic techniques for spinal oncology: a systematic literature review. Int J Spine Surg. 2023;17(3):343–9. https://doi.org/10.14444/8412.
47. Patel S, Khan MF, Gensler R, et al. Applications of endoscopic techniques in spinal oncology: a systematic review of the contemporary literature. J Clin Neurosci. 2025:136. https://doi.org/10.1016/J.JOCN.2025.111232/ATTACHMENT/87E9E99F-A329-46B4-A449-C8FCE01F723E/MMC1.DOCX.
48. Tatsui CE, Lee SH, Amini B, et al. Spinal laser interstitial thermal therapy: a novel alternative to surgery for metastatic epidural spinal cord compression. Neurosurgery. 2016;79(Suppl 1):S73–82. https://doi.org/10.1227/NEU.0000000000001444.

49. Tatsui CE, Belsuzarri TAB, Oro M, et al. Percutaneous surgery for treatment of epidural spinal cord compression and spinal instability: technical note. Neurosurg Focus. 2016;41(4) https://doi.org/10.3171/2016.8.FOCUS16175.
50. Tatsui CE, Stafford RJ, Li J, et al. Utilization of laser interstitial thermotherapy guided by real-time thermal MRI as an alternative to separation surgery in the management of spinal metastasis. J Neurosurg Spine. 2015;23(4):400–11. https://doi.org/10.3171/2015.2.SPINE141185.
51. Yang JH, Kim HJ, Chang DG, Nam Y, Suh SW. Learning curve for minimally invasive scoliosis surgery in adolescent idiopathic scoliosis. World Neurosurg. 2023;175:e201–7. https://doi.org/10.1016/J.WNEU.2023.03.053.

Chapter 7
The Multidisciplinary Management of Sacral Tumors

Max Vaynrub

Introduction

The management of sacral tumors warrants a dedicated discussion due to the unique skeletal, neurologic, vascular, soft tissue, and colorectal considerations of this anatomic region. The challenges include issues related to tumor control, structural stability, neurologic deficits, wound healing, rehabilitation, pain control, and psychiatric care. Since these domains are rarely affected in isolation, multidisciplinary care—including spine surgery, plastic surgery, colorectal surgery, radiation oncology, rehabilitation medicine, urology, pain management, and psychiatry is critical to optimizing patient outcomes.

The considerations involved in the management of sacral tumors vary greatly depending on the nature of the tumor, the systemic staging of the disease, and the patient's goals and expectations. Certain diagnoses, such as primary sarcoma, depend primarily on en bloc surgical resection for tumor control, and significant surgical morbidity is often accepted in pursuit of cure [1, 2]. In contrast, the primary goal is palliation for patients with sacral metastasis and limited life expectancy, and treatment plans should emphasize minimizing iatrogenic morbidity; tumor control is established primarily with systemic therapy and radiotherapy, and the surgical indications are more limited. Some situations require more nuanced multidisciplinary discussions and exploration of patient values [3]. For instance, although sacrectomy is the most definitive treatment for sacral chordoma [4–6], some patients are unwilling to accept the neurologic morbidity; while long-term follow-up data are needed to delineate the benefits and risks of definitive radiotherapy, short- and medium-term data suggest that this may be a viable alternative [7].

M. Vaynrub (✉)
Department of Surgery, Orthopaedic Service, Memorial Sloan Kettering Cancer Center, New York, NY, USA
e-mail: vaynrubm@mskcc.org

Y. Yamada et al. (eds.), *Multidisciplinary Spine Tumor Management*,
https://doi.org/10.1007/978-3-032-07519-2_7

Management of Primary Sacral Tumors

The management of primary tumors of the spine and sacrum is a debated topic. While many studies report outcomes following specific interventions, the data are largely from retrospective and uncontrolled studies. As with many rare diseases, prospective comparative data on the treatment of primary sacral tumors are lacking, and randomized trials are generally infeasible. Thus, most comparisons of treatment modalities have relied on systematic reviews, and treatment decisions often are based on inherently flawed comparisons of outcomes from different treatment centers, heterogeneous patient cohorts, and nonstandardized terminology to describe interventions.

A notable attempt to standardize surgical terminology was the introduction of the concept of Enneking-appropriate (EA) and Enneking-inappropriate (EI) resection [8]. Adapted from the Enneking surgical staging system for extremities [9], this system categorizes treatment as EI if a malignant tumor or an aggressive benign tumor is transgressed (intralesional excision). EA treatment involves an en bloc excision with a final pathology report that the surgical margins were marginal (outside the tumor but through the reactive zone) or wide (tumor fully surrounded by intact normal tissue). An important distinction between Enneking staging for the spine and staging for extremities is that marginal margins would not be considered acceptable in an extremity, while the anatomic constraints of the spine (e.g., dura and critical vasculature) often preclude wide resection without unreasonable morbidity.

Though the benefit to overall survival is variable, in general, EA resection leads to improved local control [4, 10–12]. For instance, in a study comparing EA and EI resection for sacral chordoma, EA surgery was associated with significantly lower local recurrence (29% vs. 64%; $p < 0.001$) and a trend toward lower mortality (28% vs. 43%; $p = 0.099$) [6]. While it is intuitive that a more complete oncologic resection will reduce the likelihood of recurrence, it is important to acknowledge the limitations of these results. First, patients who had previously undergone intralesional surgery and presented to a study center after recurrence were analyzed in the EI cohort, even if the salvage surgery had been en bloc marginal/wide. As recurrent tumors have worse outcomes, this biased the EI group to poorer outcomes. Second, while the results demonstrated that outcomes of EA surgery were superior to those of other surgical approaches, the study was not designed to make direct comparisons with other treatment modalities, such as definitive radiotherapy.

As such, the optimal treatment is not always obvious. Advances in the use of modern radiotherapy for tumor ablation have yielded oncologic outcomes on par with, if not better than, results in the surgical literature for tumors traditionally considered radioresistant (e.g., chordoma and chondrosarcoma), though comparisons between studies can be misleading and studies directly comparing modalities are lacking [13, 14]. Higher dose regimens of radiotherapy have been associated with improved tumor control [7], but the proximity of the rectum to the presacral extent of the tumor can limit the dose that can safely be administered. Temporary organ displacement—an interventional radiology technique that mobilizes the rectum anteriorly via the percutaneous introduction of a catheter that is subsequently filled with saline—creates the space necessary to administer high-dose radiosurgery safely (Fig. 7.1) [15].

Another consideration is that the treatment that offers the highest rate of tumor control is not necessarily the best treatment for each patient. When formulating a treatment plan, it is important to be familiar with the natural history of the patient's tumor, treatment-specific outcomes, salvage options, treatment-related morbidity, and the patient's goals. As an example, although sacrectomy with EA margins may provide the best oncologic outcomes for sacral chordoma, it may not be the best treatment choice for an elder who presents with a minimally symptomatic sacral chordoma and wishes to prioritize near-term quality of life.

Salvage options are important to consider. A tumor for which local recurrence is associated with decreased survival and poor local salvage may justify maximally aggressive treatment even if it results in treatment-related morbidity. For example, outcomes are frequently poor for recurrent chordoma: Salvage surgery is associated with a 5-year local recurrence-free survival rate of 47–76% and an overall survival rate of 50% [5, 16]. Salvage radiotherapy rates are also compromised, with 5-year local control rates reported as 50–57% [17].

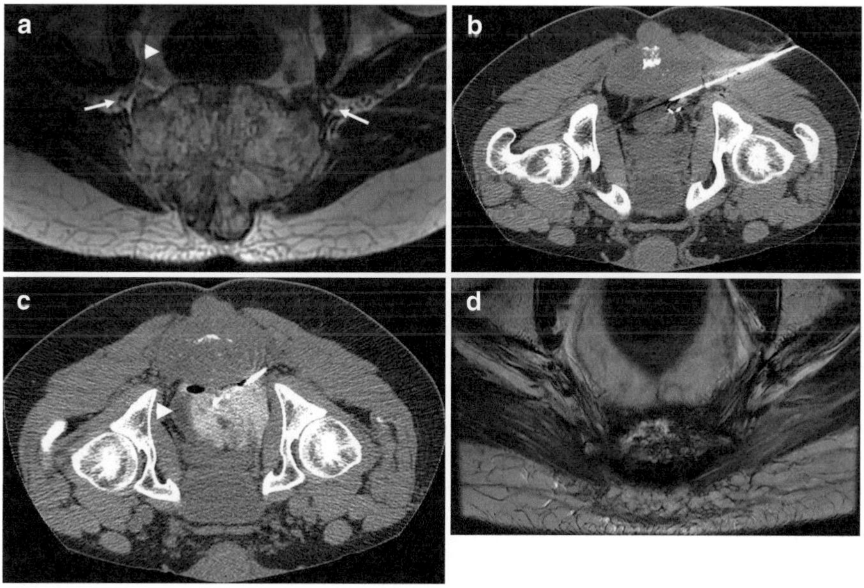

Fig. 7.1 A 52-year-old with conventional chordoma of the sacrum with lateral extension to the pudendal nerves (arrows) and close proximity to the rectum (arrowhead) on axial T2-weighted MRI (**a**). Given the anticipated morbidity of pudendal nerve sacrifice related to bladder, bowel, and sexual function, the patient was treated with definitive radiosurgery consisting of 24 Gy in a single fraction. A percutaneous catheter was introduced (**b**) and inflated with saline for temporary organ displacement, mobilizing the rectum (arrowhead) away from the tumor (**c**). At 14 months after treatment, there was a marked reduction in the size of the tumor (**d**)

In contrast, the availability of reliable salvage options would argue against morbid treatment on presentation. An excellent example of this is the giant cell tumor of bone (GCTB). While en bloc resection of GCTB is associated with lower rates of recurrence than intralesional resection (4% vs. 28%; $p = 0.029$) [18], the morbidity of en bloc sacrectomy is substantial. Since salvage treatment is usually successful, a higher rate of local recurrence in this setting can be acceptable. In a study of 24 patients who underwent nerve-sparing intralesional resection, 7 (29%) experienced local recurrence; 6 of them had successful salvage therapy with repeat nerve-sparing surgery and adjuvant treatment (e.g., radiotherapy), and the remaining patient with en bloc resection [19].

It is also important to be familiar with established and emerging medical therapies. Arguably the best-known example is denosumab, an anti-RANKL (receptor-activator of nuclear kappa B ligand) antibody, which has proven to be extremely useful in management of GCTB and aneurysmal bone cyst, though the clinical experience with the latter is much smaller and off-label [20, 21]. In the neoadjuvant setting, denosumab can facilitate surgical resection by decreasing the presacral extension of the tumor or by inducing peripheral ossification that can aid intraoperative identification of the tumor margins. Alternatively, it can be utilized as chronic therapy in lieu of surgery, though this approach carries risks of osteonecrosis of the jaw, atypical femur fracture, and rebound osteoporosis or tumor recurrence on discontinuation. The limit on the length of therapy and the optimal long-term dosing regimen are unknown.

Outcomes

While patient-centered decision-making is important in all aspects of medicine, it is especially salient when planning potentially life-altering treatment for sacral tumors. Patients differ in their prioritization of quality of life versus length of life. Realistic oncologic expectations are important to discuss. While some patients may accept the morbidity of sacrectomy even when a disease with a low survival rate is diagnosed, such as dedifferentiated chordoma or radiation-associated sarcoma, others may choose to avoid surgery [22].

It is crucial to convey realistic expectations about treatment-related morbidity and risks, the anticipated recovery process, and the impact on quality of life. The spectrum of morbidity between distal sacrectomy and total sacrectomy is large. There is no universally accepted outcome measure, which complicates comparisons between studies. Furthermore, patients should understand that quoted functional outcomes are averages and that individual neurologic outcomes are difficult to predict. Traditionally, the S4 and S5 nerve roots have been regarded as expendable, though several studies report bladder and/or bowel dysfunction even with distal sacrectomy. In studies of patients who had salvage of bilateral S3 nerve roots, Todd et al. reported bladder dysfunction in 4 of 13 patients and Ji et al. reported mean functional scores of 7.06/9 for bladder and 7.31/9 for bowel [1, 23]. Most bladder, bowel, and sexual function is associated with the S2 and S3 nerves, and all patients with bilateral S2 nerve-root sacrifice experience bladder/bowel incontinence and sexual dysfunction [23]. Pudendal nerve status is often omitted in reports, despite its contribution to continence and sexual function. While the S2 nerve roots may contribute to toe flexion and minor lower extremity sensation, lower extremity morbidity is generally not reported until S1 nerve roots are sacrificed [1]. More recently, Patient-Reported Outcomes Measurement Information System (PROMIS) scores have been reported for various levels of sacrectomy; use of this measure has demonstrated increasing levels of disability with more proximal resections and has allowed for comparisons with population norms and with other disease states.

Complications

The potential for complications in sacral tumor surgery is high. The risk of achieving a positive margin resection is significant. Dedicated imaging in the plane of the sacrum aids surgical planning. As sacral tumors often grow large prior to clinical presentation, and there is little room to maneuver within the pelvic cavity, the presacral margin is often thin and delimited only by presacral fascia. Collaboration with colorectal surgery is often helpful in dissecting and maintaining a mesorectal layer anterior to the tumor.

Tumors can also be difficult to contain in the relatively loose fatty tissue of the epidural space or in the neuroforamina. Furthermore, some tumors, such as chordoma, tend to track along the piriformis and sacrospinous ligaments, making a wide resection difficult to achieve and increasing the risk for recurrence. Collaboration with radiation oncologists is important for certain tumors to provide adjuvant therapy to reduce recurrence risk or to discuss definitive radiotherapy when surgery is not the best option [24].

Rectal injury is a risk of sacral surgery, especially when the patient has had radiotherapy or prior surgery due to the development of adhesions, or in the setting of direct tumor involvement of the rectum. In these situations, collaboration with a colorectal surgeon is helpful. A posterior-only approach also carries the risk of rectal injury during osteotomy; this risk can be mitigated in certain situations with the use of stereotactic navigation and an ultrasonic osteotomy device.

Wound complications are frequently encountered in sacral surgery and reportedly occur in 36–44% of sacral resections [25, 26]. Risk factors include prior surgery, prior radiation, hypoalbuminemia, intraoperative rectal or dural injury, prolonged operative time, and greater numbers of surgeons [25]. In contrast to the proximal sacrum, which is covered with robust paraspinal musculature, the mid-distal sacrum lacks overlying paraspinal or gluteal muscle in the midline, resulting in a subcutaneous primary closure in the absence of flaps. Following sacrectomy, there is a large dead space that is at risk of developing seroma, hematoma, and infection. High sacrectomies are often performed with internal iliac artery ligation, either due to tumor proximity or as a means of decreasing operative blood loss. This further complicates wound healing, as the gluteal vessels form the main vascular supply to the gluteal soft tissue. Many patients undergoing sacral surgery have had prior radiotherapy (either as planned neoadjuvant treatment or preceding disease recurrence), which increases the risk of wound complications to a variable extent (depending on dose, radiation modality, and timing). Common postoperative patient positions can be problematic for wound healing. For example, because supine positioning puts direct pressure on a healing primary repair or flap, the patient may need to be maintained in a lateral or prone position. Similarly, sitting requires hip flexion, which increases the tension on the gluteal repair. Patients often have postoperative positioning restrictions for weeks to months after surgery. Close collaboration with plastic surgery is essential for successful soft tissue management.

While various degrees of bladder, bowel, and sexual neurologic deficits have been correlated with the level of sacrectomy, the variability in neurologic outcomes is large [1, 2, 23, 27, 28]. The variation is likely multifactorial and related to difficult-to-quantify factors, such as individual variation in innervation patterns, degree of intraoperative dissection and traction of preserved nerve roots, history of radiation to the neurologic elements, involvement of the pudendal nerves, and dissection of the presacral and rectal neurologic plexus. For this reason, patients should be counseled preoperatively that there is a wide spectrum of possible neurologic outcomes relevant to their level of neurologic sacrifice.

Sacral Anatomy and Biomechanics

In contrast to the mobile spine, the sacrum is a rigid structure consisting of five fused vertebral segments. It is positioned between the bilateral ilia in a structurally significant wedged-keystone configuration that resists caudal migration of the sacrum and allows the transmission of body weight between the lower extremities and the rest of the axial skeleton. The sacrum interfaces with the pelvis through the sacroiliac joints, which are composed of synovial and syndesmotic components. The joints achieve a high level of stability due to reciprocally irregular surfaces between the sacrum and ilia, as well as to the robust sacroiliac, lumbosacral, and iliolumbar ligaments, which are among the strongest in the body. Distal to the sacroiliac joints, the sacrotuberous and sacrospinous ligaments provide stable links between the sacrum and the ischial tuberosities and ischial spines, respectively.

Approximately two-thirds of patients undergoing sacrectomy have tumors at or below the level of S2 [23]. When partial sacrectomy is performed just distal to the S1 foramina, 16–25% of the sacroiliac joints are sacrificed, compared with 25–72% of the joints when the resection is performed just proximal to the S1 foramina; the variability stems from the trajectory of the osteotomy lateral to the foramina (transverse versus oblique distally) [29, 30]. Partial sacrectomy resulted in a statistically significant decrease in load to failure, from 3,014 N in the intact sacrum to 2,166 N for osteotomies below the S1 foramina and 1,044 N for osteotomies above the S1 foramina. As a comparison, the greatest physiologic loads in the lumbar spine are in a position of flexion (2,105 N when standing and 1,801 N when sitting) [31]. Importantly, failures did not occur through the compromised sacroiliac joints, but rather as sagittally oriented fractures through Denis Zone II (in the plane of the foramina). The reason for nonfailure through the joints is likely related to the redundancy and strength of the spanning ligaments. To that end, there is no statistically significant difference in compressive stiffness until 72% of the joint is resected, at which point stiffness is still 83% of normal ($p < 0.05$); torsional stiffness is significantly decreased after resection of 25% and 72% of the joint (82% and 72% residual stiffness, respectively, $p < 0.05$) [30].

In load-to-failure tests, displacement occurs as forward rotation of the central lumbosacral spine in relation to the pelvis, with a moment of rotation at the posterior-superior S1 body [29, 32]. The aim of stabilization is not simply to secure the sacroiliac joints, but also to resist this flexion moment. The methods through which this goal is accomplished differ between primary and metastatic tumors, and are discussed in further detail in the ensuing sections.

Reconstruction

While this discussion and the literature focus on skeletal and soft tissue reconstruction, it is important to plan for the reconstruction of colorectal, urologic, gynecologic, and vascular structures that may require sacrifice.

The residual sacrum is thought to be potentially unstable—and skeletal reconstruction is generally considered—after en bloc resection through or above the S1 foramina [29, 30]. However, this practice is not universal, and some surgeons choose not to reconstruct even following total sacrectomy. In a series of 16 patients undergoing total sacrectomy without reconstruction, the 14 who had a relatively narrow resection (medial to or through the sacroiliac joints) achieved reasonable functional outcomes; their mean Musculoskeletal Tumor Society (MSTS) score was 19 out of 30, and 13 were ambulatory (5 without an assistive device). The two patients who underwent a wider resection (3 cm lateral to the sacroiliac joints) were both nonambulatory and had a mean MSTS score of 12.

In 2016, a systematic review by AOSpine Knowledge Forum Tumor found no difference in ambulatory function between reconstructed and nonreconstructed patients, but those undergoing reconstruction had a shorter length of stay (50 vs. 74 days) and a lower wound dehiscence rate (23% vs. 67%). The review's conclusion was a weak recommendation with very low certainty of evidence that patients who undergo total sacrectomy be stabilized with spinopelvic reconstruction [33].

The preponderance of the literature, however, has focused not on whether skeletal reconstruction should be undertaken for a high or total sacrectomy, but rather on the choice of reconstruction techniques. A number of biomechanical studies have demonstrated the benefits of dual iliac screw [34] and dual rod [35] instrumentation in terms of resisting compression and torsion forces (Fig. 7.2). In addition, a

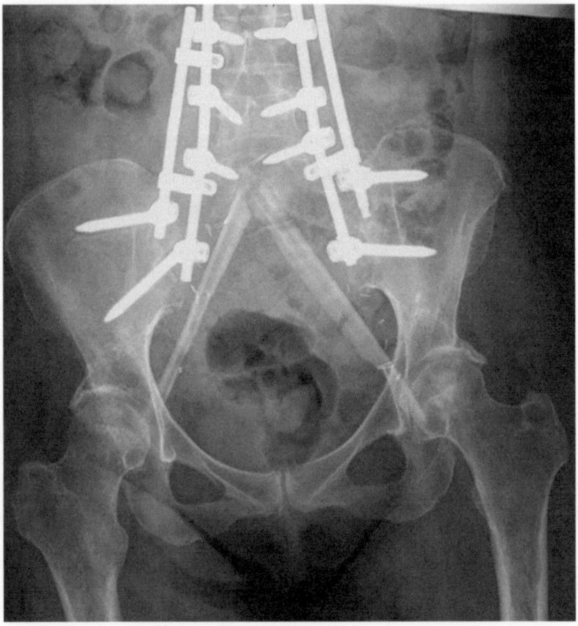

Fig. 7.2 A 50-year-old male with radiation-associated sarcoma of the sacrum who underwent total sacrectomy and reconstruction with bilateral fibula autograft and four-rod lumbopelvic instrumentation

multivariate analysis has demonstrated a clinical benefit to this construct: a decreased rate of fixation failure (hazard ratio, 3.88; $p = 0.035$) [36].

A 2014 systematic review reported a lower rate of surgical complications and a trend toward a lower rate of hardware failure with the use of anterior column reconstruction [37]. Similarly, a multivariate analysis found that anterior column fixation reduced the rate of hardware failure (hazard ratio, 3.82; $p = 0.04$) [36]. Of note, posterior pelvic ring fixation (such as with a transiliac bolt) was not a predictor of hardware failure.

The choice of anterior column fixation is also important. Compared with fibula allografts, free vascularized fibula (FVF) strut grafts lead to more rapid union (8 vs. 11 months; $p = 0.004$), a lower rate of nonunion (17 vs. 61%; $p = 0.007$, higher MSTS93 functional outcome scores (62% vs. 42%; $p = 0.003$), and a higher rate of ambulation (91% vs. 61%, $p = 0.028$) [38]. The AOSpine Knowledge Forum Tumor made a weak recommendation, with very low certainty of evidence, for the use of FVF [33].

However, FVF grafts are not universally used. One obstacle to their use is the significant prolongation of time that the patient is in the prone position during what is already a long and complex surgery. However, staging the surgery over 2 days has been shown to be associated with decreased perioperative morbidity, transfusion requirement, and cost [39, 40], and can be a useful method of allowing FVF grafts to be used more safely. A second obstacle to the use of FVF grafts is the difficulty of obtaining suitable recipient vessels at the surgical site, particularly after prior radiation or prior surgery or when the patient is in the prone position. However, many of these patients also undergo soft tissue reconstruction with a vertical rectus abdominis musculocutaneous (VRAM) pull-through flap, which can be considered as a potential flow-through source of recipient vessels [41].

As suggested above, the plastic surgery team is a crucial part of the skeletal and soft tissue reconstruction following sacrectomy. Mid-to-distal sacrectomy with limited muscle sacrifice may not require flap reconstruction, but may benefit from rectal sling reconstruction with mesh or acellular dermal matrix to prevent rectal herniation. Patients undergoing high and total sacrectomy typically benefit from flap reconstruction. Gluteus maximus advancement flaps are often used when reconstruction is performed using a posterior-only approach, while a pedicled VRAM pull-through flap is a good option when a combined anterior-posterior approach is used [42]. Data from a systematic review suggests that rates of wound complications and return to the operating room are lower, and the length of stay is shorter, in patients who undergo soft tissue reconstruction after total sacrectomy, prompting a strong recommendation with very low certainty of evidence [33].

Our practice is to use spinopelvic skeletal reconstruction for patients undergoing sacrectomy above the level of the S1 foramina, with an anterior-posterior approach staged over 2 days, vascularized free fibula graft when feasible, dual-rod and dual-screw instrumentation, and a rotational VRAM pull-through flap.

Management of Metastatic Sacral Tumors

Metastases to the sacrum represent 7–10% of all spine metastases [43]. In contrast to primary sacral tumors, there is little role for surgery for tumor control in sacral metastatic disease. Rather, surgery is reserved for skeletal stabilization and neurologic decompression, while tumor control is achieved with radiation and/or systemic therapy. As the focus is on palliation, great care should be devoted to avoid complications and to expedite the patient's return to function and to systemic therapy. Whenever possible, open surgery should be avoided in favor of minimally invasive interventions.

Pathologic and insufficiency sacral fractures are common among patients with metastatic disease due to a combination of osteopenia/osteoporosis, sacral lesions, and prior pelvic radiation. Most of these fractures are vertically oriented through the sacral ala, which represents a stable fracture pattern with minimal risk of displacement and symptoms that are likely to resolve either spontaneously or with medical intervention. The authors' preferred treatment paradigm is to offer sacroiliac steroid injection and/or cluneal-nerve block to patients with significant pain or functional disability. If palliation is insufficient or temporary, minimally invasive stabilization with sacroplasty or percutaneous screw fixation can be considered [44, 45].

Rarely, patients develop an unstable pattern of pathologic sacral fracture with a "U" or "H" orientation that effectively dissociates the spine from the rest of the pelvis, analogous to the spinopelvic dissociation pattern seen in the trauma setting. Reliable detection of this fracture pattern requires the availability and scrutiny of coronal imaging in the plane of the sacrum, which can demonstrate the transverse fracture component, and of sagittal imaging, which demonstrates any angular or translational displacement. Given the rotational instability of this fracture pattern along the moment arm through the S1 body, triangular osteosynthesis in the form of lumbopelvic fixation with transiliac-transsacral fixation is more biomechanically stable than iliosacral fixation alone (Fig. 7.3) [46, 47]. However, open surgery in metastatic sacral disease has a complication rate of 40%, or 62% with prior radiotherapy [48]. Recently, percutaneous techniques to achieve fracture reduction and triangular osteosynthesis in the trauma population have been described [49], and these techniques have been adapted successfully for use in pathologic sacral instability to avoid open surgery [50].

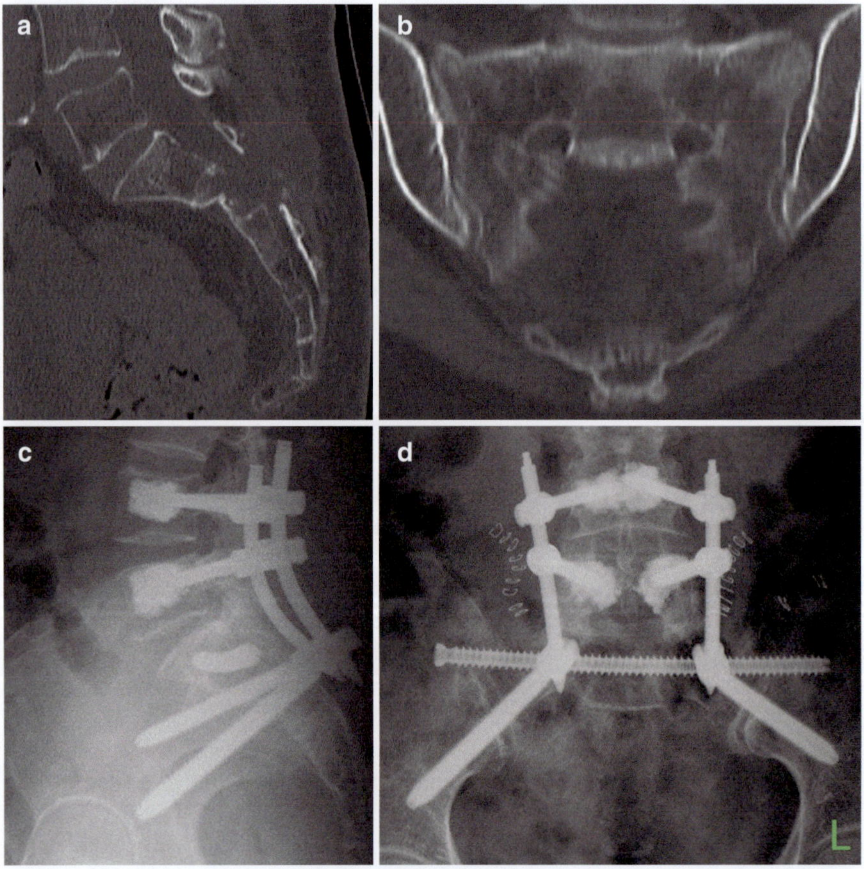

Fig. 7.3 A 59-year-old female with metastatic breast cancer at S2 vertebral body who had been treated twice with palliative radiotherapy sustained a pathologic U-type fracture with kyphotic angulation visible on sagittal CT (**a**) and vertical transforaminal fracture lines (arrows) visible on sacral-plane coronal CT (**b**). Given the multiply radiated field, the patient underwent closed reduction and percutaneous triangular osteosynthesis with a transiliac-transsacral screw and cement-augmented lumbopelvic instrumentation (**c** and **d**)

Conclusion

The management of sacral tumors requires a comprehensive approach based on an understanding of tumor characteristics, surgical and nonsurgical treatment outcomes, and salvage options. Patient-centered decision-making is crucial, as treatments can be life-altering and the potential for complications is high. The treatment of primary sacral tumors is focused on disease control and potential cure while balancing treatment morbidity. In metastatic disease to the sacrum, the focus is on palliation, and treatment-related morbidity should be avoided. Outcomes are optimized by multidisciplinary engagement with tumor control, reconstruction, and rehabilitation.

References

1. Ji T, Guo W, Yang R, Tang X, Wang Y, Huang L. What are the conditional survival and functional outcomes after surgical treatment of 115 patients with sacral chordoma? Clin Orthop Relat Res. 2017;475(3):620–30. https://doi.org/10.1007/s11999-016-4773-8.
2. Phukan R, Herzog T, Boland PJ, Healey J, Rose P, Sim FH, et al. How does the level of sacral resection for primary malignant bone tumors affect physical and mental health, pain, mobility, incontinence, and sexual function? Clin Orthop Relat Res. 2016;474(3):687–96. https://doi.org/10.1007/s11999-015-4361-3.
3. Yeung CM, Bilsky M, Boland PJ, Vaynrub M. The role of en bloc resection in the modern era for primary spine tumors. Spine. 2023; (in press)
4. Zuckerman SL, Lee SH, Chang GJ, Walsh GL, Mehran RJ, Gokaslan ZL, et al. Outcomes of surgery for sacral chordoma and impact of complications: a report of 50 consecutive patients with long-term follow-up. Global Spine J. 2021;11(5):740–50. https://doi.org/10.1177/2192568221101144
5. Stacchiotti S, Casali PG, Lo Vullo S, Mariani L, Palassini E, Mercuri M, et al. Chordoma of the mobile spine and sacrum: a retrospective analysis of a series of patients surgically treated at two referral centers. Ann Surg Oncol. 2010;17(1):211–9. https://doi.org/10.1245/s10434-009-0740-x.
6. Varga PP, Szoverfi Z, Fisher CG, Boriani S, Gokaslan ZL, Dekutoski MB, et al. Surgical treatment of sacral chordoma: prognostic variables for local recurrence and overall survival. Eur Spine J. 2015;24(5):1092–101. https://doi.org/10.1007/s00586-014-3728-6.
7. Jin CJ, Berry-Candelario J, Reiner AS, Laufer I, Higginson DS, Schmitt AM, et al. Long-term outcomes of high-dose single-fraction radiosurgery for chordomas of the spine and sacrum. J Neurosurg Spine. 2019:1–10. https://doi.org/10.3171/2019.7.SPINE19515.
8. Fisher CG, Saravanja DD, Dvorak MF, Rampersaud YR, Clarkson PW, Hurlbert J, et al. Surgical management of primary bone tumors of the spine: validation of an approach to enhance cure and reduce local recurrence. Spine (Phila Pa 1976). 2011;36(10):830–6. https://doi.org/10.1097/BRS.0b013e3181e502e5.
9. Enneking WF. A system of staging musculoskeletal neoplasms. Clin Orthop Relat Res. 1986;204:9–24.
10. Dekutoski MB, Clarke MJ, Rose P, Luzzati A, Rhines LD, Varga PP, et al. Osteosarcoma of the spine: prognostic variables for local recurrence and overall survival, a multicenter ambispective study. J Neurosurg Spine. 2016;25(1):59–68. https://doi.org/10.3171/2015.11.SPINE15870.

11. Charest-Morin R, Dirks MS, Patel S, Boriani S, Luzzati A, Fehlings MG, et al. Ewing sarcoma of the spine: prognostic variables for survival and local control in surgically treated patients. Spine (Phila Pa 1976). 2018;43(9):622–9. https://doi.org/10.1097/BRS.0000000000002386.
12. Fisher CG, Versteeg AL, Dea N, Boriani S, Varga PP, Dekutoski MB, et al. Surgical management of spinal chondrosarcomas. Spine (Phila Pa 1976). 2016;41(8):678–85. https://doi.org/10.1097/BRS.0000000000001485.
13. De Amorim BK, DeLaney T. Chordomas and chondrosarcomas-The role of radiation therapy. J Surg Oncol. 2016;114(5):564–9. https://doi.org/10.1002/jso.24368.
14. Imai R, Kamada T, Tsuji H, Yanagi T, Baba M, Miyamoto T, et al. Carbon ion radiotherapy for unresectable sacral chordomas. Clin Cancer Res. 2004;10(17):5741–6. https://doi.org/10.1158/1078-0432.CCR-04-0301.
15. Maybody M, Soliman MM, Yamada Y, Tahour D, Hsu M, Moskowitz CS, et al. Temporary organ displacement to escalate radiation dose to retroperitoneal tumors and decrease toxicity to organs at risk. J Vasc Interv Radiol. 2020;31(10):1578–86. https://doi.org/10.1016/j.jvir.2020.01.011.
16. Stacchiotti S, Gronchi A, Fossati P, Akiyama T, Alapetite C, Baumann M, et al. Best practices for the management of local-regional recurrent chordoma: a position paper by the Chordoma Global Consensus Group. Ann Oncol. 2017;28(6):1230–42. https://doi.org/10.1093/annonc/mdx054.
17. Ailon T, Torabi R, Fisher CG, Rhines LD, Clarke MJ, Bettegowda C, et al. Management of locally recurrent chordoma of the mobile spine and sacrum: a systematic review. Spine (Phila Pa 1976). 2016;41(Suppl 20):S193–S8. https://doi.org/10.1097/BRS.0000000000001812.
18. Charest-Morin R, Fisher CG, Varga PP, Gokaslan ZL, Rhines LD, Reynolds JJ, et al. En bloc resection versus intralesional surgery in the treatment of giant cell tumor of the spine. Spine (Phila Pa 1976). 2017;42(18):1383–90. https://doi.org/10.1097/BRS.0000000000002094.
19. Domovitov SV, Chandhanayingyong C, Boland PJ, McKeown DG, Healey JH. Conservative surgery in the treatment of giant cell tumor of the sacrum: 35 years' experience. J Neurosurg Spine. 2016;24(2):228–40. https://doi.org/10.3171/2015.4.SPINE13215.
20. Bukata SV, Blay JY, Rutkowski P, Skubitz K, Henshaw R, Seeger L, et al. Denosumab treatment for giant cell tumor of the spine including the sacrum. Spine (Phila Pa 1976). 2021;46(5):277–84. https://doi.org/10.1097/BRS.0000000000003728.
21. Raux S, Bouhamama A, Gaspar N, Brugieres L, Entz-Werle N, Mallet C, et al. Denosumab for treating aneurysmal bone cysts in children. Orthop Traumatol Surg Res. 2019;105(6):1181–5. https://doi.org/10.1016/j.otsr.2019.04.028.
22. Hung YP, Diaz-Perez JA, Cote GM, Wejde J, Schwab JH, Nardi V, et al. Dedifferentiated chordoma: clinicopathologic and molecular characteristics with integrative analysis. Am J Surg Pathol. 2020;44(9):1213–23. https://doi.org/10.1097/PAS.0000000000001501.
23. Todd LT Jr, Yaszemski MJ, Currier BL, Fuchs B, Kim CW, Sim FH. Bowel and bladder function after major sacral resection. Clin Orthop Relat Res. 2002;397:36–9. https://doi.org/10.1097/00003086-200204000-00006.
24. Rotondo RL, Folkert W, Liebsch NJ, Chen YL, Pedlow FX, Schwab JH, et al. High-dose proton-based radiation therapy in the management of spine chordomas: outcomes and clinicopathological prognostic factors. J Neurosurg Spine. 2015;23(6):788–97. https://doi.org/10.3171/2015.3.SPINE14716.
25. Dea N, Charest-Morin R, Sciubba DM, Bird JE, Disch AC, Mesfin A, et al. Optimizing the adverse event and HRQOL profiles in the management of primary spine tumors. Spine (Phila Pa 1976). 2016;41(Suppl 20):S212–S7. https://doi.org/10.1097/BRS.0000000000001821.
26. Ruggieri P, Angelini A, Pala E, Mercuri M. Infections in surgery of primary tumors of the sacrum. Spine (Phila Pa 1976). 2012;37(5):420–8. https://doi.org/10.1097/BRS.0b013e3182213a44.
27. van Wulfften Palthe OD, Houdek MT, Rose PS, Yaszemski MJ, Sim FH, Boland PJ, et al. How does the level of nerve root resection in en bloc sacrectomy influence patient-reported outcomes? Clin Orthop Relat Res. 2017;475(3):607–16. https://doi.org/10.1007/s11999-016-4794-3.

28. Gunterberg B. Effects of major resection of the sacrum. Clinical studies on urogenital and anorectal function and a biomechanical study on pelvic strength. Acta Orthop Scand Suppl. 1976;162:1–38. https://doi.org/10.3109/ort.1976.47.suppl-162.01.
29. Hugate RR Jr, Dickey ID, Phimolsarnti R, Yaszemski MJ, Sim FH. Mechanical effects of partial sacrectomy: when is reconstruction necessary? Clin Orthop Relat Res. 2006;450:82–8. https://doi.org/10.1097/01.blo.0000229331.14029.44.
30. Yu B, Zheng Z, Zhuang X, Chen H, Xie D, Luk KD, et al. Biomechanical effects of transverse partial sacrectomy on the sacroiliac joints: an in vitro human cadaveric investigation of the borderline of sacroiliac joint instability. Spine (Phila Pa 1976). 2009;34(13):1370–5. https://doi.org/10.1097/BRS.0b013e3181a3d440.
31. Sato K, Kikuchi S, Yonezawa T. In vivo intradiscal pressure measurement in healthy individuals and in patients with ongoing back problems. Spine (Phila Pa 1976). 1999;24(23):2468–74. https://doi.org/10.1097/00007632-199912010-00008.
32. McCord DH, Cunningham BW, Shono Y, Myers JJ, McAfee PC. Biomechanical analysis of lumbosacral fixation. Spine (Phila Pa 1976). 1992;17(8 Suppl):S235–S43. https://doi.org/10.1097/00007632-199208001-00004.
33. Reynolds JJ, Khundkar R, Boriani S, Williams R, Rhines LD, Kawahara N, et al. Soft tissue and bone defect management in total sacrectomy for primary sacral tumors: a systematic review with expert recommendations. Spine (Phila Pa 1976). 2016;41(Suppl 20):S199–204. https://doi.org/10.1097/BRS.0000000000001834.
34. Yu BS, Zhuang XM, Zheng ZM, Li ZM, Wang TP, Lu WW. Biomechanical advantages of dual over single iliac screws in lumbo-iliac fixation construct. Eur Spine J. 2010;19(7):1121–8. https://doi.org/10.1007/s00586-010-1343-8.
35. Mindea SA, Chinthakunta S, Moldavsky M, Gudipally M, Khalil S. Biomechanical comparison of spinopelvic reconstruction techniques in the setting of total sacrectomy. Spine (Phila Pa 1976). 2012;37(26):E1622–E7. https://doi.org/10.1097/BRS.0b013e31827619d3.
36. Tang X, Yang R, Qu H, Cai Z, Guo W. Factors associated with spinopelvic fixation mechanical failure after total sacrectomy. Spine (Phila Pa 1976). 2018;43(18):1268–74. https://doi.org/10.1097/BRS.0000000000002635.
37. Bederman SS, Shah KN, Hassan JM, Hoang BH, Kiester PD, Bhatia NN. Surgical techniques for spinopelvic reconstruction following total sacrectomy: a systematic review. Eur Spine J. 2014;23(2):305–19. https://doi.org/10.1007/s00586-013-3075-z.
38. Wellings EP, Houdek MT, Owen AR, Bakri K, Yaszemski MJ, Sim FH, et al. Comparison of free vascularized fibular flaps and allograft fibular strut grafts to supplement spinopelvic reconstruction for sacral malignancies. Bone Joint J. 2021;103-B(8):1414–20. https://doi.org/10.1302/0301-620X.103B8.BJJ-2020-2302.R1.
39. Ramamurthy R, Bose JC, Muthusamy V, Natarajan M, Kunjithapatham D. Staged sacrectomy – an adaptive approach. J Neurosurg Spine. 2009;11(3):285–94. https://doi.org/10.3171/2009.3.SPINE08824.
40. Brown MJ, Kor DJ, Curry TB, Warner MA, Rodrigues ES, Rose SH, et al. Sacral tumor resection: the effect of surgical staging on patient outcomes, resource management, and hospital cost. Spine (Phila Pa 1976). 2011;36(19):1570–8. https://doi.org/10.1097/BRS.0b013e3181f6137d.
41. Garvey PB, Clemens MW, Rhines LD, Sacks JM. Vertical rectus abdominis musculocutaneous flow-through flap to a free fibula flap for total sacrectomy reconstruction. Microsurgery. 2013;33(1):32–8. https://doi.org/10.1002/micr.21990.
42. Kim JE, Pang J, Christensen JM, Coon D, Zadnik PL, Wolinsky JP, et al. Soft-tissue reconstruction after total en bloc sacrectomy. J Neurosurg Spine. 2015;22(6):571–81. https://doi.org/10.3171/2014.10.SPINE14114.
43. Charest-Morin R, Fisher CG, Versteeg AL, Sahgal A, Varga PP, Sciubba DM, et al. Clinical presentation, management and outcomes of sacral metastases: a multicenter, retrospective cohort study. Ann Transl Med. 2019;7(10):214. https://doi.org/10.21037/atm.2019.04.88.

44. Moussazadeh N, Laufer I, Werner T, Krol G, Boland P, Bilsky MH, et al. Sacroplasty for cancer-associated insufficiency fractures. Neurosurgery. 2015;76(4):446–50. https://doi.org/10.1227/NEU.0000000000000658.
45. Hoch A, Pieroh P, Henkelmann R, Josten C, Bohme J. In-screw polymethylmethacrylate-augmented sacroiliac screw for the treatment of fragility fractures of the pelvis: a prospective, observational study with 1-year follow-up. BMC Surg. 2017;17(1):132. https://doi.org/10.1186/s12893-017-0330-y.
46. Jazini E, Weir T, Nwodim E, Tannous O, Saifi C, Caffes N, et al. Outcomes of lumbopelvic fixation in the treatment of complex sacral fractures using minimally invasive surgical techniques. Spine J. 2017;17(9):1238–46. https://doi.org/10.1016/j.spinee.2017.04.032.
47. Schildhauer TA, Ledoux WR, Chapman JR, Henley MB, Tencer AF, Routt ML Jr. Triangular osteosynthesis and iliosacral screw fixation for unstable sacral fractures: a cadaveric and biomechanical evaluation under cyclic loads. J Orthop Trauma. 2003;17(1):22–31. https://doi.org/10.1097/00005131-200301000-00004.
48. Feiz-Erfan I, Fox BD, Nader R, Suki D, Chakrabarti I, Mendel E, et al. Surgical treatment of sacral metastases: indications and results. J Neurosurg Spine. 2012;17(4):285–91. https://doi.org/10.3171/2012.7.SPINE09351.
49. Williams SK, Quinnan SM. Percutaneous lumbopelvic fixation for reduction and stabilization of sacral fractures with spinopelvic dissociation patterns. J Orthop Trauma. 2016;30(9):e318–e24. https://doi.org/10.1097/BOT.0000000000000559.
50. Baksh N, Yeung C, Vaynrub M. Percutaneous lumbopelvic fixation for pathologic sacral fractures and spinopelvic dissociation: patient series. J Neurosurg Case Lessons. 2023;6(6):CASE23205.

Chapter 8
Radiotherapy for Primary Tumors of the Spine

Daniel Higginson

Chordomas

Background Chordomas are thought to arise from notochordal remnants and can involve any area of the spine, though clival and sacral chordomas are most common. Classic chordomas generally occur in adults whereas dedifferentiated chordomas, often associated with *SMARCB1* loss, can occur in children and adults. Multidisciplinary discussion is needed to address the complex issues involving resectability, functional outcomes after surgery, and the indication, mode, and dose of radiotherapy. Different centers frequently recommend different treatment regimens for the same lesion, and this section will provide the current thinking of our center while describing some alternative approaches.

Workup MRI spine w/wo contrast. A biopsy is needed to confirm the diagnosis since a hamartoma called notochordal rests can have the appearance of a chordoma on imaging, but does not need treatment [1]. If dedifferentiated chordoma is detected, then systemic staging for metastases is indicated, such as CT C/A/P.

Treatment All parties generally agree that *en bloc* resection with wide margins is the best treatment in terms of tumor control. However, this approach is often precluded by anatomic constraints and prohibitive morbidity. Generally partial sacrectomies at or below the level of S3 are well tolerated while more proximal sacrifices involve incremental loss of function, considerations of skeletal stability, and greater operative risk. For lesions within the mobile spine, there remains debate as to the optimal approach, with some centers advocating aggressive *en bloc* resections

D. Higginson (✉)
Department of Radiation Oncology, Memorial Sloan Kettering Cancer Center, New York, NY, USA
e-mail: higginsd@mskcc.org

Y. Yamada et al. (eds.), *Multidisciplinary Spine Tumor Management*,
https://doi.org/10.1007/978-3-032-07519-2_8

combined with radiotherapy. However, most such cases involve close or positive margins at the thecal sac, prompting adjuvant radiotherapy, and can involve a high surgical complication risk. Nevertheless, surgery may improve outcomes based on SEER/Medicare data [2], and therefore, subtotal resections (STR) are commonly performed.

Following STR or biopsy, adjuvant radiotherapy may consist of fractionated radiotherapy with the goal of achieving a dose of >70 Gy in 2 Gy fractions [3–6]. In our practice, when a fractionated radiotherapy course is pursued, proton radiotherapy is the preferred approach to limit dose to organs-at-risk such as lung and bowel. We aim to reach a total dose of 75.6–77.4 Gy RBE in 1.8 Gy RBE fractions (see Figs. 8.2 and 8.3) [7–14]. Another approach can be to use pre-operative photon and post-operative proton radiation as described by Delaney et al. in a phase II trial with total doses to 70.2 Gy RBE to the high-risk CTV and possibly further boosts to residual disease to 73.8–77.4 Gy RBE [15]. Finally, carbon ions in some centers can be similarly used and prescribed to a total dose of >70.4 Gy in 2.2–4.4 Gy RBE fractions [9].

At our center, our approach in many cases has been to pursue surgery if needed to decompress the spinal canal and/or stabilize the spine prior to radiotherapy. Carbon-based hardware is placed if it is anticipated that the subsequent radiotherapy will involve proton radiation. If decompression of the canal or stabilization is not needed, then a primary radiation approach is often selected. One emerging paradigm has been to use single fraction SRS to 24 Gy [16]. For sacral cases, organ displacement with a saline bolus inserted through a catheter can be used to reduce dose to the adjacent bowel if needed (see Fig. 8.1) [17]. We initially used this dose as a pre-operative regimen, followed by surgery 3–4 months later after patient recovery, and found that 50% of cases had pathological complete responses [18]. Now our approach is to use single fraction SRS if anatomically feasible and reserve surgery for the time of progression. For mobile spine cases, single fraction SRS is applicable to diseases involving 1–2 levels (Figs. 8.2 and 8.3).

The management of non-metastatic dedifferentiated chordoma is largely similar to the above, with the added tool of the EZH2 inhibitor tazemetostat, which we have used in some cases to reduce the extent of disease prior to local therapy as well as to manage metastatic cases.

Outcomes In patients undergoing surgery, the surgical margin status is the driving factor of outcomes [19, 20]. However, local relapse occurs in 16–50% of cases even when margins are pathologically negative [7, 11, 19, 21, 22]. While often slow growing, chordomas are notorious for relentless recurrences years after initial therapy and lack of local control can eventually lead to patient deaths. In our view, there are three promising radiation strategies that are better than historical local control

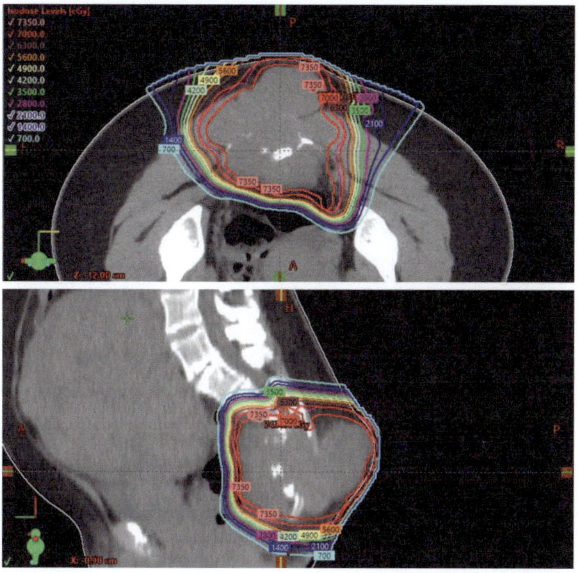

Fig. 8.1 Sacral chordoma. 52 year old with biopsy proven sacral chordoma encompassing S2-S3 with extensive soft tissue component. She was offered pre-operative or definitive single fraction SRS (24 Gy × 1), surgery with pre- and post-operative radiotherapy components, or definitive protons radiotherapy alone. Surgery would have involved colostomy and urinary diversion and thus she elected a primary radiotherapy approach. The extensive soft tissue was felt to increase risk of soft tissue injury with single fraction SRS and thus proton RT to 70 Gy RBE in 2Gy fractions was employed. Dmax to cauda was 7242 cGy RBE and Dmax to rectum was 7439 cGy RBE

data. First, proton therapy to 74 Gy (RBE) in a series of 100 patients resulted in a 3-year local control of 94% [23]. Second, carbon ion therapy in a series of 188 patients has also produced local control data of 80% at 5 years and 56% at 10 years [24, 25]. Third, the single fraction SRS experience for chordoma at our center has found that in 32 patients receiving 24 Gy in a single fraction, the 5-year local recurrence-free survival was 89.9% [16], suggesting the radio surgery may provide curative therapy. The addition of surgery for these patients did not improve the probability of local control. Thus patients who present with disease unsuitable for en bloc resection (ie high grade epidural cord compression) may still be achieve a cure if intralesional resection is combined with high dose radio surgery. In 8 other retrospective series describing outcomes for SBRT or SRS, the median local recurrence-free survival was 71% [9].

Follow-up MRI spine for surveillance on a q4–6 month basis for 2 years, followed by q6 months until year 5 and then indefinite annual follow-up [16].

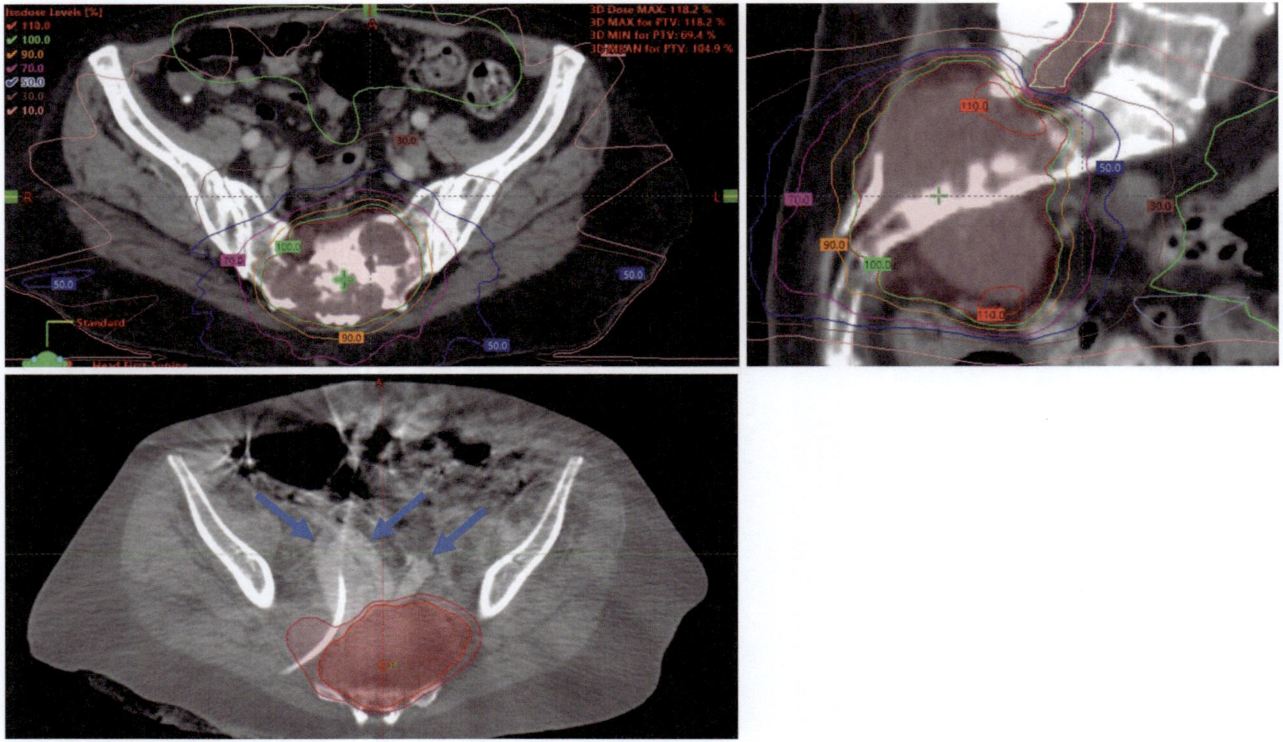

Fig. 8.2 78 year old female with history of atrial fibrillation, CVA, CKD, rectal bleeding, who was diagnosed with S2-S4 sacral chordoma after months of worsening sacral pain, rectal pressure, left leg pain/numbness. She was offered a primary radiotherapy approach due to poor surgical candidacy. 24 Gy × 1 was prescribed with an overall plan Dmax of 118.2%. At the time of treatment, a catheter was placed to fill a balloon adjacent to the mass, displacing bowel (see PMID: 32861570). Blue arrows highlight the opaque saline bolus. The Dmax to bowel was 2607 cGy without displacement and 886 cGy (estimated) with displacement

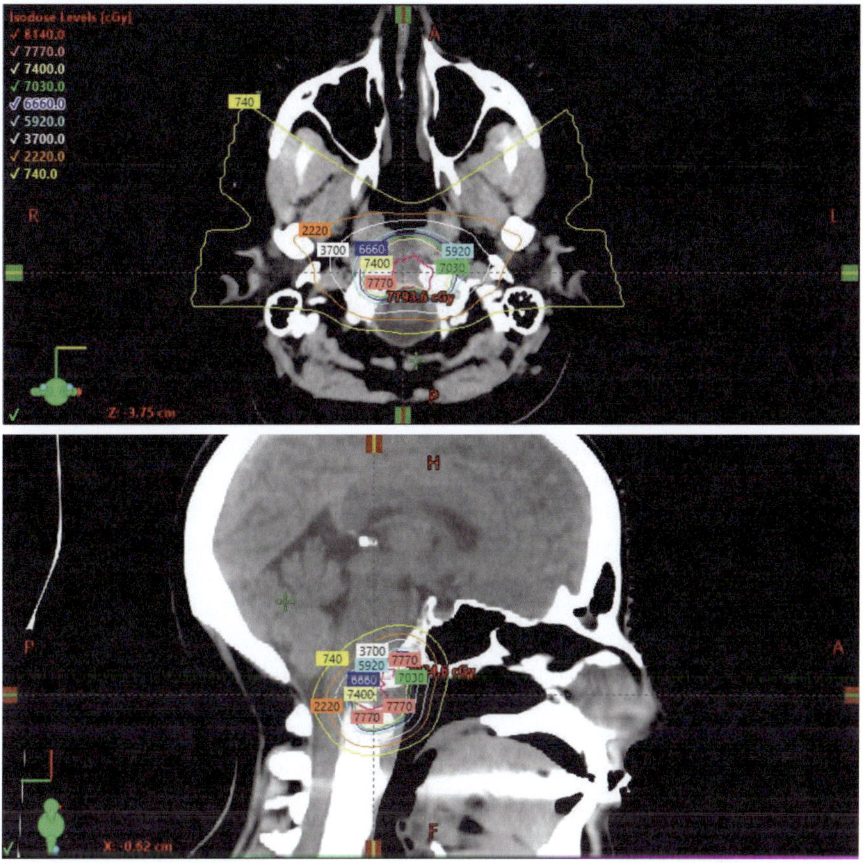

Fig. 8.3 42 year old with an inferior clivus chordoma which was subtotally resected with an anterior craniofacial approach. Postoperative proton radiotherapy was administered to 74 Gy RBE in 2 Gy fractions. Dmax to brainstem was 6482 cGy RBE and spinal cord 4564 cGy RBE

Primary Sarcomas of the Spine

Background Although sarcomas are a highly diverse group of mesenchymal tumors, they have typically been studied together in the spine because of their rarity and common treatment approaches. Chondrosarcomas and osteosarcomas are most common in adult patients with other possibilities including myxofibrosarcoma, fibrosarcomas, undifferentiated pleomorphic sarcoma, or unspecified high-grade sarcomas. Ewing's sarcoma, a blue cell primitive neuroectodermal tumor most common in children, will be discussed in a separate section. Each of these tumors occurs rarely and management principles are largely similar to chordoma. As with chordoma, they are usually unresectable and radiation doses can be limited by spinal cord tolerances.

Workup MRI spine w/wo contrast. A biopsy is needed to confirm the diagnosis. Metastatic workup should include CT C/A/P.

Treatment For resectable cases, such as primarily paraspinal disease without dural involvement or only limited bony involvement, a wide margin resection is first-line treatment. Post-operative radiation would be conventionally fractionated and involve >60 Gy. For true spinal lesions, some centers have recommended *en bloc* resections with corpectomies and placement of cages to replace 1–2 vertebral levels, but the common approach at our center is to pursue primary radiation approaches instead. For unresectable disease, surgery may still be indicated for decompression of the disease and resolution of mechanical instability.

There are a variety of radiation approaches with no clear indication of superiority of one over the other. For conventional fractionation, it is seemingly important to achieve doses >70–74 Gy for local control, and for this reason, proton-based radiotherapy is favored to spare organs-at-risk such as the lung and bowel. As with chordoma, another approach is to utilize single-fraction SRS for smaller lesions involving 1–2 levels. High-dose hypofractionated SBRT, such as 12 Gy × 3 or 8 Gy × 5, can also be considered. Lower-dose SBRT, such as 6 Gy × 5 or 9 Gy × 3, likely provides insufficient dose for cure. Finally, carbon ion therapy resulted in impressive local control in a series of sarcoma and chordomas [26–30].

For osteosarcoma, pre- and post-operative chemotherapy is well established. For resectable tumors with wide margins, radiotherapy would not be indicated. In the spine, however, radiation is often needed as primary local control therapy or adjuvant treatment for positive margins. This is in contrast to other bony sites of osteosarcoma wherein radiation is not frequently needed.

Another separate consideration is low-grade chondrosarcoma, which has much better outcomes than high-grade sarcomas. Many of these tumors are indolent, and for instance, low-grade chondrosarcomas in the skull base can achieve durable local control with radiotherapy [31].

Outcomes Several manuscripts describe a local control difference between cases able to achieve margin-negative resection compared to cases with intralesional resection, though of course these differences could also be explained by case selection [32–34]. It is also difficult to precisely estimate local control and survival data following radiotherapy because of the rarity of these tumors and frequent inclusion of low-grade chondrosarcomas and Ewing's sarcomas along with high-grade sarcomas in many studies. In general, adult osteosarcoma [35] and high-grade chondrosarcomas [36, 37] exhibit a poor prognosis relative to pediatric patients and also relative to other anatomic sites of disease. In a SEER Medicare analysis, high-grade chondrosarcoma of the spine results only in a 1.9-year median overall survival when including all cases, with only ~20% of patients achieving durable disease control. For cases with local-only disease at presentation, long-term disease control is only achieved in ~60% [37].

Follow-up MRI spine for surveillance every 3 months for 2 years, followed by 6-month intervals until year 5 and then indefinite annual follow-up. Adult osteosarcomas, high-grade chondrosarcomas, and other high-grade sarcomas frequently metastasize to the lungs and therefore 3–6 month interval CT chest × 2 years and annual CT C/A/P would be reasonable.

Ewing's Sarcoma

Background Ewing's sarcoma (EWS) is a small round blue cell tumor with very different management from chordomas and primary sarcomas of the spine. While the median age at presentation is 14 years, these tumors are diagnosed in humans of any age. Only a small percentage of EWS arise in the spine (estimated 12–17%) [38, 39].

Workup MRI spine w/wo contrast. CT chest and head to toe PET/CT scan for detection of metastatic disease. Additional labs include LDH and ESR, which have prognostic significance, LFTs, and CBC.

Treatment Systemic therapy is a key component of management, irrespective of presentation, since survival after local therapy alone historically was only 10% [40, 41]. Chemotherapy involves vincristine, doxorubicin, cyclophosphamide and actinomycin-D (VDC(A)) alternating with ifosphamide and etoposide (IE) for 48 weeks. Local therapies to the primary site and also to limited sites of metastatic disease are indicated as well, such as lung metastases. The timing of the local therapy for spinal primary or metastasis depends on presentation. For cord compression or spinal instability, surgery might be recommended upfront for rapid symptomatic relief [42]. Surgery can also be a standalone local therapy for cases amenable to en bloc resection with wide margins and in non-emergent cases, this would typically occur at week 12–18 of chemotherapy. However, as with chordomas and primary sarcomas of the spine, most spinal EWS cases are not amenable to *en bloc* wide margin resections, and primary radiotherapy may also be used as the local therapy either without surgery at 12–18 weeks or as treatment following a subtotal resection or decompression surgery. The pre-chemotherapy/pre-surgical GTV plus a 1.5–2 cm margin to CTV1 is treated in 1.8 Gy fractions to 45 Gy, followed by a boost to 55.8 Gy to osseous GTV and post-chemotherapy/post-surgical paraspinal disease plus a 1.5 cm margin to CTV2. Other studies have reduced the GTV to CTV margins to 1 cm with excellent local control results [43, 44]. Proton beam radiotherapy should be highly considered for this disease, and if surgery is performed, then carbon-based hardware is highly preferred for proton compatibility. The cord constraint used in cooperative group studies has been 45 in AEWS0031 to 50.4 Gy in AEWS1031 [43]. Delineation of the cord through fusion of a T2 MRI spine sequence or through a myelogram prior to simulation may be advantageous for achieving adequate dose while respecting cord constraints.

Outcomes Both surgery and radiotherapy can be effective local control therapies. In a review of 1058 patients treated on protocol, local failure was only 7.5% with surgery, with or without adjuvant radiotherapy, and there was no difference between marginal resections with post-operative RT compared to surgery alone [45]. Local failure was 26% in those receiving radiotherapy alone, but these were primarily larger tumors [45]. Over 90% local control results are seen in modern series with radiotherapy alone [43, 44]. In a modern series of 32 patients with spinal and para-spinal EWS treated with protons at the University of Florida, gross total resections were performed in 14 patients and 18 patients had biopsy only or subtotal resections. All patients then received proton-based radiotherapy (50.4 Gy RBE following GTR or 55.8 Gy RBE for gross disease). Local control was 92% and progression free survival was 79% at 5 years [43]. However, very large tumors may have worse local control following radiotherapy alone and a prospective phase II trial at St. Jude's Hospital found that dose escalation to 64.8Gy for tumors larger than 8 cm improved local control to 100% compared to the historical reference of 52% [44]. Thus, both surgery and radiotherapy can be highly effective local control modalities and the choice between them involves multidisciplinary discussion. Late toxicities from radiotherapy can involve growth abnormalities and kyphosis in pediatric patients and vertebral body fractures.

Follow-up MRI spine for surveillance on a q3-month basis for 2 years, followed by q6 months until year 5 and then indefinite annual follow-up. Systemic surveillance includes head-to-toe PET and CT chest every 3 months × 2 years, then spaced out to every 4–6 months to 5 years.

Ependymoma

Background Pediatric ependymomas are mostly intracranial and will not be discussed here. Adult ependymomas conversely arise mostly within the spine and represent the most common intramedullary tumor in adults [46]. Fortunately, most (89%) are benign-grade II ependymomas termed myxopapillary ependymomas that commonly arise within the filum terminale. Grade III anaplastic ependymomas are much less common (11%) [47]. Patients can present with pain, sensory or motor symptoms and occasionally these lesions are discovered incidentally in asymptomatic patients.

Workup MRI spine w/wo contrast of the spine and of the brain. These lesions are isotense or slightly hypointense on T1, typically contrast-enhancing with relatively homogenous signal compared to astrocytomas. They are well circumscribed, often in contrast to astrocytomas. Like astrocytomas, they can involve cysts and a syrinx. The adjacent bone may demonstrate widening of the canal and scalloping of the vertebral body. Myxopapillary ependymomas do not typically seed the CSF, but can cause drop metastases into the lower thecal sac in the sacrum. Anaplastic ependymoma can seed the CSF and CSF sampling is indicated.

Treatment Surgery is the mainstay of treatment, and in contrast to astrocytoma, clear resection planes lead to a high percentage of cases with gross total resections [46, 48]. For myxopapillary cases, however, surgery can be deferred initially for asymptomatic patients with stable lesions since the clinical course may be indolent. For symptomatic cases or for growing myxopapillary lesions, surgery is indicated. For patients who achieve a gross total resection, adjuvant RT is not indicated for grade II myxopapillary cases. After a subtotal resection of grade II myxopapillary cases, adjuvant RT may be indicated on a case-by-case basis with the understanding that these are slow-growing, benign tumors. In many cases, such as younger patients at risk of second malignancy, adjuvant RT can be delayed until progression. For instance, in a French series of 101 patients with spinal myxopapillary ependymoma, approximately 50% of patients with subtotal resections and no initial radiotherapy recurred, but all recurrences were successfully salvaged with radiotherapy and/or surgery at the time of recurrence [49].

For grade III anaplastic ependymoma, outcomes are less favorable and adjuvant RT is indicated for all cases. The dose typically used would be 45 Gy to CTV1 in 1.8 Gy fractions, defined as the T1 plus contrast volume and T2 edema, and a cone down to 50.4–55.8 Gy to the T1 post contrast volume only (see Fig. 8.4). The preoperative MRIs would be used to define tumor extent. In anaplastic ependymoma, there can be CSF seeding, and proton-based craniospinal irradiation could be considered to a total dose of 30–36 Gy in these cases. However, this situation would be extremely rare.

Outcomes For grade II myxopapillary tumors, survival is rarely affected by the disease. The cause-specific survival at 5 years is 87–97% [46]. Tumor progression was only 7% in a systematic review of 457 patients in 69 studies [46]. Outcomes for anaplastic ependymoma, however, are not as favorable, with estimates ranging from 27–71% overall survival at 5 years [46, 50]. In patients who recur, possible salvage treatments include repeat resection and re-irradiation.

Follow-up MRI spine for surveillance on a q3-month basis for 2 years, followed by q6 months until year 5 and then indefinite annual follow-up.

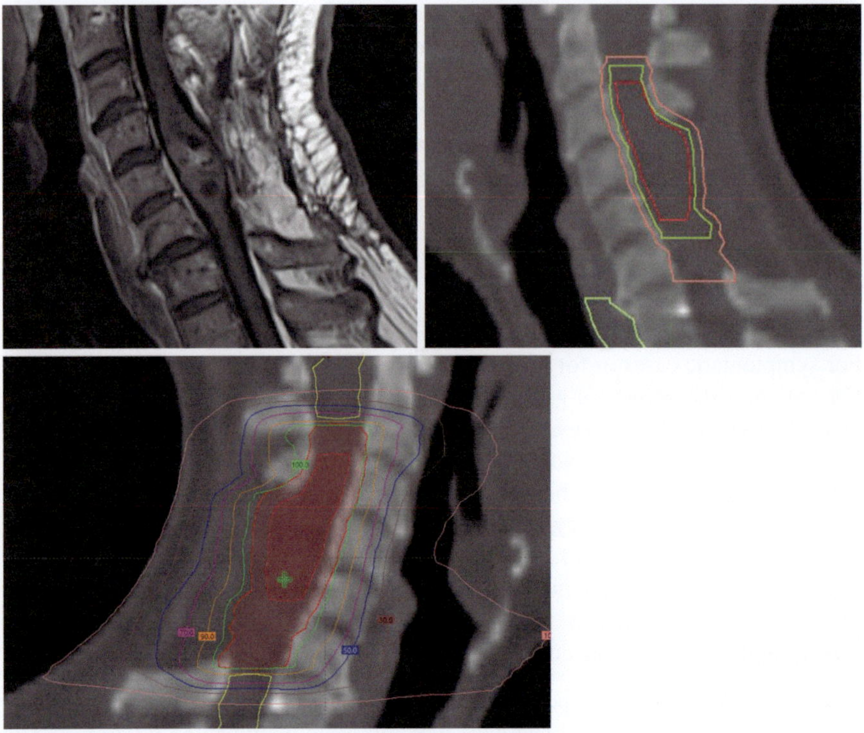

Fig. 8.4 Grade II conventional ependymoma. 62 year old who underwent a previous resection, followed by stable symptoms for 5 years until he developed right hand numbness, leading to discovery of a recurrence. The recurrence involved intramedullary cystic structures. GTV (red) was outlined through fusion of the T1 postcontrast sequence. PTV (peach) was a 3 mm radial and ~2 cm superior-inferior expansion on GTV. Prescription dose was 55.8 Gy in 1.8 fractions. The cord was not constrained within the PTV and the overall Dmax of the plan was 104%. Please note an aggressive approach was used here, whereas 54 Gy or 50.4Gy prescription might also be used

Spinal Cord Astrocytomas

Background Similar to gliomas in the brain, spinal cord gliomas can range from low-grade astrocytomas to grade IV glioblastomas, with grade affecting outcomes. Most spinal astrocytomas in both adults and children are less than grade IV and many are low-grade or juvenile pilocytic astrocytomas [51–53]. A plurality of spinal cord gliomas have H3K27M mutations typical of midline gliomas (20–40%), though the prognostic significance of this mutation in grade III/IV spinal cord gliomas is uncertain [54–57]. Biopsy can provide valuable information in terms of determining tumor grade and prognosis. However, there are situations in which cord biopsy is not worth its risks and treatment decisions are made empirically without knowing tumor grade. Patients typically present with motor and sensory deficits consistent with the levels of involvement or more subtle symptoms such as back pain. Occasionally low-grade spinal cord astrocytomas are incidentally discovered in asymptomatic patients.

Workup MRI spine w/wo contrast. Lesions can be isotense on T1 and hyperintense on T2 with contrast enhancement in most but not all astrocytomas [58]. Contrast enhancement is likely inhomogeneous, in contrast to ependymomas. Higher-grade lesions may involve areas of necrosis without contrast enhancement and possibly intratumoral cysts. There may also be an associated syrinx.

Treatment For patients with incidentally discovered lesions with a radiographic appearance most consistent with low-grade disease, the best timing of surgery is unclear and patients are typically followed expectantly to monitor for growth or emergence of symptoms. While in the brain, there is a rationale for delaying radiotherapy for low-grade gliomas due to a desire to avoid cognitive neurotoxicity, radiation for spinal lesions does not involve neurocognitive risk, but does involve a small risk of radiation myelitis and second malignancies. For patients with symptoms or with radiographic appearance consistent with high-grade glioma, surgery is the initial consideration, but gross total resection is rarely achieved due to a lack of dissection planes [59–63]. Adjuvant radiotherapy is therefore often used following maximal safe resection. In young patients—especially young children—with low-grade histology, expectant management initially instead of immediate adjuvant radiotherapy is a possibility [64, 65]. Concurrent temozolomide is used on a case-by-case basis for many patients, analogously to its use for brain gliomas.

While the seminal Walker studies in brain gliomas found survival benefits of dose escalation to 60 Gy, no equivalent data is available for spinal gliomas. In addition, the generally accepted cord constraints limit dose. Two retrospective series suggest adjuvant radiotherapy improves overall survival compared to surgery alone [66, 67]. Patients in one study received 45 Gy in 1.8 Gy fractions, well below the traditional TD5/5 of 50 Gy for the cord [9]. In the second study, the median dose used in 57 patients was 50 Gy in 1.8 Gy fractions [10]. The MSK approach has been to offer 50.4–54 Gy in 1.8 Gy fractions with concurrent temozolomide. The areas of enhancement, T1 hypointensity, and/or edema on T2 are generally contoured; however, cord edema can extend across a very broad superior/inferior extent of cord, not all of which is actually tumor-involved. Therefore, we use case-by-case judgment on how much of the edema to cover.

Outcomes Overall survival depends mostly on tumor grade, with grade IV glioblastomas with very poor survival [66, 68]. In the SEER/Medicare analysis from 664 patients, the 5-year OS was only 14% for grade III/IV astrocytomas, 70% for grade II and 82% for grade I pilocytic astrocytomas. Within a grade, there is some evidence that the extent of resection [69] and provision of adjuvant RT improves progression-free survival or OS [66, 67]. The additional value of concurrent and adjuvant temozolomide is unknown for spinal astrocytomas, but is used in our center, extrapolating from the brain glioma data.

Follow-up Adjuvant temozolomide can continue following radiotherapy in an analogous fashion to high-grade gliomas in the brain. MRI spine for surveillance on a q3-month basis for 2 years, followed by q6 months until year 5 and then indefinite annual follow-up.

Schwannoma

Background Schwannonas and meningiomas are by far the most common intradural extramedullary tumors and share many similarities in their diagnosis, workup and treatment. They can be associated with neurofibromatosis type II, the clinical syndrome schwannomatosis, or develop as isolated lesions. They typically present with pain, motor or sensory syndromes corresponding to the location.

Workup MRI spine w/wo contrast. These appear as T2 hyperintense lesions that can be entirely intradural within the canal or extend through the neuroforamen and present with a dumbbell-like appearance. In contrast to meningioma, they do not display dural tails or calcification. They can enhance with contrast. Referral to clinical genetics for workup of genetic schwannomatosis if patients have >2 non-intradermal schwannomas and have no history of vestibular schwannomas or have a family history of schwannomatosis [70].

Treatment The treatment with the fastest resolution of symptoms is gross total resection. Radiation can be used for medically or surgically inoperable cases. Both conventional fractionation and radiosurgery approaches are justified and draw from data for vestibular schwannomas [71, 72], but SRS or hypofractionated SBRT are most frequently used [72–75]. The doses selected included 14–16 Gy × 1, 8 Gy × 3, or 5 Gy × 5. Interestingly, over the years the SRS dose used for vestibular schwannoma has been reduced to 12.5 Gy × 1 with excellent local control, and analogously, a lesser SRS dose may also be effective in schwannomas in the spine [71, 72]. A typical middle ground dose selected at our center is 8 Gy × 3 (see Fig. 8.5).

Outcomes Recurrence is unusual following gross total resection, but can be significant in those lesions subtotally resected [76]. Local control following SRS or hypofractionated SBRT is excellent, with 80–90% local control in most series [71–75].

Follow-up MRI spine q6 months for 2 years and then annual follow-up. Of note, vestibular schwannomas can exhibit pseudoprogression at 6 months and up to 3 years after treatment. However, it is unclear whether this phenomenon also occurs with spinal schwannomas [77, 78].

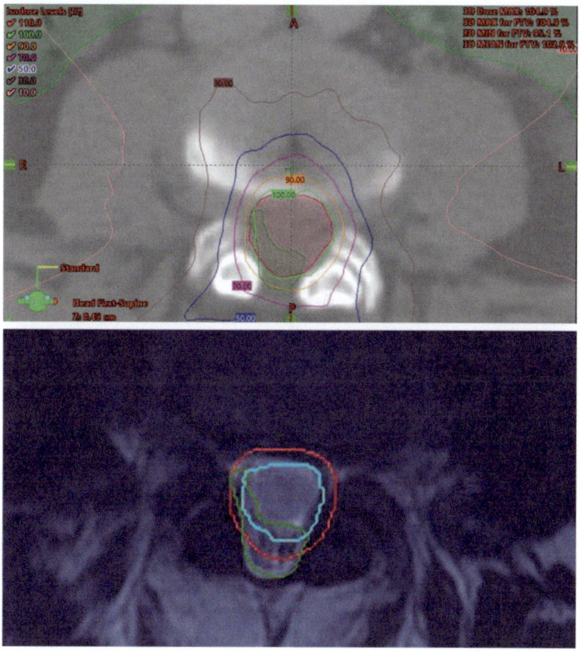

Fig. 8.5 Recurrent schwannoma at L4 after a previous resection. The GTV (teal) directly contacted the cauda (green). CTV = GTV in the case. Fusion of an MRI scan was used to outline these structures. A 2 mm GTV-PTV margin was used. Prescription dose was 8 Gy × 3 and an SBRT technique used for patient setup and imaging verification. Overall Dmax of the plan was 104.9% and the cauda Dmax was 25.17 Gy

Meningioma

Background Meningiomas of the spine can arise from the dural layers of the thecal sac. In the brain, they arise within the 40–70 year old age group with a 2 to 1 female predominance. They can also arise within the context of neurofibromatosis type 2. Prior radiation for other cancers is a risk factor. There are three grades of meningiomas, grades I–III, representing ~90%, 7%, and 2% of cases, respectively. Grade 1 (benign) meningiomas are defined as those with <4 mitoses per 10 high-powered fields. Atypical or grade 2 meningiomas have 4–19 mitoses per 10 high-powered fields and malignant or grade 3 meningiomas have 20 or more mitoses and can metastasize. The Simpson grading system is used to define the completeness of resection of both tumor and dural attachments, with grade IV and V tumors demonstrating higher recurrence rates secondary to incomplete tumor resection.

In the brain, they can be found incidentally in asymptomatic patients, and in fact, the majority of meningiomas can be observed with minimal or no growth [79–82]. However, in the spine there can be less of a window to monitor growth before cord compression develops. Biologic, tumor-related pain followed by level-dependent neurologic deficits are frequent presentations.

Workup These are intradural, extramedullary masses that are well defined, bright on T2 and demonstrate homogeneous enhancement with contrast on both CT and MRI. Calcified meningiomas may represent those that are slower growing. Dural tails can be more difficult to observe in spinal meningiomas compared to the brain due to constrained anatomy.

Management Spinal meningiomas can generally be completely excised (Simpsons grade I–II), most are WHO grade I meningiomas, recurrence is rare, and so usually adjuvant radiotherapy is usually not needed. Adjuvant RT should be delivered for grade 2 and 3 meningiomas. Since many patients present with symptoms, surgery is more likely to rapidly resolve symptoms and is therefore preferred.

Radiation can consist of conventional fractionated radiation or stereotactic radiosurgery, analogous to meningiomas in the brain. For adjuvant radiation, we recommend performing a myelogram for cord delineation using IMRT to prescribe 50–54 Gy while keeping the Dmax to cord <50 Gy. In the brain, grade 2–3 cases are typically treated with 54–60 Gy, but these doses are not practical to achieve in the spine due to cord constraints. Volumes should be generated through image registration of the pre-operative and post-operative MRI studies. CTV should consist of the pre-operative tumor volumes with 5 mm margins along every dural surface radially and in superior/inferior directions. PTV expansion of 3 mm with daily kV imaging would be a reasonable approach.

Radiosurgery is also an option and typical single fraction doses are 12–16 Gy or 21–24 Gy in 3 fractions or 25 Gy in 5 fractions. The Dmax to cord at our center is 14 Gy using a myelogram-defined cord and thus cases with extensive tumor contact with the cord may be best addressed surgically or with a conventionally fractionated approach.

Outcomes Local control following surgery is quite good, with >90% control reported in most series. Possible risk factors for recurrence include Simpson's grade II–III resection, WHO grade 2–3, anterior dural attachment, presence of calcifications, and dural tail.

Follow-up MRI spine q6 months for 2 years and then annual follow-up.

Aggressive Hemangiomas

Background Benign hemangiomas are extremely common and typically recognized incidentally as T1 and T2 hyperintense lesions on MRI. Aggressive hemangiomas are large benign tumors resulting in bone destruction/replacement, back pain, and/or spinal canal compromise. The Enneking staging system can divide them into Stage I-III. Stage I hemangiomas grow slowly, involve sharp borders within the bone, and rarely recur after resection. Stage II hemangiomas, or atypical hemangiomas, have sharp borders within the bone and cortical erosion of bone at the edges. Stage III hemangiomas, also known as aggressive hemangiomas, are more tumor-like with extension of the tumor outside the bone into the spinal canal or paraspinal tissue. Stages I-II are managed with intralesional resection if treatment is needed at all for symptomatic relief. Aggressive hemangiomas can be managed with surgery, conventionally fractionated radiation, radiosurgery or other techniques such as radiofrequency ablation, definitive onyx arterial embolization or even intralesional injection of ethanol.

Workup CT and MRI imaging. CT will help evaluate the borders of the lesion to discriminate between stages and evaluate for extraosseous spread or cortical thinning. CT can also exhibit the "polka dot" pattern of speckled bone within the hemangioma. MRI also helps distinguish hemangioma types. Stage I-II are hyperintense on T1 whereas aggressive hemangiomas are hypointense on T1. Lesions can be biopsied, but more frequently surgery is the first source of a pathologic specimen if needed.

Treatment For stage I (typical) and stage II (atypical) hemangioma, no treatment is necessary if there are no symptoms or medically manageable symptoms. For stage III aggressive hemangioma, treatment can involve decompression and/or instrumentation based on the presence of epidural disease or mechanical instability. Pre-operative embolization is used to reduce hemorrhage risk. For partial resections, adjuvant radiotherapy can be used to reduce the risk of recurrence or radiotherapy can be used as primary treatment in the absence of high-grade cord compression or mechanical instability. For patients without significant epidural disease or instability and for those medically high risk for surgery, a primary RT approach can be pursued.

A large range of conventionally fractionated radiation doses from 20 to 50 Gy have been used [83–89]. There are two respective studies of 117 and 84 patients that found a dose response in terms of pain relief for regimens above 34–36 Gy [84, 86]. A 45 Gy regimen in 1.8 Gy fractions is recommended by one group [90]. SRS/SBRT approaches include 6 Gy × 5 or 9 Gy × 3 or 18 Gy × 1 [91–95].

Outcomes Many series primarily report pain relief as the outcomes rather than radiographic control. In one of the larger series, when doses >36Gy were used, complete pain relief was seen in 82% of patients. A recent systematic review for outcomes following SRS/SBRT similarly found 88% pain relief with 46% complete pain relief [94]. Fewer series report local control data, though for SRS/SBRT local control was 100% in 18 patients, with most patients having stable or partial response rather than complete resolution [94].

Follow-up MRI spine 3 months following radiation and then spaced to q6-month imaging per physician judgment.

Aneurysmal Bone Cysts

Background Aneurysmal bone cysts are benign tumors that can be locally aggressive in the spine and cause pain or neurologic compromise. They are true tumors as most involve a t(16,17) translocation that activates the USP6 oncogene involved in osteoblast maturation. Radiologically they appear as cyst-like structures with a light rim of bone and internal blood-filled cavities. They can arise as single entities but also as secondary structures next to other primary tumors of the bone, such as giant cell tumors, chondrosarcomas, and osteosarcomas.

Workup Both MRI w/wo contrast of the spine and CT spine provide insight. The CT can better show the bony rims and septa of the cysts. The MRI can demonstrate the blood-filled cysts, which may exhibit fluid levels with bright T1, T2 signals and also differential signal intensity within the fluid reflecting blood products of varying age.

Management The primary management is surgical—either *en bloc* resection or intralesional gross total resection, unless surgery would involve excessive morbidity. Intralesional resections are most common. The reported recurrence rate following surgery ranges from 19 to 26% [96]. Many recurrences occur within the first year of follow-up and are usually salvaged with repeat surgery. ABCs involve overexpression of RANKL and there is some evidence of the benefit of denosumab, though the current data are not as robust or mature as denosumab for giant cell tumors of bone. In a systematic review of 43 cases reported in 17 manuscripts, denosumab resulted in pain relief in most cases and either resulted in volume reduction or re-ossification in 36 of 39 cases, with a 19% recurrence rate while on denosumab [97]. As of now, typically denosumab may be attempted for unresectable or recurrent lesions with no other options. It can also be used as a bridge therapy initially to improve resectability [98].

Radiotherapy can also be effective for ABCs. Typical doses involve 26–30.6 Gy in 1.8 or 2.0 Gy fractions with reported local control of ~90% [99–105]. ABCs commonly occur in young patients and thus surgical management is preferable. If radiotherapy is deemed needed due to the unresectability of the disease in a young patient, then proton-based radiation would be a reasonable approach to limit integral dose.

Outcomes A systematic review of 771 ABC lesions found similar local control of 86–88% with radiotherapy, curettage plus radiotherapy, or curettage plus cryotherapy. Patients who received curettage and a bone graft had a 31% risk of recurrence [106].

Follow-up Recurrence often happens within the first year of treatment. Thus, q3-month imaging for the first year makes sense, followed by q6-month imaging. Patients who receive radiotherapy should have ongoing, lifelong imaging for monitoring of second malignancies.

Giant Cell Tumors

Background Giant cell tumors of bone are classified as intermediate malignant, but exhibit a large range in growth kinetics, ranging from indolent to locally aggressive. In some cases, GCTB can metastasize to the lungs and yet remain clinically indolent. The etiology is secondary to aberrant RANKL signaling between stromal cells and osteoclastic giant cells, and a recent discovery that the RANKL inhibitory monoclonal antibody denosumab is highly effective [107–110].

Workup MRI and CT of the involved lesion.

Treatment Surgery is historically the mainstay of treatment for these tumors, with radiotherapy reserved for unresectable cases. Surgery can involve intralesional curettage approaches to improve functional outcomes though the local recurrence rates can be as high as 27–31% and en bloc resection is associated with lower recurrence rates [111–115]. Radiotherapy is additionally avoided as many of these patients are young and at risk for secondary malignancies long term [116]. Denosumab can be used as neoadjuvant therapy to reduce tumor size and improve resectability [107, 117] and also to improve clinical symptoms such as pain. In an analysis of 24 patients, denosumab resulted in re-ossification in 92% and reduced symptoms, but invoked a small degree of regression of tumor burden (maximum diameter 52.5 to 48.2 mm) [117]. Thus, a typical outcome of denosumab has been re-ossification of lytic areas, stabilization of disease, and small regressions.

If surgery is feasible at initial presentation, it is not currently clear whether neoadjuvant denosumab is beneficial. In a small randomized trial with 18 patients, preoperative denosumab was not associated with relapse-free survival compared to surgery alone and RFS was only 60–63% at 2 years in both arms [107].

Finally, denosumab as primary treatment can also induce durable responses. In a large phase II trial involving 267 patients with unresectable disease, only 11% of patients had disease progression with a median of 65 months of follow-up [118]. However, discontinuation of denosumab results in high rates of secondary recurrence and thus patients are maintained on therapy permanently [119].

Based on superb responses to denosumab with or without resection, radiation therapy for GCTB is now less commonly used at our center. First-line options, such as surgery, denosumab alone, or neoadjuvant denosumab plus surgery, have dominated the management of nearly all patients. When considered, the local control benefits of radiotherapy have been balanced against a non-negligible risk of malignant transformation [120]. When radiotherapy is used, the local control estimates are 80–85% with 5 years of follow-up [121–125]. A range of radiation doses between 45 and 55 Gy have been recommended; in the largest series of 122 patients, the authors recommend conventionally fractionated 50 Gy [124].

Follow-up q3–6 month per the physician discretion.

Hemangioblastomas

Background Hemangioblastomas(HB) are slow-growing tumors that can arise within the cerebellum, brain stem, or spinal cord. They can be associated with Von Hippel-Lindau syndrome (VHL, 25%) or arise sporadically (75%). Sporadic cases can occasionally be detected incidentally or following symptoms, such as pain, weakness or numbness. They can also hemorrhage, leading to the sudden onset of neurologic symptoms. Patients with VHL are commonly diagnosed with intramedullary spinal cord hemangioblastomas as part of work-up. They appear as highly contrast-enhancing lesions that appear discrete, subpial and can have an associated syrinx [126].

Workup MRI total spine and MRI brain w/wo contrast. Additional workup/management of VHL is nicely reviewed elsewhere [127, 128]. Referral to medical genetics for patients with 2 or more HB lesions or patients with other tumors such as pheochromacytomas, pancreatic lesions, renal cell carcinomas, or neuroendocrine tumors. Also refer patients diagnosed <30 years of age or those with a relative with VHL or history of pheochromocytoma.

Treatment Options vary according to location. For limited disease in the cerebellum, surgical resection is preferred. For asymptomatic patients, the indication for resection is to prevent future hemorrhage and symptoms. Recently a HIF 2-alpha inhibitor, Belzutifan, has demonstrated good tumor control and a reduction in size for VHL-associated hemangioblastoma, renal cell carcinomas and pancreatic neuroectodermal tumors [129]. Consideration can be made for SRS or hypofractionated SBRT and many series report outcomes of spinal HBs and intracranial HBs together [130–133]. Conventionally fractionated RT (50–55 Gy) can also be used in circumstances where SRS is infeasible [134]. For small lesions, our typical approach is hypofractionated SBRT, 8 Gy × 3, with 1 mm PTV margins and a cord Dmax limited to 24 Gy outside PTV (See Fig. 8.6).

Outcomes A pooled systematic review of outcomes of 660 lesions in 15 studies found a 5-year local control rate of 92% following SRS [135]. A separate systematic review specifically of spinal hemangioblastoma found long-term control of 96% following surgical resection [136].

Follow-up Follow-up by MRI at q6-month intervals initially, then annual.

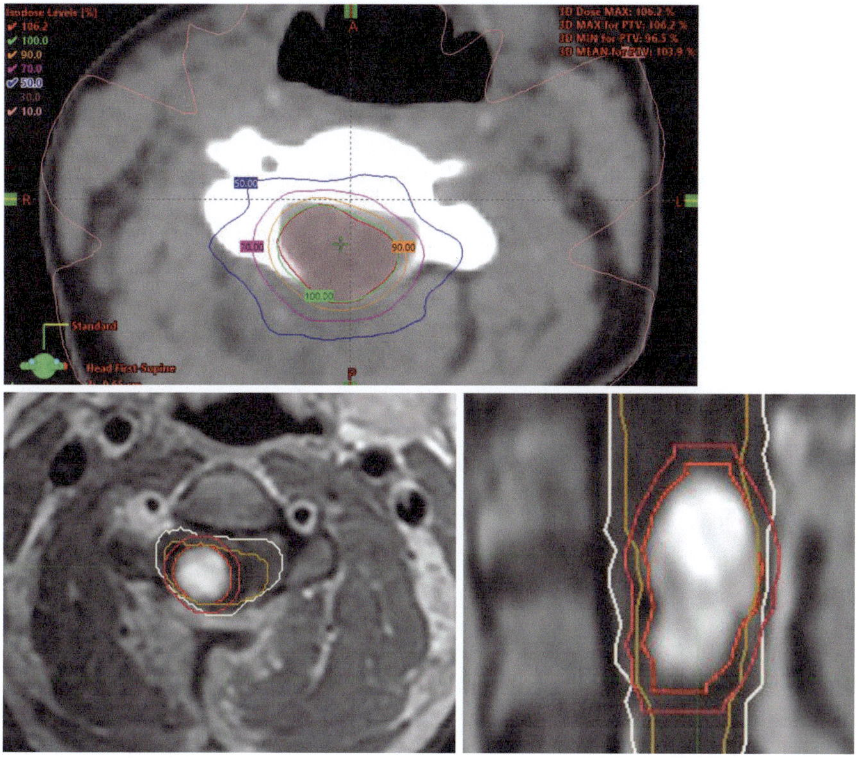

Fig. 8.6 Hemangioblastoma. 22 year old with new diagnosis of VHL s/p laminectomy at C4 for biopsy. GTV is outlined by fusion of T1 post contrast MRI sequence (red). CTV = GTV. A 2 mm GTV-PTV margin was added and an SBRT technique was used for patient setup and verification. Prescription dose was 8 Gy × 3. Overall Dmax of the plan was 106%. The cord (brown) is indistinguishable from the GTV and therefore envelops the GTV. Dmax to cord was 25.48 Gy, above our general cord constrain of 24 Gy, which was viewed as necessary under the circumstances for this unresectable tumor

Paragangliomas

Background Paragangliomas are neuroendocrine tumors that rarely can involve the spine when they arise from adjacent structures such as the glossopharyngeal or vagus nerves, carotid body, or sympathetic nerves in the abdomen abutting the anterior vertebrae. They can also present within the spinal canal, arising directly from the cauda equina [137–142]. Paragangliomas can be divided into sympathetic and parasympathetic gangliomas. Sympathetic gangliomas typically arise in the sympathetic paravertebral ganglia and are often functional secretors of catecholamines, resulting in episodic hypertension, headache, sweating and tachycardia similar to pheochromacytomas. Parasympathetic gangliomas are typically in the head and neck and are nonfunctional. Most are sporacic, but some are associated more broadly with MEN2, NF1, or VHL genetic syndromes. This section will focus on the treatment of known, benign lesions associated with the spine while the reader can consult other excellent reviews on diagnosis and work-up of genetic syndromes and more specifics about PGs in the head and neck [143]. In addition, while most paragangliomas are benign tumors, they can metastasize. For the treatment of malignant paraganglioma metastases, please refer to the excellent chapter on radiosurgery for bone metastases.

Work-up MRI spine w/wo contrast. The lesions exhibit a "salt and pepper" appearance, with signal voids on T2 and a bright overall appearance. Within the cauda, there can be highly prominent vessels supplying the tumor. Additional imaging tests such as FDG-PET, MIBG, or Ga-68 DOTATATE scans may be useful for staging and in some circumstances when tumor localization is unknown. However, radiation planning is typically designed on the basis of the spine MRI. 24-h urine fractionated metanephrines and catecholamines to diagnose functional tumors.

Treatment These tumors can often be observed initially in many asymptomatic patients to determine growth kinetics and behavior. For symptomatic patients, resection more rapidly and completely resolves symptoms and radiation is typically used for unresectable cases or for post-operative treatment [144]. For cauda lesions, surgery alone, if feasible, would be expected to more rapidly relieve symptoms, but may not be possible in all cases and primary or adjuvant radiotherapy may be considered.

Dosing and planning parameters are largely derived from what is known about paragangliomas of the head and neck since these tumors are rare in the spine. Both conventionally fractionated regimens [145–149] and SRS/SBRT dose regimens can be successful [144, 150–157]. Conventionally fractionated radiation should involve a dose of 45–56 Gy. Common single fraction regimens are 12–16 Gy whereas hypofractionated SBRT can be 30 Gy in 5 fractions or 24 Gy in 3 fractions. Of note, our center's Dmax constraint for the cauda is 30 Gy in 5 fractions, which enables SBRT dosing of lesions in close proximity to the cauda.

Outcomes Local control is generally >80% in most primary radiation series. There is at least one study suggesting a dose response. One series found that those cases treated with $BED_{10} \geq 53$ Gy exhibited 91% local control at 5 years compared to 62% for those treated with a lower dose [144]. Other radiosurgery series report >90% long-term local control [158]. In a systematic review of all head and neck PG series, in 1144 total cases in 37 manuscripts, the overall local control was 94.2% with a median follow-up of 44 months with single fraction SRS [158]. Symptoms improved in 49% of patients and permanent sequelae were limited.

Follow-up MRI spine w/wo contrast 3 months after radiotherapy or resection and then spaced to every 6–12 months. For secreting tumors, annual testing of urine metanephrines and catecholamines is indicated and thus ongoing follow-up with endocrinology is indicated.

Solitary Plasmacytomas

Background Solitary plasmacytomas of bone (SBP) in the spine are defined as plasma cell neoplasms, histologically confirmed by biopsy of the lesion and yet without evidence of systemic myeloma. Criteria for absence of systemic myeloma include (1) ≤10% plasma cells on bone marrow biopsy, (2) absence of additional lesions by skeletal survey or PET/CT, and (3) absence of end-organ damage attributable to the plasma cell dyscrasia such as Hgb <10 g/dL or 2 g/dL below normal, serum calcium >11.5 mg/dL, or serum creatinine >2 mg/dL. Patients can have ≤10% bone marrow involvement and/or monoclonal urinary light chains (ULC); however, these findings are prognostic for eventual relapse into multiple myeloma.

A high-risk cohort of patients with SBP has been identified by the International Myeloma Working Group as those with detectable but <10% bone marrow involvement. These SBP patients with "minimal marrow involvement" have a much higher risk of multiple myeloma—60–70% risk with a median time to progression of 18–26 months [159–161]. Conversely, patients without any detectable occult marrow disease by multiparameter flow cytometry or any ULC, have a better prognosis with 88–92% of patients with durable disease-free survival [160, 161].

An M-spike on serum protein electrophoresis at the time of diagnosis, not meeting criteria for myeloma, is not necessarily prognostic [161] and may or may not resolve following radiotherapy. However, resolution after RT is associated with improved outcomes [162].

Work-up CBC, serum chemistries including Cr, Ca, LFTs, SPEP with immunofixation and 24-hr UPEP, LDH, Beta-2 microglobulin, skeletal survey or PET/CT, bone marrow biopsy with multiparameter flow cytometry, MRI spine w/wo contrast.

Treatment Surgery followed by post-operative radiation may be indicated for mechanical instability, but otherwise, radiation alone is the primary modality. Typical radiation doses for plasmacytomas in bone or extramedullary tissues have been 45–50 Gy historically. Spine lesions have an additional consideration in terms of the cord dose constraint, which could be conservatively kept to below 46 Gy for plans without cord-sparing IMRT with a 45 Gy in 1.8 Gy fraction plan (see Fig. 8.7). With IMRT and cord sparing, 50.4 Gy in 1.8 Gy fractions is an alternative with the cord dose Dmax constrained to 46 Gy. Which strategy to use would depend on the position of the lesion and the presence of epidural disease. At our center, IMRT is preferred for limiting the dose to bowel, lung and other anterior structures. Prior reports have treated lesions with coverage of one vertebral level above and below the lesion as margin; however, our approach is currently to treat the vertebral level involved, including the full posterior elements and any paraspinal disease and add a 1 cm CTV expansion into bone and involved paraspinal tissues above and below the involved level, respecting anatomic boundaries such as lung and esophagus. Then, with daily kV imaging, we use a 3 mm PTV expansion.

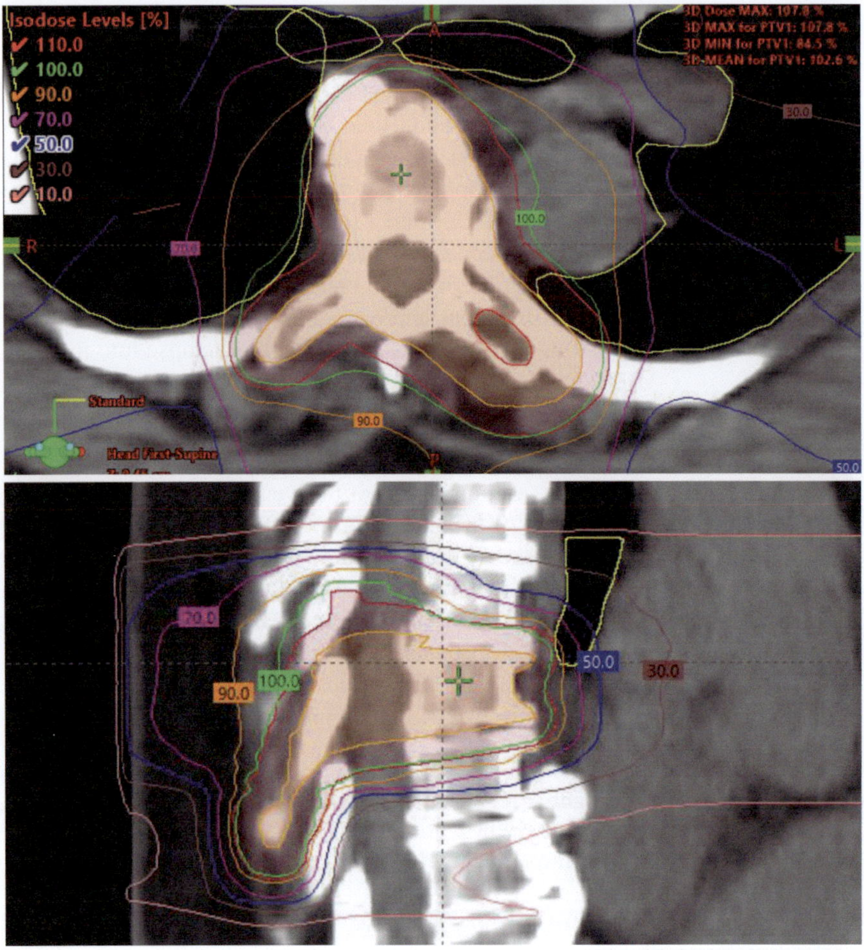

Fig. 8.7 Solitary plasmacytoma in the left pedicle of T6. CTV (orange) includes the entire vertebral body plus at least 1 cm margin around GTV, which in this case was limited to small area in the pedicle (red). A 3 mm PTV (red) was used with daily kV orthogonal imaging for setup verification. Prescription dose was 45 Gy in 1.8 Gy fractions and overall Dmax was 107.8%. Dmax to the spinal cord (defined by fused MRI) was 46.8 Gy

Special Situations For patients with slightly more than 10% clonal plasma cells on BM and no other signs of end-organ damage or additional lesions, then primary RT could be considered as a temporizing measure though systemic progression is likely within 2 years. In a few cases, our center has treated 2 lesions that seem to be behaving as solitary lesions or in some cases metachronous lesions one after the other if there are still no signs of systemic myeloma. Finally, while the local control following RT is excellent (~90%), we have treated a few local-only recurrences with re-irradiation SBRT using techniques similar to metastatic disease with doses such as 27 Gy in 3 fractions with an aggressively limited cord Dmax to 16 Gy.

Outcomes Local control is typically very high, but reported outcomes do vary between 80% and 100% [163–168]. There is retrospective evidence of improved local control when doses >40 Gy are used compared to <40 Gy [165, 169]. However, a Princess Margaret hospital cohort did not find a local control difference with patients treated with 30–40 Gy or >40 Gy [164]. They did find, however, that lesions >5 cm in diameter had considerably worse outcomes. Finally, the cohort from the Rare Cancer Network study group did not find either a dose response or dependence on lesion size [170]. Thus, there remains uncertainty about the optimal dose. For lesions <5 cm in size, the NCCN recommends 40 Gy and for larger lesions 40–50 Gy is recommended. At our center, we feel 45–50.4 Gy is easily achievable with IMRT and is typically used.

Follow-up Myeloma labs on a q3-month basis for 2 years, then spaced to q6 months. MRI spine q3 months for 2 years, then spaced to q6 months. PET/CT for overall surveillance at 6 months, then as indicated by myeloma labs.

	Prescription doses	GTV/CTV notes
Chordoma	*Protons*: 74–77.4 Gy RBE in 1.8 Gy fractions *SRS*: 24 Gy × 1; alternative 12 Gy × 3	For SRS, CTV follows the general rules of coverage for spine SBRT for bone metastases (see PMID: 22608954). For proton fractionated radiotherapy, the entire involved vertebrae are covered with paraspinal expansions of CTV, which are utilized per the physician's discretion to account for microscopic "skip" lesions (see PMID: 29181683)
Primary sarcomas of the spine	*Protons*: 70–74 Gy RBE in 2.0 Gy fractions; 60 Gy RBE considered for R1 resections *SRS*: 24 Gy × 1; 8 Gy × 5	For proton radiotherapy, CTV should generally cover the entire vertebral body and the involved paraspinal disease. While treatment of extremity sarcomas has involved 1.5–2.0 radial and 4 cm superior-inferior margins for microscopic coverage, in the spine natural anatomic barriers limit areas at risk and CTV coverage into the paraspinal tissues is at least 1 cm and per physician judgment. For SRS, CTV follows the general rules of coverage for spine SBRT for bone metastases (see PMID: 22608954)
Ewing's sarcoma	*Protons*: 55.8 Gy RBE for gross disease; consider escalation to 64.8 Gy RBE for tumors >8 cm; 45 Gy RBE for R1 resections of paraspinal lesions (rare)	CTV1 = Pre-chemotherapy/pre-surgical GTV + 1–1.5 cm, which is treated to 45 Gy RBE; CTV2 = Post-chemotherapy/post-surgical GTV + 1–1.5 cm = CTV2, which is boosted to 55.8 Gy RBE

	Prescription doses	GTV/CTV notes
Ependymoma	*EBRT*: 50.4–55.8 Gy in 1.8 Gy fractions; *Proton CSI*: 30–36 Gy if needed for positive CSF cytology (rare)	GTV1: T1 + C enhancing plus T2 edema, treated to 45 Gy; GTV2 = T1 + contrast only, boosted to 50.4–55.8 Gy. 1–2 cm GTV to CTV margins. Evaluate for drop metastases in the sacrum, which we do not view as evidence of CSF involvement if CSF cytology is negative.
Spinal cord astrocytomas	*EBRT*: Grade 1: 45–50.4 in 1.8 Gy fractions; grade 2: 50.4–54 Gy in 1.8 Gy fractions; grade 3–4: 54–55.8 Gy	For grade I, GTV includes the T1 + C with a 0.5–1.0 cm margin to CTV. For grade 2, GTV1 includes T1 + C plus T1 hypointense or isointense widened areas plus T2 edema to 45 Gy followed by cone down to GTV2 T1 + C only to 50.1–54 Gy. 1–2 cm GTV to PTV margins are included. For grade 3–4, GTV1 includes T1 + C enhancing plus T2 edema treated to 45–50.4 Gy and GTV2 includes T1 + C only, which is boosted to 54–55.8Gy. 1.5–2.0 cm GTV to CTV margins are used.
Schwannoma	*SBRT*: 14–16 Gy × 1, 8 Gy × 3, or 5Gy × 5 *EBRT*: for large tumors 45 Gy in 1.8 Gy fractions	For most cases CTV = GTV since these tumors are highly discrete.
Meningioma	*SRS*: 12–16 Gy × 1 or 7–8 Gy × 3 or 5 Gy × 5 *EBRT*: 50.4–54 Gy in 1.8 Gy fractions	CTV = GTV plus 5 mm margins along every dural surface radially and in the superior/inferior directions
Aggressive hemangiomas	*SBRT*: 6 Gy × 5, 9 Gy × 3, or 18 Gy × 1 *EBRT*: 45 Gy in 1.8 Gy fractions	CTV follows the general rules of coverage for spine SBRT for bone metastases (see PMID: 22608954).
Aneurysmal bone cysts	*EBRT*: 30.6 Gy in 1.8 Gy fractions	CTV = Involved cysts with coverage of the entire involved vertebrae. 5 mm margin into paraspinal soft tissue.
Giant cell tumors	*EBRT*: 50 Gy in 2 Gy fractions	CTV follows the general rules of coverage for spine SBRT for bone metastases (see PMID: 22608954).
Hemangioblastomas	*SBRT*: 8 Gy × 3 *EBRT* for large lesions: 50–55 Gy in 1.8–2.0Gy fractions	CTV = GTV. 1 mm CTV to PTV margins. Dmax to cord outside PTV limited to 24Gy.
Paragangliomas	*SBRT*: 6 Gy × 5 or 8 Gy × 3 or 12–16 Gy × 1	CTV follows the general rules of coverage for spine SBRT for bone metastases (see PMID: 22608954).

	Prescription doses	GTV/CTV notes
Solitary plasmacytomas	*EBRT*: 45–50.4 Gy in 1.8 Gy fractions	CTV: entire involved vertebral level and paraspinal tissue plus 1 cm expansion, respecting anatomic boundaries such as lung and esophagus.

Technique: IMRT or VMAT is used in every situation above, either when referring to conventionally fractionated external beam radiotherapy (EBRT) or stereotactic body radiotherapy (SBRT).
Total organ displacement: This complex approach involves simulation and then insertion of a balloon catheter at the time of treatment to displace the bowel from the sacral chordoma mass. It is considered for single fraction SRS (24 Gy × 1) if the bowel is directly adjacent to the mass. See previous publications for additional details [17].
PTV margins for SBRT: CTV to PTV margins depend upon setup and image guidance. For SBRT cases, we utilize a "CDR frame" consisting of an alpha cradle and lateral support paddles. A mask is used for metastases at T5 and above. Daily orthogonal kV pairs and CBCTs are performed with MD verification of films prior to treatment. A 6-degree-of-freedom couch (Varian) improves alignment. ExacTrac (Brainlab) or Intrafraction motion review (IMR, Varian) is used to monitor intrafraction motion. For spinal cord delineation, the spinal cord is outlined using the contrast on the simulation CT from a prior myelogram. Or we use a fusion of a specialized MRI sequence and add a 1 mm PRV. Under these ideal conditions, we use only a 2 mm CTV to PTV margin but exclude the thecal sac from PTV.
PTV margins for fractionated RT: For fractionated radiotherapy cases with anatomy and prescription doses that allow for dose to the cord to be well below the spinal cord constraint, then a 3–4 mm PTV margin with daily kV imaging and weekly CBCT would be sufficient. If there is epidural disease and the cord constraint limits coverage, then elements of SBRT setup and planning can be incorporated such as a CDR frame immobilization, myelogram for cord delineation, and even daily CBCT if needed.

References

1. Iorgulescu JB, et al. Benign notochordal cell tumors of the spine: natural history of 8 patients with histologically confirmed lesions. Neurosurgery. 2013;73:411–6. https://doi.org/10.1227/01.neu.0000431476.94783.c6.
2. Jawad MU, Scully SP. Surgery significantly improves survival in patients with chordoma. Spine (Phila Pa 1976). 2010;35:117–23. https://doi.org/10.1097/BRS.0b013e3181b44387.
3. Fuller DB, Bloom JG. Radiotherapy for chordoma. Int J Radiat Oncol Biol Phys. 1988;15:331–9. https://doi.org/10.1016/s0360-3016(98)90012-8.
4. Romero J, et al. Chordoma: results of radiation therapy in eighteen patients. Radiother Oncol. 1993;29:27–32. https://doi.org/10.1016/0167-8140(93)90169-9.
5. Magrini SM, et al. Chordoma-natural history, treatment and prognosis. The Florence Radiotherapy Department experience (1956-1990) and a critical review of the literature. Acta Oncol. 1992;31:847–51. https://doi.org/10.3109/02841869209089717.
6. Klekamp J, Batzdorf U, Samii M, Bothe HW. The surgical treatment of Chiari I malformation. Acta Neurochir. 1996;138:788–801. https://doi.org/10.1007/BF01411256.
7. Stacchiotti S, Sommer J, Chordoma Global Consensus, G. Building a global consensus approach to chordoma: a position paper from the medical and patient community. Lancet Oncol. 2015;16:e71–83. https://doi.org/10.1016/S1470-2045(14)71190-8.

8. Ares C, et al. Effectiveness and safety of spot scanning proton radiation therapy for chordomas and chondrosarcomas of the skull base: first long-term report. Int J Radiat Oncol Biol Phys. 2009;75:1111–8. https://doi.org/10.1016/j.ijrobp.2008.12.055.
9. Redmond KJ, et al. Radiotherapy for mobile spine and sacral Chordoma: a critical review and practical guide from the Spine Tumor Academy. Cancers (Basel). 2023;15 https://doi.org/10.3390/cancers15082359.
10. Akiyama T, et al. Analysis of the infiltrative features of Chordoma: the relationship between micro-skip metastasis and postoperative outcomes. Ann Surg Oncol. 2018;25:912–9. https://doi.org/10.1245/s10434-017-6268-6.
11. Amichetti M, Amelio D, Cianchetti M, Enrici RM, Minniti G. A systematic review of proton therapy in the treatment of chondrosarcoma of the skull base. Neurosurg Rev. 2010;33:155–65. https://doi.org/10.1007/s10143-009-0235-z.
12. Hug EB, Slater JD. Proton radiation therapy for chordomas and chondrosarcomas of the skull base. Neurosurg Clin N Am. 2000;11:627–38.
13. Munzenrider JE, Liebsch NJ. Proton therapy for tumors of the skull base. Strahlenther Onkol. 1999;175(Suppl 2):57–63. https://doi.org/10.1007/BF03038890.
14. Castro JR, et al. Experience in charged particle irradiation of tumors of the skull base: 1977-1992. Int J Radiat Oncol Biol Phys. 1994;29:647–55. https://doi.org/10.1016/0360-3016(94)90550-9.
15. DeLaney TF, et al. Long-term results of phase II study of high dose photon/proton radiotherapy in the management of spine chordomas, chondrosarcomas, and other sarcomas. J Surg Oncol. 2014;110:115–22. https://doi.org/10.1002/jso.23617.
16. Jin CJ, et al. Long-term outcomes of high-dose single-fraction radiosurgery for chordomas of the spine and sacrum. J Neurosurg Spine. 2019;1–10 https://doi.org/10.3171/2019.7.SPINE19515.
17. Maybody M, et al. Temporary organ displacement to escalate radiation dose to retroperitoneal tumors and decrease toxicity to organs at risk. J Vasc Interv Radiol. 2020;31:1578–86. https://doi.org/10.1016/j.jvir.2020.01.011.
18. Wu AJ, Bilsky MH, Edgar MA, Yamada Y. Near-complete pathological response of chordoma to high-dose single-fraction radiotherapy: case report. Neurosurgery. 2009;64:E389–90; discussion E390. https://doi.org/10.1227/01.NEU.0000338073.49649.1A.
19. Radaelli S, et al. The sacral chordoma margin. Eur J Surg Oncol. 2020;46:1415–22. https://doi.org/10.1016/j.ejso.2020.04.028.
20. Yu X, et al. Comparison of wide margin and inadequate margin for recurrence in Sacral Chordoma: a meta-analysis. Spine (Phila Pa 1976). 2020;45:814–9. https://doi.org/10.1097/BRS.0000000000003386.
21. Stacchiotti S, et al. Best practices for the management of local-regional recurrent chordoma: a position paper by the Chordoma Global Consensus Group. Ann Oncol. 2017;28:1230–42. https://doi.org/10.1093/annonc/mdx054.
22. Varga PP, et al. Surgical treatment of sacral chordoma: prognostic variables for local recurrence and overall survival. Eur Spine J. 2015;24:1092–101. https://doi.org/10.1007/s00586-014-3728-6.
23. Chhabra AM, et al. Clinical outcomes and toxicities of 100 patients treated with proton therapy for chordoma on the proton collaborative group prospective registry. Radiother Oncol. 2023;183:109551. https://doi.org/10.1016/j.radonc.2023.109551.
24. Lu VM, O'Connor KP, Mahajan A, Carlson ML, Van Gompel JJ. Carbon ion radiotherapy for skull base chordomas and chondrosarcomas: a systematic review and meta-analysis of local control, survival, and toxicity outcomes. J Neuro-Oncol. 2020;147:503–13. https://doi.org/10.1007/s11060-020-03464-1.
25. Imai R, Kamada T, Araki N, Working Group for, B. & Soft Tissue, S. Carbon ion radiation therapy for unresectable Sacral Chordoma: an analysis of 188 cases. Int J Radiat Oncol Biol Phys. 2016;95:322–7. https://doi.org/10.1016/j.ijrobp.2016.02.012.

26. Kamada T, et al. Efficacy and safety of carbon ion radiotherapy in bone and soft tissue sarcomas. J Clin Oncol. 2002;20:4466–71. https://doi.org/10.1200/JCO.2002.10.050.
27. Serizawa I, et al. Carbon ion radiotherapy for unresectable retroperitoneal sarcomas. Int J Radiat Oncol Biol Phys. 2009;75:1105–10. https://doi.org/10.1016/j.ijrobp.2008.12.019.
28. Matsunobu A, et al. Impact of carbon ion radiotherapy for unresectable osteosarcoma of the trunk. Cancer. 2012;118:4555–63. https://doi.org/10.1002/cncr.27451.
29. Shiba S, et al. Impact of carbon ion radiotherapy on inoperable bone Sarcoma. Cancers (Basel). 2021;13 https://doi.org/10.3390/cancers13051099.
30. Pennington Z, et al. Systematic review of charged-particle therapy for chordomas and sarcomas of the mobile spine and sacrum. Neurosurg Focus. 2021;50:E17. https://doi.org/10.3171/2021.2.FOCUS201059.
31. Ravindran PK, et al. Skull-base chondrosarcoma: a systematic review of the role of postoperative radiotherapy. Cancers (Basel). 2024;16 https://doi.org/10.3390/cancers16050856.
32. Abunimer AM, et al. Gross total resection of spinal chondrosarcoma is associated with improved locoregional relapse-free survival and overall survival. Eur Spine J. 2023;32:994–1002. https://doi.org/10.1007/s00586-022-07505-3.
33. Boriani S, et al. Chondrosarcoma of the mobile spine: report on 22 cases. Spine (Phila Pa 1976). 2000;25:804–12. https://doi.org/10.1097/00007632-200004010-00008.
34. Yang X, et al. Chondrosarcomas of the cervical and cervicothoracic spine: surgical management and long-term clinical outcome. J Spinal Disord Tech. 2012;25:1–9. https://doi.org/10.1097/BSD.0b013e31820bb085.
35. Longhi A, Errani C, Gonzales-Arabio D, Ferrari C, Mercuri M. Osteosarcoma in patients older than 65 years. J Clin Oncol. 2008;26:5368–73. https://doi.org/10.1200/JCO.2007.14.9104.
36. Sun Y, et al. Development and validation of a nomogram for predicting prognosis of high-grade chondrosarcoma: a surveillance, epidemiology, and end results-based population analysis. J Orthop Surg (Hong Kong). 2023;31:10225536231174255. https://doi.org/10.1177/10225536231174255.
37. Arshi A, et al. Chondrosarcoma of the Osseous spine: an analysis of epidemiology, patient outcomes, and prognostic factors using the SEER registry from 1973 to 2012. Spine (Phila Pa 1976). 2017;42:644–52. https://doi.org/10.1097/BRS.0000000000001870.
38. Gupta AA, et al. Clinical outcome of children and adults with localized Ewing sarcoma: impact of chemotherapy dose and timing of local therapy. Cancer. 2010;116:3189–94. https://doi.org/10.1002/cncr.25144.
39. Hesla AC, Bruland OS, Jebsen N, Styring E, Eriksson S, Tsagozis P. Ewing sarcoma of the mobile spine; predictive factors for survival, neurological function and local control. A Scandinavian sarcoma group study with a mean follow-up of 12 years. J Bone Oncol. 2019;14:100216. https://doi.org/10.1016/j.jbo.2018.100216.
40. Falk S, Alpert M. Five-year survival of patients with Ewing's sarcoma. Surg Gynecol Obstet. 1967;124:319–24.
41. Martin RC 2nd, Brennan MF. Adult soft tissue Ewing sarcoma or primitive neuroectodermal tumors: predictors of survival? Arch Surg. 2003;138:281–5. https://doi.org/10.1001/archsurg.138.3.281.
42. Mirzaei L, Kaal SE, Schreuder HW, Bartels RH. The neurological compromised spine due to Ewing Sarcoma. What first: surgery or chemotherapy? therapy, survival, and neurological outcome of 15 cases with primary Ewing Sarcoma of the vertebral column. Neurosurgery. 2015;77:718–24; discussion 724–715. https://doi.org/10.1227/NEU.0000000000000903.
43. Indelicato DJ, et al. Modern therapy for spinal and Paraspinal Ewing Sarcoma: an update of the University of Florida experience. Int J Radiat Oncol Biol Phys. 2022;113:161–5. https://doi.org/10.1016/j.ijrobp.2022.01.007.
44. Talleur AC, et al. Limited margin radiation therapy for children and young adults with Ewing Sarcoma achieves high rates of local tumor control. Int J Radiat Oncol Biol Phys. 2016;96:119–26. https://doi.org/10.1016/j.ijrobp.2016.04.001.

45. Schuck A, et al. Local therapy in localized Ewing tumors: results of 1058 patients treated in the CESS 81, CESS 86, and EICESS 92 trials. Int J Radiat Oncol Biol Phys. 2003;55:168–77. https://doi.org/10.1016/s0360-3016(02)03797-5.
46. Farooqi S, et al. Clinical characteristics, management, and outcomes of intramedullary spinal cord Ependymomas in adults: a systematic review. World Neurosurg. 2023;173:237–250 e238. https://doi.org/10.1016/j.wneu.2023.02.098.
47. Wu J, Armstrong TS, Gilbert MR. Biology and management of ependymomas. Neuro-Oncology. 2016;18:902–13. https://doi.org/10.1093/neuonc/now016.
48. Oh MC, et al. Adjuvant radiotherapy delays recurrence following subtotal resection of spinal cord ependymomas. Neuro-Oncology. 2013;15:208–15. https://doi.org/10.1093/neuonc/nos286.
49. Montero AS, et al. Clinical characteristics and long-term surgical outcome of spinal myxopapillary ependymoma: a French cohort of 101 patients. J Neuro-Oncol. 2021;152:491–9. https://doi.org/10.1007/s11060-021-03717-7.
50. Liu X, et al. Outcomes in treatment for primary spinal anaplastic ependymomas: a retrospective series of 20 patients. J Neurosurg Spine. 2013;19:3–11. https://doi.org/10.3171/2013.3.SPINE12183.
51. Fakhreddine MH, et al. Treatment, prognostic factors, and outcomes in spinal cord astrocytomas. Neuro-Oncology. 2013;15:406–12. https://doi.org/10.1093/neuonc/nos309.
52. Milano MT, et al. Primary spinal cord glioma: a surveillance, epidemiology, and end results database study. J Neuro-Oncol. 2010;98:83–92. https://doi.org/10.1007/s11060-009-0054-7.
53. Houten JK, Cooper PR. Spinal cord astrocytomas: presentation, management and outcome. J Neuro-Oncol. 2000;47:219–24. https://doi.org/10.1023/a:1006466422143.
54. Chai RC, et al. The molecular characteristics of spinal cord gliomas with or without H3 K27M mutation. Acta Neuropathol Commun. 2020;8:40. https://doi.org/10.1186/s40478-020-00913-w.
55. Alvi MA, et al. Spinal cord high-grade infiltrating gliomas in adults: clinico-pathological and molecular evaluation. Mod Pathol. 2019;32:1236–43. https://doi.org/10.1038/s41379-019-0271-3.
56. Sun T, et al. Deep learning based on preoperative magnetic resonance (MR) images improves the predictive power of survival models in primary spinal cord astrocytomas. Neuro-Oncology. 2023;25:1157–65. https://doi.org/10.1093/neuonc/noac280.
57. Ogunlade J, Wiginton JG, Elia C, Odell T, Rao SC. Primary spinal Astrocytomas: a literature review. Cureus. 2019;11:e5247. https://doi.org/10.7759/cureus.5247.
58. Seo HS, et al. Nonenhancing intramedullary astrocytomas and other MR imaging features: a retrospective study and systematic review. AJNR Am J Neuroradiol. 2010;31:498–503. https://doi.org/10.3174/ajnr.A1864.
59. Hersh AM, et al. Perioperative outcomes and survival after surgery for intramedullary spinal cord tumors: a single-institution series of 302 patients. J Neurosurg Spine. 2022;1–11 https://doi.org/10.3171/2022.1.SPINE211235.
60. Adams H, Avendano J, Raza SM, Gokaslan ZL, Jallo GI, Quinones-Hinojosa A. Prognostic factors and survival in primary malignant astrocytomas of the spinal cord: a population-based analysis from 1973 to 2007. Spine (Phila Pa 1976). 2012;37:E727–35. https://doi.org/10.1097/BRS.0b013e31824584c0.
61. Haque W, Verma V, Barber S, Tremont IW, Brian Butler E, Teh BS. Management, outcomes, and prognostic factors of adult primary spinal cord gliomas. J Clin Neurosci. 2021;84:8–14. https://doi.org/10.1016/j.jocn.2020.12.015.
62. Parker F, et al. Intramedullary astrocytomas: a French retrospective multicenter study. Neurochirurgie. 2017;63:402–9. https://doi.org/10.1016/j.neuchi.2016.09.007.
63. Minehan KJ, Brown PD, Scheithauer BW, Krauss WE, Wright MP. Prognosis and treatment of spinal cord astrocytoma. Int J Radiat Oncol Biol Phys. 2009;73:727–33. https://doi.org/10.1016/j.ijrobp.2008.04.060.

64. Guss ZD, Moningi S, Jallo GI, Cohen KJ, Wharam MD, Terezakis SA. Management of pediatric spinal cord astrocytomas: outcomes with adjuvant radiation. Int J Radiat Oncol Biol Phys. 2013;85:1307–11. https://doi.org/10.1016/j.ijrobp.2012.11.022.
65. Scheinemann K, et al. Survival and functional outcome of childhood spinal cord low-grade gliomas. Clinical article. J Neurosurg Pediatr. 2009;4:254–61. https://doi.org/10.3171/2009.4.PEDS08411.
66. Corradini S, et al. Radiotherapy of spinal cord gliomas : a retrospective mono-institutional analysis. Strahlenther Onkol. 2016;192:139–45. https://doi.org/10.1007/s00066-015-0917-0.
67. Abdel-Wahab M, et al. Spinal cord gliomas: a multi-institutional retrospective analysis. Int J Radiat Oncol Biol Phys. 2006;64:1060–71. https://doi.org/10.1016/j.ijrobp.2005.09.038.
68. Epstein FJ, Farmer JP, Freed D. Adult intramedullary astrocytomas of the spinal cord. J Neurosurg. 1992;77:355–9. https://doi.org/10.3171/jns.1992.77.3.0355.
69. Basheer A, Rammo R, Kalkanis S, Felicella MM, Chedid M. Multifocal intradural extramedullary Pilocytic Astrocytomas of the spinal cord: a case report and review of the literature. Neurosurgery. 2017;80:E178–84. https://doi.org/10.1093/neuros/nyw029.
70. Kehrer-Sawatzki H, Farschtschi S, Mautner VF, Cooper DN. The molecular pathogenesis of schwannomatosis, a paradigm for the co-involvement of multiple tumour suppressor genes in tumorigenesis. Hum Genet. 2017;136:129–48. https://doi.org/10.1007/s00439-016-1753-8.
71. Gerszten PC, Quader M, Novotny J Jr, Flickinger JC. Radiosurgery for benign tumors of the spine: clinical experience and current trends. Technol Cancer Res Treat. 2012;11:133–9. https://doi.org/10.7785/tcrt.2012.500242.
72. Kalash R, et al. Stereotactic body radiation therapy for benign spine tumors: is dose de-escalation appropriate? J Neurosurg Spine. 2018;29:220–5. https://doi.org/10.3171/2017.12.SPINE17920.
73. Dodd RL, Ryu MR, Kamnerdsupaphon P, Gibbs IC, Chang SD Jr, Adler JR Jr. CyberKnife radiosurgery for benign intradural extramedullary spinal tumors. Neurosurgery. 2006;58:674–85; discussion 674-685. https://doi.org/10.1227/01.NEU.0000204128.84742.8F.
74. Gerszten PC, Burton SA, Ozhasoglu C, McCue KJ, Quinn AE. Radiosurgery for benign intradural spinal tumors. Neurosurgery. 2008;62:887-895; discussion 895-886. https://doi.org/10.1227/01.neu.0000318174.28461.fc.
75. Sachdev S, et al. Stereotactic radiosurgery yields long-term control for benign intradural, extramedullary spinal tumors. Neurosurgery. 2011;69:533–9; discussion 539. https://doi.org/10.1227/NEU.0b013e318218db23.
76. Seppala MT, Haltia MJ, Sankila RJ, Jaaskelainen JE, Heiskanen O. Long-term outcome after removal of spinal neurofibroma. J Neurosurg. 1995;82:572–7. https://doi.org/10.3171/jns.1995.82.4.0572.
77. Woodson E. Radiation for sporadic vestibular Schwannoma: an update on modalities, emphasizing hearing loss, side effects, and tumor control. Otolaryngol Clin N Am. 2023;56:521–31. https://doi.org/10.1016/j.otc.2023.02.011.
78. Breshears JD, et al. Temporal dynamics of Pseudoprogression after Gamma Knife radiosurgery for vestibular Schwannomas-a retrospective volumetric study. Neurosurgery. 2019;84:123–31. https://doi.org/10.1093/neuros/nyy019.
79. Nakamura M, Roser F, Michel J, Jacobs C, Samii M. The natural history of incidental meningiomas. Neurosurgery. 2003;53:62–70; discussion 70–61. https://doi.org/10.1227/01.neu.0000068730.76856.58.
80. Herscovici Z, Rappaport Z, Sulkes J, Danaila L, Rubin G. Natural history of conservatively treated meningiomas. Neurology. 2004;63:1133–4. https://doi.org/10.1212/01.wnl.0000138569.45818.50.
81. Olivero WC, Lister JR, Elwood PW. The natural history and growth rate of asymptomatic meningiomas: a review of 60 patients. J Neurosurg. 1995;83:222–4. https://doi.org/10.3171/jns.1995.83.2.0222.

82. Go RS, Taylor BV, Kimmel DW. The natural history of asymptomatic meningiomas in Olmsted County, Minnesota. Neurology. 1998;51:1718–20. https://doi.org/10.1212/wnl.51.6.1718.
83. Wang B, et al. Intraoperative vertebroplasty during surgical decompression and instrumentation for aggressive vertebral hemangiomas: a retrospective study of 39 patients and review of the literature. Spine J. 2018;18:1128–35. https://doi.org/10.1016/j.spinee.2017.11.003.
84. Heyd R, et al. Radiotherapy for symptomatic vertebral hemangiomas: results of a multicenter study and literature review. Int J Radiat Oncol Biol Phys. 2010;77:217–25. https://doi.org/10.1016/j.ijrobp.2009.04.055.
85. Miszczyk L, Tukiendorf A. Radiotherapy of painful vertebral hemangiomas: the single center retrospective analysis of 137 cases. Int J Radiat Oncol Biol Phys. 2012;82:e173–80. https://doi.org/10.1016/j.ijrobp.2011.04.028.
86. Rades D, Bajrovic A, Alberti W, Rudat V. Is there a dose-effect relationship for the treatment of symptomatic vertebral hemangioma? Int J Radiat Oncol Biol Phys. 2003;55:178–81. https://doi.org/10.1016/s0360-3016(02)03734-3.
87. Miszczyk L, Ficek K, Trela K, Spindel J. The efficacy of radiotherapy for vertebral hemangiomas. Neoplasma. 2001;48:82–4.
88. Brackrock S, Krull A, Schwarz R, Alberti W. Results of radiotherapy for vertebral hemangioma. Strahlenther Onkol. 1999;175:405–8. https://doi.org/10.1007/s000660050029.
89. Winkler C, Dornfeld S, Baumann M, Christen N, Herrmann T, Eberhardt HJ. The efficacy of radiotherapy in vertebral hemangiomas. Strahlenther Onkol. 1996;172:681–4.
90. Sharma S, Kamal R, Rathi AK. Vertebral hemangioma - the current radiation therapy perspective. Rep Pract Oncol Radiother. 2023;28:93–101. https://doi.org/10.5603/RPOR.a2023.0009.
91. Chen Y, Zhang E, Wang Q, Yuan H, Zhuang H, Lang N. Early response assessment after CyberKnife stereotactic radiosurgery for symptomatic vertebral hemangioma by quantitative parameters from dynamic contrast-enhanced MRI. Eur Spine J. 2021;30:2867–73. https://doi.org/10.1007/s00586-021-06742-2.
92. Yu NY, et al. Linear accelerator-based single-fraction stereotactic body radiotherapy for symptomatic vertebral body hemangiomas: the Mayo Clinic experience. J Clin Neurosci. 2020;80:74–8. https://doi.org/10.1016/j.jocn.2020.07.060.
93. Zhang M, Chen YR, Chang SD, Veeravagu A. CyberKnife stereotactic radiosurgery for the treatment of symptomatic vertebral hemangiomas: a single-institution experience. Neurosurg Focus. 2017;42:E13. https://doi.org/10.3171/2016.9.FOCUS16372.
94. Conti A, Starnoni D, Barges-Coll J, Papadimitriou K, Levivier M, Tuleasca C. Radiosurgery for Benign vertebral body hemangiomas of the spine: a systematic review and meta-analysis. World Neurosurg. 2022;164:97–105. https://doi.org/10.1016/j.wneu.2022.03.120.
95. Sung KS, et al. Hypofractionated stereotactic radiosurgery for aggressive vertebral haemangioma and useful follow-up imaging modality: case report and review of the literature. Br J Neurosurg. 2019;1–5 https://doi.org/10.1080/02688697.2019.1648756.
96. Hauschild O, et al. Aneurysmal bone cyst (ABC) : treatment options and proposal of a follow-up regime. Acta Orthop Belg. 2016;82:474–83.
97. Maximen J, Robin F, Tronchot A, Rossetti A, Ropars M, Guggenbuhl P. Denosumab in the management of Aneurysmal bone cyst. Joint Bone Spine. 2022;89:105260. https://doi.org/10.1016/j.jbspin.2021.105260.
98. Giantini-Larsen AM, Chakravarthy VB, Barzilai O, Newman WC, Wexler L, Bilsky MH. The role of neoadjuvant denosumab in the treatment of aneurysmal bone cysts: a case series and review of the literature. J Neurosurg Pediatr. 2022;30:547–54. https://doi.org/10.3171/2022.8.PEDS22314.
99. Mendenhall WM, Zlotecki RA, Gibbs CP, Reith JD, Scarborough MT, Mendenhall NP. Aneurysmal bone cyst. Am J Clin Oncol. 2006;29:311–5. https://doi.org/10.1097/01.coc.0000204403.13451.52.

100. Nobler MP, Higinbotham NL, Phillips RF. The cure of aneurysmal bone cyst. Irradiation superior to surgery in an analysis of 33 cases. Radiology. 1968;90:1185–92. https://doi.org/10.1148/90.6.1185.
101. Feigenberg SJ, Marcus RB Jr, Zlotecki RA, Scarborough MT, Berrey BH, Enneking WF. Megavoltage radiotherapy for aneurysmal bone cysts. Int J Radiat Oncol Biol Phys. 2001;49:1243–7. https://doi.org/10.1016/s0360-3016(00)01462-0.
102. Vergel De Dios AM, Bond JR, Shives TC, McLeod RA, Unni KK. Aneurysmal bone cyst. A clinicopathologic study of 238 cases. Cancer. 1992;69:2921–31. https://doi.org/10.1002/1097-0142(19920615)69:12<2921::aid-cncr2820691210>3.0.co;2-e.
103. Boriani S, et al. Aneurysmal bone cyst of the mobile spine: report on 41 cases. Spine (Phila Pa 1976). 2001;26:27–35. https://doi.org/10.1097/00007632-200101010-00007.
104. Marks RD Jr, Scruggs HJ, Wallace KM, Fenn JO. Megavoltage therapy in patients with aneurysmal bone cysts. Radiology. 1976;118:421–4. https://doi.org/10.1148/118.2.421.
105. Elsayad K, et al. Radiotherapy for aneurysmal bone cysts : a rare indication. Strahlenther Onkol. 2017;193:332–40. https://doi.org/10.1007/s00066-016-1085-6.
106. Schreuder HW, Veth RP, Pruszczynski M, Lemmens JA, Koops HS, Molenaar WM. Aneurysmal bone cysts treated by curettage, cryotherapy and bone grafting. J Bone Joint Surg Br. 1997;79:20–5. https://doi.org/10.1302/0301-620x.79b1.7097.
107. Jamshidi K, Gharehdaghi M, Hajialiloo SS, Mirkazemi M, Ghaffarzadehgan K, Izanloo A. Denosumab in patients with giant cell tumor and its recurrence: a systematic review. Arch Bone Joint Surg. 2018;6:260–8.
108. Singh AS, Chawla NS, Chawla SP. Giant-cell tumor of bone: treatment options and role of denosumab. Biologics. 2015;9:69–74. https://doi.org/10.2147/BTT.S57359.
109. Thomas D, et al. Denosumab in patients with giant-cell tumour of bone: an open-label, phase 2 study. Lancet Oncol. 2010;11:275–80. https://doi.org/10.1016/S1470-2045(10)70010-3.
110. Ueda T, et al. Objective tumor response to denosumab in patients with giant cell tumor of bone: a multicenter phase II trial. Ann Oncol. 2015;26:2149–54. https://doi.org/10.1093/annonc/mdv307.
111. Balke M, et al. Giant cell tumor of bone: treatment and outcome of 214 cases. J Cancer Res Clin Oncol. 2008;134:969–78. https://doi.org/10.1007/s00432-008-0370-x.
112. Arbeitsgemeinschaft K, et al. Local recurrence of giant cell tumor of bone after intralesional treatment with and without adjuvant therapy. J Bone Joint Surg Am. 2008;90:1060–7. https://doi.org/10.2106/JBJS.D.02771.
113. Kivioja AH, et al. Cement is recommended in intralesional surgery of giant cell tumors: a Scandinavian Sarcoma Group study of 294 patients followed for a median time of 5 years. Acta Orthop. 2008;79:86–93. https://doi.org/10.1080/17453670710014815.
114. Algawahmed H, Turcotte R, Farrokhyar F, Ghert M. High-speed burring with and without the use of surgical adjuvants in the Intralesional management of giant cell tumor of bone: a systematic review and meta-analysis. Sarcoma. 2010;2010 https://doi.org/10.1155/2010/586090.
115. Errani C, et al. Giant cell tumor of the extremity: a review of 349 cases from a single institution. Cancer Treat Rev. 2010;36:1–7. https://doi.org/10.1016/j.ctrv.2009.09.002.
116. Palmerini E, Picci P, Reichardt P, Downey G. Malignancy in giant cell tumor of bone: a review of the literature. Technol Cancer Res Treat. 2019;18:1533033819840000. https://doi.org/10.1177/1533033819840000.
117. Yuan B, et al. Radiologic and clinical changes after denosumab treatment for giant cell tumors of the mobile spine: a quantitative study. Insights Imaging. 2022;13:93. https://doi.org/10.1186/s13244-022-01226-3.
118. Chawla S, et al. Denosumab in patients with giant-cell tumour of bone: a multicentre, open-label, phase 2 study. Lancet Oncol. 2019;20:1719–29. https://doi.org/10.1016/S1470-2045(19)30663-1.
119. Perrin DL, et al. The role of Denosumab in joint preservation for patients with giant cell tumour of bone. Bone Joint J. 2021;103-B:184–91. https://doi.org/10.1302/0301-620X.103B1.BJJ-2020-0274.R1.

120. Rock MG, et al. Secondary malignant giant-cell tumor of bone. Clinicopathological assessment of nineteen patients. J Bone Joint Surg Am. 1986;68:1073–9.
121. Caudell JJ, et al. Radiotherapy in the management of giant cell tumor of bone. Int J Radiat Oncol Biol Phys. 2003;57:158–65. https://doi.org/10.1016/s0360-3016(03)00416-4.
122. Shi W, et al. Radiotherapy in the management of giant cell tumor of bone. Am J Clin Oncol. 2013;36:505–8. https://doi.org/10.1097/COC.0b013e3182568fb6.
123. Feigenberg SJ, Marcus RB Jr, Zlotecki RA, Scarborough MT, Berrey BH, Enneking WF. Radiation therapy for giant cell tumors of bone. Clin Orthop Relat Res. 2003;207–216 https://doi.org/10.1097/01.blo.0000069890.31220.b4.
124. Ruka W, et al. The megavoltage radiation therapy in treatment of patients with advanced or difficult giant cell tumors of bone. Int J Radiat Oncol Biol Phys. 2010;78:494–8. https://doi.org/10.1016/j.ijrobp.2009.07.1704.
125. Miszczyk L, Wydmanski J, Spindel J. Efficacy of radiotherapy for giant cell tumor of bone: given either postoperatively or as sole treatment. Int J Radiat Oncol Biol Phys. 2001;49:1239–42. https://doi.org/10.1016/s0360-3016(00)01520-0.
126. Roonprapunt C, Silvera VM, Setton A, Freed D, Epstein FJ, Jallo GI. Surgical management of isolated hemangioblastomas of the spinal cord. Neurosurgery. 2001;49:321–7; discussion 327–328. https://doi.org/10.1097/00006123-200108000-00012.
127. van Leeuwaarde RS, Ahmad S, van Nesselrooij B, Zandee W, Giles RH. In GeneReviews((R)), eds M. P. Adam et al. 1993.
128. Larcher A, et al. Multidisciplinary management of patients diagnosed with von Hippel-Lindau disease: a practical review of the literature for clinicians. Asian J Urol. 2022;9:430–42. https://doi.org/10.1016/j.ajur.2022.08.002.
129. Jonasch E, et al. Belzutifan for renal cell carcinoma in von Hippel-Lindau disease. N Engl J Med. 2021;385:2036–46. https://doi.org/10.1056/NEJMoa2103425.
130. Moss JM, Choi CY, Adler JR Jr, Soltys SG, Gibbs IC, Chang SD. Stereotactic radiosurgical treatment of cranial and spinal hemangioblastomas. Neurosurgery. 2009;65:79–85; discussion 85. https://doi.org/10.1227/01.NEU.0000348015.51685.D2.
131. Kano H, Niranjan A, Mongia S, Kondziolka D, Flickinger JC, Lunsford LD. The role of stereotactic radiosurgery for intracranial hemangioblastomas. Neurosurgery. 2008;63:443–50; discussion 450–441. https://doi.org/10.1227/01.NEU.0000313120.81565.D7.
132. Hanakita S, et al. The long-term outcomes of radiosurgery for intracranial hemangioblastomas. Neuro-Oncology. 2014;16:429–33. https://doi.org/10.1093/neuonc/not201.
133. Palmer K, et al. Stereotactic radiosurgery for spinal Haemangioblastoma: a Retrospective Single-Centre Experience from the United Kingdom. Stereotact Funct Neurosurg. 2023;101:22–9. https://doi.org/10.1159/000527943.
134. Koh ES, Nichol A, Millar BA, Menard C, Pond G, Laperriere NJ. Role of fractionated external beam radiotherapy in hemangioblastoma of the central nervous system. Int J Radiat Oncol Biol Phys. 2007;69:1521–6. https://doi.org/10.1016/j.ijrobp.2007.05.025.
135. Qiu J, et al. Stereotactic radiosurgery for central nervous system hemangioblastoma in von Hippel-Lindau disease: a systematic review and meta-analysis. Clin Neurol Neurosurg. 2020;195:105912. https://doi.org/10.1016/j.clineuro.2020.105912.
136. Bridges KJ, Jaboin JJ, Kubicky CD, Than KD. Stereotactic radiosurgery versus surgical resection for spinal hemangioblastoma: a systematic review. Clin Neurol Neurosurg. 2017;154:59–66. https://doi.org/10.1016/j.clineuro.2017.01.012.
137. Matsumoto M, et al. Paraganglioma of the cauda equina: a report of two cases with unusual histopathological features. Clin Neuropathol. 2012;31:39–43. https://doi.org/10.5414/np300379.
138. Singh NG, et al. Paraganglioma of cauda equina: report of seven cases. Brain Tumor Pathol. 2005;22:15–20. https://doi.org/10.1007/s10014-004-0170-1.
139. Yang SY, Jin YJ, Park SH, Jahng TA, Kim HJ, Chung CK. Paragangliomas in the cauda equina region: clinicopathoradiologic findings in four cases. J Neuro-Oncol. 2005;72:49–55. https://doi.org/10.1007/s11060-004-2159-3.

140. Corinaldesi R, Novegno F, Giovenali P, Lunardi T, Floris R, Lunardi P. Paraganglioma of the cauda equina region. Spine J. 2015;15:e1–8. https://doi.org/10.1016/j.spinee.2014.10.021.
141. Aghakhani N, George B, Parker F. Paraganglioma of the cauda equina region—report of two cases and review of the literature. Acta Neurochir. 1999;141:81–7. https://doi.org/10.1007/s007010050269.
142. Yoshida A, Umekita Y, Ohi Y, Hatanaka S, Yoshida H. Paraganglioma of the cauda equina. A case report and review of the literature. Acta Pathol Jpn. 1991;41:305–10.
143. Lloyd S, Obholzer R, Tysome J, Group, B. C. British Skull Base Society clinical consensus document on management of head and neck Paragangliomas. Otolaryngol Head Neck Surg. 2020;163:400–9. https://doi.org/10.1177/0194599820915490.
144. Breen W, et al. External beam radiation therapy for advanced/unresectable malignant paraganglioma and pheochromocytoma. Adv Radiat Oncol. 2018;3:25–9. https://doi.org/10.1016/j.adro.2017.11.002.
145. Hinerman RW, Amdur RJ, Morris CG, Kirwan J, Mendenhall WM. Definitive radiotherapy in the management of paragangliomas arising in the head and neck: a 35-year experience. Head Neck. 2008;30:1431–8. https://doi.org/10.1002/hed.20885.
146. Chino JP, Sampson JH, Tucci DL, Brizel DM, Kirkpatrick JP. Paraganglioma of the head and neck: long-term local control with radiotherapy. Am J Clin Oncol. 2009;32:304–7. https://doi.org/10.1097/COC.0b013e318187dd94.
147. Krych AJ, Foote RL, Brown PD, Garces YI, Link MJ. Long-term results of irradiation for paraganglioma. Int J Radiat Oncol Biol Phys. 2006;65:1063–6. https://doi.org/10.1016/j.ijrobp.2006.02.020.
148. Lightowlers S, et al. Excellent local control of paraganglioma in the head and neck with fractionated radiotherapy. Clin Oncol (R Coll Radiol). 2010;22:382–9. https://doi.org/10.1016/j.clon.2010.02.006.
149. Vogel J, et al. External beam radiation therapy in treatment of malignant pheochromocytoma and paraganglioma. Front Oncol. 2014;4:166. https://doi.org/10.3389/fonc.2014.00166.
150. Foote RL, et al. Glomus jugulare tumor: tumor control and complications after stereotactic radiosurgery. Head Neck. 2002;24:332–8; discussion 338-339. https://doi.org/10.1002/hed.10005.
151. Henzel M, et al. Fractionated stereotactic radiotherapy of glomus jugulare tumors. Local control, toxicity, symptomatology, and quality of life. Strahlenther Onkol. 2007;183:557–62. https://doi.org/10.1007/s00066-007-1701-6.
152. Wegner RE, Rodriguez KD, Heron DE, Hirsch BE, Ferris RL, Burton SA. Linac-based stereotactic body radiation therapy for treatment of glomus jugulare tumors. Radiother Oncol. 2010;97:395–8. https://doi.org/10.1016/j.radonc.2010.09.004.
153. Guss ZD, et al. Radiosurgery of glomus jugulare tumors: a meta-analysis. Int J Radiat Oncol Biol Phys. 2011;81:e497–502. https://doi.org/10.1016/j.ijrobp.2011.05.006.
154. Jordan JA, Roland PS, McManus C, Weiner RL, Giller CA. Stereotastic radiosurgery for glomus jugulare tumors. Laryngoscope. 2000;110:35–8. https://doi.org/10.1097/00005537-200001000-00007.
155. Chen PG, Nguyen JH, Payne SC, Sheehan JP, Hashisaki GT. Treatment of glomus jugulare tumors with gamma knife radiosurgery. Laryngoscope. 2010;120:1856–62. https://doi.org/10.1002/lary.21073.
156. Lieberson RE, Adler JR, Soltys SG, Choi C, Gibbs IC, Chang SD. Stereotactic radiosurgery as the primary treatment for new and recurrent paragangliomas: is open surgical resection still the treatment of choice? World Neurosurg. 2012;77:745–61. https://doi.org/10.1016/j.wneu.2011.03.026.
157. Liscak R, et al. Leksell Gamma Knife radiosurgery of the jugulotympanic glomus tumor: long-term results. J Neurosurg. 2014;121(Suppl):198–202. https://doi.org/10.3171/2014.7.GKS14923.

158. Fatima N, Pollom E, Soltys S, Chang SD, Meola A. Stereotactic radiosurgery for head and neck paragangliomas: a systematic review and meta-analysis. Neurosurg Rev. 2021;44:741–52. https://doi.org/10.1007/s10143-020-01292-5.
159. Rajkumar SV, et al. International Myeloma Working Group updated criteria for the diagnosis of multiple myeloma. Lancet Oncol. 2014;15:e538–48. https://doi.org/10.1016/S1470-2045(14)70442-5.
160. Paiva B, et al. Multiparameter flow cytometry for staging of solitary bone plasmacytoma: new criteria for risk of progression to myeloma. Blood. 2014;124:1300–3. https://doi.org/10.1182/blood-2014-04-567909.
161. Hill QA, Rawstron AC, de Tute RM, Owen RG. Outcome prediction in plasmacytoma of bone: a risk model utilizing bone marrow flow cytometry and light-chain analysis. Blood. 2014;124:1296–9. https://doi.org/10.1182/blood-2014-04-566521.
162. Wilder RB, Ha CS, Cox JD, Weber D, Delasalle K, Alexanian R. Persistence of myeloma protein for more than one year after radiotherapy is an adverse prognostic factor in solitary plasmacytoma of bone. Cancer. 2002;94:1532–7. https://doi.org/10.1002/cncr.10366.
163. Weber DM. Solitary bone and extramedullary plasmacytoma. Hematology Am Soc Hematol Educ Program. 2005;373–376 https://doi.org/10.1182/asheducation-2005.1.373.
164. Tsang RW, et al. Solitary plasmacytoma treated with radiotherapy: impact of tumor size on outcome. Int J Radiat Oncol Biol Phys. 2001;50:113–20. https://doi.org/10.1016/s0360-3016(00)01572-8.
165. Mendenhall CM, Thar TL, Million RR. Solitary plasmacytoma of bone and soft tissue. Int J Radiat Oncol Biol Phys. 1980;6:1497–501. https://doi.org/10.1016/0360-3016(80)90006-1.
166. Frassica DA, Frassica FJ, Schray MF, Sim FH, Kyle RA. Solitary plasmacytoma of bone: Mayo Clinic experience. Int J Radiat Oncol Biol Phys. 1989;16:43–8. https://doi.org/10.1016/0360-3016(89)90008-4.
167. Mendenhall WM, Mendenhall CM, Mendenhall NP. Solitary plasmacytoma of bone and soft tissues. Am J Otolaryngol. 2003;24:395–9. https://doi.org/10.1016/s0196-0709(03)00092-9.
168. Reed V, et al. Solitary plasmacytomas: outcome and prognostic factors after definitive radiation therapy. Cancer. 2011;117:4468–74. https://doi.org/10.1002/cncr.26031.
169. Goyal G, et al. Treatment approaches and outcomes in plasmacytomas: analysis using a national dataset. Leukemia. 2018;32:1414–20. https://doi.org/10.1038/s41375-018-0099-8.
170. Knobel D, et al. Prognostic factors in solitary plasmacytoma of the bone: a multicenter Rare Cancer Network study. BMC Cancer. 2006;6:118. https://doi.org/10.1186/1471-2407-6-118.

Chapter 9
Stereotactic Radiotherapy for Spine Metastases

Christopher Jackson, E. Christopher Dee, and Yoshiya Yamada

Introduction

Perhaps the greatest innovation in the field of radiation oncology in the twenty-first Century has been the advent of stereotactic body radiation therapy (SBRT). This paradigm is made possible by the marriage of three-dimensional imaging technology that can be applied in near-real-time with highly precise radiation treatment planning capabilities that provide highly conformal radiotherapy. Image guidance is typically provided by on-board imagers that perform cone beam CT and KV imaging of the target area. These scans can provide three-dimensional information about the location of the target with very high precision, as well as the location of nearby critical tissues such as the spinal cord and esophagus. By greatly reducing the uncertainty of positioning with image guidance, the additional margin on the target volume necessary for treatment can be reduced to a matter of several millimeters or less, significantly decreasing the volume of normal tissue that is necessarily treated. By limiting the volume of normal tissue exposed to high-dose radiation, side effects are also much less likely, and the biologically effective dose (BED) of radiation can be increased within the tumor without significantly increasing the risk of toxicity to other vital body organs. This marriage has allowed the safe delivery of high-dose/ablative radiotherapy in the spine, despite close proximity to the spinal cord or esophagus.

This paradigm is now commonly referred to as stereotactic therapy. The term “stereo” comes from the Greek stereos, meaning “solid,” and “taxis,” meaning arrangement or order. In modern medicine, *stereotactic* has come to mean relating to the precise localization of a tissue. Stereotactic biopsies were the first medical

C. Jackson · E. C. Dee · Y. Yamada (✉)
Department of Radiation Oncology, Memorial Sloan Kettering Cancer Center, New York, NY, USA
e-mail: yamadaj@mskcc.org

Y. Yamada et al. (eds.), *Multidisciplinary Spine Tumor Management*,
https://doi.org/10.1007/978-3-032-07519-2_9

application of this concept. Stereotactic radiosurgery (SRS)—or the use of multiple, precisely positioned radiation beams to target tumors—delivers an entire course of treatment in a single session and has been used as routine treatment of brain metastases for over 60 years. More recently, this technology has been applied to the treatment of spinal tumors. SBRT refers to extracranial stereotactic treatment of high-dose-per-fraction radiotherapy in 2–5 fractions. SRS is biologically more potent than SBRT but also carries a higher risk of complications. SBRT is radiobiologically less potent than SRS because the dose is broken up into smaller amounts and given over a longer time, but SBRT is therefore less likely to injure normal tissues. Hence, SBRT is commonly preferred over SRS in cases of larger target volumes or in the setting of previous radiation therapy to the same site. Both SRS and SBRT are best suited for discrete, well-defined targets.

In stark contrast, conventionally fractionated palliative radiotherapy, typically using opposing radiation fields, makes no attempt to spare normal tissues and often delivers higher doses of radiation to the surrounding normal tissues than the actual tumor. Because of the greater amount of normal tissue that is irradiated with conventional palliative radiation, radiation dose schedules are necessarily low-dose-per-fraction treatment delivered to a moderate or lower total dose compared to hypofractionated radiotherapy. This tradeoff is necessary to allow for normal tissue tolerance. Tumor doses are likewise lower; therefore, conventional palliative treatment is often less durable and less effective compared to hypofractionated radiotherapy. The advantage of conventional palliative radiotherapy for spinal metastases is that it is a relatively uncomplicated technique, can be done quickly with minimum preparation, and can treat larger volumes. It is also much less expensive than SRS or SBRT.

Stereotactic Radiosurgery and Stereotactic Body Radiation Therapy

There has been a relative plethora of evidence for SRS and SBRT of the spine in the past 10 years, including prospective randomized trials. For the local treatment of spinal metastases, both SRS and SBRT have been utilized as stand-alone treatment, but the modalities are also utilized in combination with surgery and as salvage treatment for recurrences after both conventional palliative radiotherapy and hypofractionated radiotherapy.

Radiobiology

Numerous peer-reviewed publications have described the very high rates of durable tumor control that can be achieved with the SRS/SBRT paradigm. In general, SRS provides higher probabilities of local control and more durable treatment responses compared to SBRT. This may be due to the higher biologic effectiveness of high-dose SRS. For example, linear quadratic modeling would predict that 24Gy in a single fraction for radioresistant disease ($\alpha/\beta = 3$) would give a BED of 216 Gy_3 and a corresponding 2 Gy equivalent dose (EQD2) of 129 Gy. The same calculation for 24Gy in two fractions (or 12Gy per fraction) would result in a BED of 120 Gy and EQD2 of 72 Gy, suggesting significantly less biologic impact when fractionation is utilized. When 30Gy is prescribed over 3 fractions, the same calculation results in a BED of 130 Gy_3 and an EQD2 of 78 Gy, suggesting that 12Gy × 2 and 10Gy × 3 would be expected to give similar probabilities of tumor control, but inferior to 24Gy × 1. In fact, if we accept the linear quadratic model at these ultra-high doses per fraction, even adding an additional fraction of 12 Gy (12Gy × 3) would still not be biologically equivalent to 24Gy × 1. Although the relevance of linear quadratic modeling can be debated at these high-dose levels, clinical data would suggest that SRS provides superior tumor outcomes compared to hypofractionated treatment schedules.

High-Dose Stereotactic Radiosurgery

The long-term results of spine SRS have been reported for 811 lesions in 657 patients treated at a single institution. The median follow-up was 27 months, with the longest follow-up extending to 141 months. In this retrospective report, 24Gy × 1 was found to be superior to doses lower than 24Gy × 1, and the cumulative incidence of local failure at 4 years was 2.3% for the 24Gy cohort [1]. A retrospective report of 279 de novo metastases in 145 patients treated with 12Gy × 2 found local recurrence in 17.6% at 2 years [2]. Although comparisons between these two studies can be no more than hypothesis-generating, differing fractionation schemes result in a >7-fold difference in local control rates, even with the differences in follow-up. Because of the greater biologic impact of 24Gy × 1, it is reasonable to consider such therapy as ablative.

In a randomized trial of oligometastatic patients comparing outcomes of 9Gy × 3 vs 24Gy × 1, where the majority of patients had spinal metastases, 59 patients received 24Gy × 1 and 58 patients received 9Gy × 3. The cumulative incidence of local failure was 2.7% and 5.8% at 2 and 3 years for the 24Gy × 1 cohort, and 9.1% and 22.5% for the 9Gy × 3 cohort ($p = 0.005$). This experience further suggests that SRS has an advantage in biological effectiveness over SBRT. The authors also reported that more durable local control was associated with reduced likelihood of distant metastases (5% vs 22% at 3 years, $p = 0.01$), an important finding in oligometastatic patients [3].

Another recent series of 1502 patients treated to 2134 lesions with 3-fraction SBRT to a prescription dose of either 27 or 30 Gy in 3 fractions showed 2-year local failure rates of 17 vs 11%, respectively ($p < 0.001$) [4]. These data again highlight the importance of an increased BED in providing durable local control.

Radioresistant solid tumor histologies such as renal cell carcinoma, melanoma, and most sarcomas appear to respond equally well to 24Gy × 1 compared to histologies traditionally thought to be radiation sensitive, such as breast cancer, highlighting the ablative nature of this approach. The National Cancer Center Network (NCCN) guidelines also recommend considering SRS/SBRT for radioresistant spine metastases. Tumor size also does not seem to matter in terms of the likelihood of local control when 24Gy × 1 is utilized [1]. Thus, the NOMS framework recommends SRS (24Gy × 1) for radioresistant histologies when feasible [5]. Ablative SRS should also be considered for oligometastatic patients, who may benefit the most from locally ablative treatment [6].

SRS Toxicity

Stereotactic Body Radiation Therapy

SBRT is frequently considered when patients require high BED therapy but are not suitable for SRS. Although SRS provides an excellent chance of tumor control, there are many situations where SRS is not feasible. The most common scenarios where SRS is not appropriate are when the normal tissue constraints such as the spinal cord prevent the delivery of effective doses of radiotherapy, or when there are concerns about serious toxicity when using 24Gy × 1. Surgical intervention can be helpful in these situations (Tables 9.1, 9.2, and 9.3).

Myelopathy with spine SRS is exceedingly rare. In a report of spine SRS of 811 lesions with a median follow-up of 26 months, 2 cases of radiation myelitis were noted when the spinal cord maximum dose was kept to within 14Gy, using a CT myelogram-defined spinal cord contour [7]. A retrospective review of 270 spine radiosurgery cases with a median follow-up of 46 months found one case of grade 2 radiation myelopathy, and reported a cumulative incidence of radiation myelopathy of 0.3%, suggesting that the D0.03cc to the spinal cord be limited to 14Gy or less in a single fraction [8]. In an analysis of 1423 patients treated to 1904 lesions with 3-fraction SBRT, 30 cases of grade 1–4 radiation myelopathy were identified, for a cumulative incidence of 1.8% at 2 years. There were 19 cases of grade 3–4 radiation myelopathy, corresponding to a 2-year cumulative incidence of 1.1%. A D0.1cc of 19.1 Gy to the spinal cord in 3 fractions is associated with a 1% risk of grade 3–4 radiation myelopathy 2 years after spine SBRT [9].

Neuropathy has also been observed in patients after receipt of SRS/SBRT. Stubblefield et al. reported the results of 557 lesions treated with high-dose

Table 9.1 Series reporting on reirradiation with spine SBRT over the past decade

Author/ citation	# patients	# lesions	Histology	Prior RT	Fractionation	LC rate	Pain control	RT myelitis	Other AEs
Lucido (ASTRO abstract 2023) [24]	91	107	Kidney (27%), lung (15%), prostate (14%), breast (12%)	Median 30Gy (IQR 24–30Gy)	High-risk PTV: 20–24Gy/1fx or 27–39Gy/3fx Low-risk PTV: 16–18Gy/1fx or 21–24Gy/3fx 50Gy/5fx single level	1 yr LC: 88% (81–94%) 2 yr LC: 85% (78–91%)	Not reported in abstract publication	1 patient (cumulative risk 1% [0–4%])	Vertebral compression fracture 7% at 1 yr, 9% at 2 yrs
Serrand (Cureus 2016) [25]	55	61	Breast (35.5%), kidney (21%) and lung (12.9%)	Not reported in abstract publication	25Gy/5fx	At median FU 11mo, 79.7%had local control	76.3% of painful lesions were improved	None reported (0%)	Not reported in abstract publication
Ito (JNS Spine 2018) [26]	28	28	Thyroid (7), lung (6), renal (3), colorectal (3), others (9)	30Gy/10fx (15 patients)	Decompression followed by 24Gy/2fx	1 yr LC: 70%	Not reported	1 patient	Vertebral compression fracture in 3 patients
Hashmi (JNS Spine 2016) [27]	215	247	Breast (291%), NSCLC (16.6%), kidney (13.1%), prostate (7.3%)	Median: 30Gy/10	Included 18Gy/1fx, 24Gy/3fx	6mo LC: 93% 12mo LC: 83%	Not reported	None reported (0%)	Vertebral compression fracture: 4.5%

(continued)

Table 9.1 (continued)

Author/ citation	# patients	# lesions	Histology	Prior RT	Fractionation	LC rate	Pain control	RT myelitis	Other AEs
Thibault (IJROBP 2015) [23]	40	56	RCC (23.2%), NSCLC (12.5%), thyroid (12.5%), prostate (8.9%)	SBRT median 24Gy/2fx, (range, 20–35 Gy in 1–5 fractions); 43% with conventional RT before initial SBRT	Mostly 30Gy/4fx; range: 20–35 Gy in 2–5 fractions	1 yr LC: 81%	Not reported	None reported (0%)	No vertebral compression fractures reported
Sasamura (*Journal of Radiation Research 2020*) [28]	40	42	Kidney (21%), lung (19%), liver (17%)	Median: 30Gy/10fx	25Gy/5fx to all	1 yr LC: 67% 2 yr LC: 51%	60% with pain relief after reirradiation	None reported (0%)	1 with grade 3 pain; 1 with spinal fracture
Ito (Jpn JCO 2021) [29]	123	133	Lung: 19.5%; colorectal: 19.5%; thyroid: 15.0%; renal cell: 13.5%	58 (43.6%) had previous irradiation doses of 40Gy or more	24Gy/2fx	1 yr LC: 74.2%	3-month pain response rate: 75% 12-month pain response rate: 59%	4 patients (3%)	Radiculopathy in 2 patients (1.5%), vertebral compression fracture in 17 (13.8%)
Patel (ASTRO abstract 2023) [30]	90	225	NSCLC: 17.7%; kidney: 15.6%; prostate: 14.4%; breast: 7.8%	Most common: 30Gy, median 5 fractions	Median dose 27Gy (range: 14–40Gy); median 3 fractions (range: 1–5)	6mo LC: 88.9% 1 yr LC: 83.4% 2 yr LC: 78.9%	Not reported in abstract publication	None reported (0%)	All toxicities were grade ≤2

Author/ citation	# patients	# lesions	Histology	Prior RT	Fractionation	LC rate	Pain control	RT myelitis	Other AEs
Detsky (ASTRO abstract 2019) [31]	43	83	Lung (23%), RCC (21%), prostate (19%)	29pts with prior cEBRT, 9pts with two prior cEBRT courses, 5pts with prior SBRT	24–35Gy in 2–5fx	6mo LC: 93% 12moLC: 86% 24mo LC: 81%	Not reported in paper	None reported (0%)	Vertebral compression fracture: one spinal level with new VCF, two with progression of existing VCF
Boyce-Fappiano (PRO 2017) [32]	162	237	Lung: 21%; breast: 16%; prostate: 15%; CNS: 10%; kidney: 8%	Median: 30Gy/10fx Range: 6Gy/1fx–66Gy/48fx)	Median: 16Gy/1fx Range: 10Gy/1fx–35Gy/5fx	71% at a median follow-up time of 4 months	Improved in 81%	1 with RT myelitis (0.6%)	9.3% with vertebral compression fracture attributed to RT

Table 9.2 Series reporting on spine SRS over the past decade

Author/ citation	# patients	# lesions	Histology (% radioresistant)	Dose	Median follow-up (months)	LC Rate	Pain control	RT myelitis	Other AEs
Yamada et al. (2017) [1]	657	811	Mixed (46% radioresistant)	24 (median, range 16–26)	26.9 (mean)	1 yr LC: 99% 2 yr LC: 97.7%	Not reported	0.42%	Not reported
Bate et al. (2015) [33]		24	Mixed	22 (median, range 16–23)	9.8	1 yr LC: 95.8%	Not reported	Not reported	Not reported
Sellin et al. (2015) [34]	37	40	RCC (100%)	24 (median)	49.0	Actuarial LC: 57%	Not reported	Not reported	37% VCF and/or kyphosis
Laufer et al. (2013) [21]	40	40	Mixed	24	7.6	1 yr LC: 91% 2 yr LC: 87%	Not reported	Not reported	Not reported
Ghia et al. (2016) [35]	21	21	RCC (100%)	24	23	1 yr LC: 95% 2 yr LC: 86%	Not reported	Not reported	7/21 patients (33%) had a pain flare. 6/21 patients (28%) had a VCF
Bernard et al. (2017) [36]	34	34	Mixed	18	Not Reported	2 yr LC: 76%	Not reported	Not reported	Not reported

Table 9.3 Series reporting on hypofractionated spine SBRT over the past decade

Author/ citation	# patients	# lesions	Histology	Fractionation	Median follow-up	LC rate	Pain control	RT myelitis	Other AEs
Jackson et al. (2024) [4]	1502	2134	Mixed	27 or 30 Gy in 3 fractions	14 months	2 yr LC: 89% (30 Gy) vs 83% (27 Gy)	Not reported	See separate series [9]	4.6% VCF 2 years after spine SBRT
Park et al. (2015) [37]	39	59 (14 were reirradiated)	Mixed, ≥8.5% radioresistant	Median 27 Gy in 3 fractions (range 18–35 Gy)	7.4 months	1 yr LC: 93.2% 2 yr LC: 93.2%	Not reported	None	Not reported
Anand et al. (2015) [38]	52	76	Mixed (≥13.5%)	24 Gy (median, range 24–27 Gy in 1–3 fractions)	8.48 months	1 yr LC: 94%	90% of patients without malignant epidural compression, 93.75% of patients with epidural compression (actuarial)	Not reported	Not reported
Bishop et al. (2015) [39]	285	332	Mixed (49% radioresistant)	43 Gy median in 1–3 fractions	19 months	1 yr LC: 88% 3 yr LC: 82%	Not reported	Not reported	Not reported
Bate et al. (2015) [33]		24	Mixed	20–30 Gy in 2–5 fractions	9.8	1 yr LC: 87.5%	Not reported	Not reported	7.2% VCF (including single fraction patients)

(continued)

Table 9.3 (continued)

Author/ citation	# patients	# lesions	Histology	Fractionation	Median follow-up	LC rate	Pain control	RT myelitis	Other AEs
Guckenberger et al. (2014) [40]	301	387	Mixed (≥35%)	24 Gy in 3 fx median, range 8–60 Gy 1–20 fx	11.8	1 yr LC: 89.9	Not reported	None	4.1% progression of VCF; 3.6% de novo VCF
Thibault et al. (2014) [41]	37	71	RCC (100%)	18–30 Gy in 1–5 fx	12.3	1 yr LC: 83% 2 yr LC: 66.2%	Not reported	None	9% VCFs
Sohn et al. (2014) [42]	13	13	RCC (100%)	38 (mean) Gy in 4 fx (median)	Not reported	1 yr LC: 85.7%	Complete pain relief in 3/13 (23%) patients, partial pain relief in 7/13 (53%) patients	None	0% VCFs
Folkert et al. (2014) [43]	52	52	High-grade Sarcoma (100%)	28.5 Gy (median) in 3–6 fx	12.3	1 yr LC: 84.1% 2 yr LC: 65.7%	Not reported	Not reported	Not reported
Laufer et al. (2013) [21]	146	146	Mixed	24–30 Gy in 3 fractions (high-dose hypofractionated) [37 patients] or 18–36 Gy in 5–6 fractions (low-dose hypofractionated [109 patients]	Not reported	1 yr LC for high-dose hypo-fractionated: 95.9% 1 yr LC for low-dose hypo-fractionated: 78.4%	Not reported	Not reported	Not reported

Author/ citation	# patients	# lesions	Histology	Fractionation	Median follow-up	LC rate	Pain control	RT myelitis	Other AEs
Al-Omair et al. (2013) [44]	45	45	Mixed	18–40 Gy in 3–5 fractions	3.3	2 yr LC: 44%	Not reported	Not reported	Not reported
Chang et al. (2014) [45]	27	39	HCC (100%)	28.7 Gy mean in 1–5 fractions	11	2 yr LC: 89%	Pain related to lesions controlled in 84.6% of patients 1 month post tx	None	5/27 patients had VCF (18.5%)
Bahig et al. (2016) [46]	35	49	Mixed (≥37%)	23.9 Gy in 3 fractions	23	1 yr LC: 87% 2 yr LC: 64%	Not reported	Not reported	Not reported
Bernard et al. (2017) [36]	127	148	Mixed (≥35.8%)	27/3	22.6	1 yr LC: 82.6% 2 yr LC: 76%	Not reported	None	10/148 VCF (7%)
Guckenberger et al. (2018) [47]	24	24	Mixed	35 Gy in 5 fractions	12	1 yr LC: 78.1%	Overall pain response observed in 87% of lesions	None	15% new VCFs 1 patient (2%) experienced
Tseng et al. (2018) [2]	145	279	Mixed (≥25%)	24/2	15	1 yr LC: 90.3% 2 yr LC: 82.4%	Not reported	None	Risk of VCF at 1 year: 8.5% Risk of VCF at 2 years: 13.8%

(continued)

Table 9.3 (continued)

Author/ citation	# patients	# lesions	Histology	Fractionation	Median follow-up	LC rate	Pain control	RT myelitis	Other AEs
Ghia et al. (2016) [35]	26	26	RCC (100%)	27/3 or 30/5	23	1 yr LC: 71% 2 yr LC: 55%	Not reported	Not reported	6/26 (23%) patients had a pain flare; 1/26 (4%) patients had a VCF
Rothrock et al. (2020) [48]	29	31	Mixed (100%; ESCC 2 only)	27 Gy in 3 fx (83.9% of patients)	Not reported	1 yr LC: 89.6% 2 yr LC: 78%	Not reported	None	None
Zeng et al. (2023) [49]	159	301	Mixed (68.6%)	28 Gy in 2 fx	23.5	1 yr LC: 94.6% 2 yr LC: 88.9%	Not reported	None	VCF risk at 2 yrs: 8.8%

radiosurgery in 447 patients. Neuropathy was defined electrophysiologically. Pain and weakness were present in almost all cases. The overall rate of neuropathic injury was noted to be 2.5% with a median time to onset of 10.5 months. Of these cases, 3 (21%) were grade 3 injuries [10].

Vertebral body fractures can result from spine SRS/SBRT. High-dose radiation can cause a loss of mineralization of the bone, potentially resulting in osteoporotic-type compression fractures [11]. These effects can be seen in the diseased vertebral body as well as the adjacent superior or inferior endplates of the targeted vertebral body. A 39% rate of radiographic fractures was initially reported after spine SRS [12]. Fortunately, the majority of radiographic fractures are not symptomatic. The same group reported that less than 8% of patients actually became symptomatic and required an intervention. In this study of 323 patients treated with 24Gy × 1 radiosurgery, the 5-year cumulative incidence of symptomatic fractures was found to be 7.2% [13]. In a multicenter randomized trial of 24Gy × 1 vs 9Gy × 3 for oligometastatic disease, the rate of fracture was found to be equal at 2% for both arms [3]. SC 24, a randomized trial of 12Gy × 2 vs 4Gy × 5 for the palliation of spine metastasis, reported a 1% risk of vertebral body fracture in both arms [14]. In an analysis of 1502 patients treated to 2134 lesions with 27 or 30 Gy in 3 fractions with spine SBRT, the cumulative incidence of any vertebral body compression fracture was 5.6% for 30 Gy and 3.8% for 27 Gy at 2 years ($p = 0.022$). The cumulative incidence of vertebral body compression fracture requiring kyphoplasty or surgery was 3.1% for 30 Gy and 2% for 27 Gy 2 years after spine SBRT ($p = 0.2$) [4].

In summary, while spine SRS and SBRT can result in significant toxicity, the rate of serious complications appears to be quite low, and in most cases the benefit of improved tumor response and durable tumor control of SRS/SBRT outweighs the potential risks.

Surgery and SRS/SBRT

Based upon the NOMS framework, surgery and SRS/SBRT can have an important role in the management of spine metastases [5]. A primary role for surgical intervention is mechanical stabilization. The importance of considering mechanical spinal instability is a crucial aspect of managing spine disease and is discussed in great detail in other chapters.

Separation surgery has been coined as a procedure that provides mechanical stability and allows for definitive SRS/SBRT in cases where epidural disease adjacent to the spinal cord would preclude the delivery of a tumoricidal dose of radiation without surgical separation. When prescribing a dose of 24Gy × 1, limiting the minimum dose to the gross tumor to less than 14Gy (spinal cord tolerance) has been shown to increase the risk of local recurrence, particularly in the epidural space. With stereotactic radiation therapy, the dose falls off over a few millimeters. By removing epidural disease and separating the gross tumor from the spinal cord—even by a few millimeters—separation surgery can dramatically improve target coverage. Without separation surgery, epidural disease near or abutting the cord would prevent effective SRS/SBRT because the rigid dose constraints of the spinal cord would limit the radiation dose to the tumor and thereby lessen the probability of durable tumor control.

Because of the high-dose-per-fraction and steep dose fall-off over a few millimeters, spinal SRS/SBRT can be utilized in the reirradiation setting. As the spinal cord has even lower constraints in the setting of reirradiation, separation surgery is often critical to maximize the distance between gross tumor volume and the spinal cord, thereby allowing for an additional round of high-dose-per-fraction radiation therapy. Thus, separation surgery can provide the conditions necessary for the delivery of effective doses of radiation.

Reirradiation

The most common indication for spine SBRT in the United States is reirradiation of tumors that have recurred after a prior course of radiotherapy. Randomized trials have demonstrated that after conventional palliative radiotherapy for bone metastases, up to 50% of treated tumors will experience local palliative failure within 12 months of treatment [15]. In a recently published series, Zeng et al. showed that the risk of local failure at 2 years for spinal metastases was 14.8% for SBRT (24 Gy in 2 fractions) compared to 35.6% for conventional palliative radiation therapy (20 Gy in 5 fractions) [16]. As patients are surviving longer with stage IV disease, the probability of local recurrence increases with extended follow-up and survival. This is because conventional palliative radiotherapy is not ablative therapy. In a study of patients who received conventional palliative radiation for solid tumor spine metastases with relatively long-term follow-up, both favorable and unfavorable histologies exhibited less than a 20% actuarial probability of palliation benefit at 5 years [17]. Thus, it is clear that conventional palliative radiotherapy is designed primarily for short-term pain palliation and not long-term tumor control, nor long-term pain palliation. With improvement in systemic therapy and with enhanced tools to identify good-prognosis patients such as those with oligometastatic disease, patients with metastatic disease are now outliving the benefit that conventional palliative radiotherapy can provide. Greater numbers of patients are now presenting with recurrent spine metastases after conventional therapy.

SRS/SBRT is an excellent method for effectively treating tumors that have recurred after conventional palliative radiation because it is ablative in nature and therefore more likely to eliminate otherwise radioresistant tumor cells. It is also highly conformal, limiting radiation dose to previously irradiated normal tissue, another benefit in the setting of reirradiation.

Spinal cord injury has long been a concern for reirradiation of spinal disease. Although there have been no randomized trials in human subjects assessing spinal cord tolerance, preclinical data is available to guide the judicious use of SBRT in the reirradiation setting. Medin et al. performed a dose escalation exercise in pigs using stereotactic techniques. The pigs were initially subjected to conventional radiation

(30Gy in 10 fractions) and then a year later underwent radiosurgery to the same site using stereotactic radiosurgery, mimicking the rapid dose fall-off across the spinal cord characteristic of this treatment approach. A dose-escalation exercise was performed, delivering a cord maximum dose of 14Gy to 24 Gy in a single fraction. The animals were observed for an additional year and then sacrificed. The authors then performed a detailed histopathologic examination of the twice-irradiated spinal cord and constructed a complication probability curve. Interestingly, the complication probability curve of animals that were reirradiated was almost identical to those animals that had never had the initial course of radiation, suggesting that after 1 year, the cord had completely recovered from the initial course of radiation [18]. The finding that the spinal cord dose tolerance recovers over time has also been demonstrated in both rats and primates [19, 20].

Clinically, increasing numbers of publications in the literature have described excellent tumor control and an extremely low rate of myelopathy when using SBRT for reirradiation. Tumor control rates are typically more than 80%, while the observed rates of myelopathy are less than 2%. Even in the setting of locally advanced metastases that require surgical decompression with separation surgery and postoperative SBRT, there appears to be no difference in the probability of local control between tumors treated with SBRT, whether or not they had been previously irradiated, suggesting that SBRT reirradiation can provide the same high probability of local control as de novo SBRT [21].

Optimal management of spine tumors that recur after initial SBRT is a clinical conundrum, since such lesions are likely extremely radioresistant, and nearby normal tissues have received high biological effective doses of radiation. Outcomes of salvage SBRT for spine metastases that had recurred after an initial course of SBRT have also been described. A recently reported series of 63 consecutive patients with metastases that had recurred after initial SBRT (6Gy × 5, 9–10Gy × 3, 24Gy × 1) were salvaged with 8Gy × 5 daily. The median time between courses of radiation was 13.4 months. With a median follow-up of 11.9 months, 12.7% of lesions demonstrated local failure. A cohort of 42 adjacent segment recurrences were also reported. These patients had prior SBRT to an adjacent segment, but then developed a new metastasis at an immediately adjacent segment. Because of partial overlap with the prior treatment, these patients were treated with SBRT using the same reirradiation constraints as same-segment salvage treatment. The local recurrence rate for these patients was 4.8%, with no statistically significant difference between the two groups, suggesting that 8Gy × 5 can provide local control to metastases previously given SBRT equal to lesions not previously irradiated [22]. For the entire cohort, a 4% rate of grade 3 or higher late, non-fracture complications were noted, and 17% of patients developed de novo fractures or progression of pre-existing fractures. A retrospective study of 40 patients who underwent salvage SBRT (30Gy/4 fx) was reported by the Princess Margaret group, with a median FU of 6.8 months, reporting a 12-month local control rate of 81% [23]. Hence, the SBRT paradigm of ultra-conformal high-dose radiobiologically potent radiotherapy can be applied successfully even in the setting of prior SBRT.

Summary

Spine SRS and SBRT are highly conformal, image-guided, radiobiologically potent forms of radiotherapy. Incorporation of spine SBRT into the management of spinal tumors is changing the landscape of spine oncology. Definitive and ablative durable treatment can be given to the most radioresistant tumors without having to resort to highly morbid surgery such as *en bloc* resection. It is also an effective way to provide salvage options to tumors that recur after a prior course of radiation. Significant toxicity is uncommon, even in the reirradiation setting. A growing body of evidence, which includes prospective randomized trials, favors the use of SRS/SBRT. Tantalizing prospective data for the benefit of ablative radiation for oligometastatic patients is also emerging. A multidisciplinary environment is the best approach to incorporate spinal SRS/SBRT into the treatment paradigm for the optimal management of spine tumors.

References

1. Yamada Y, et al. The impact of histology and delivered dose on local control of spinal metastases treated with stereotactic radiosurgery. Neurosurg Focus. 2017;42(1):E6.
2. Tseng CL, et al. Imaging-based outcomes for 24 Gy in 2 daily fractions for patients with de Novo spinal metastases treated with Spine Stereotactic Body Radiation Therapy (SBRT). Int J Radiat Oncol Biol Phys. 2018;102(3):499–507.
3. Zelefsky MJ, et al. Phase 3 multi-center, prospective, randomized trial comparing single-dose 24 Gy radiation therapy to a 3-fraction SBRT regimen in the treatment of Oligometastatic cancer. Int J Radiat Oncol Biol Phys. 2021;110(3):672–9.
4. Jackson C, et al. The effect of histology and delivered dose on local failure rates with three-fraction spine SBRT. Int J Radiat Oncol Biol Phys. 2024;120(2):S213.
5. Laufer I, et al. The NOMS framework: approach to the treatment of spinal metastatic tumors. Oncologist. 2013;18(6):744–51.
6. Barzilai O, et al. Survival, local control, and health-related quality of life in patients with oligometastatic and polymetastatic spinal tumors: a multicenter, international study. Cancer. 2019;125(5):770–8.
7. Katsoulakis E, et al. A detailed Dosimetric analysis of spinal cord tolerance in high-dose spine radiosurgery. Int J Radiat Oncol Biol Phys. 2017;99(3):598–607.
8. Lucido JJ, et al. Single and multifraction spine stereotactic body radiation therapy and the risk of radiation induced myelopathy. Adv Radiat Oncol. 2022;7(6):101047.
9. Jackson C, et al. Risk of radiation myelitis after Hypofractionated spine stereotactic body radiation therapy. Int J Radiat Oncol Biol Phys. 2024;120(2):S38–9.
10. Stubblefield MD, et al. Peripheral nervous system injury after high-dose single-fraction image-guided stereotactic radiosurgery for spine tumors. Neurosurg Focus. 2017;42(3):E12.
11. Katsoulakis E, et al. Pathological characteristics of spine metastases treated with high-dose single-fraction stereotactic radiosurgery. Neurosurg Focus. 2017;42(1):E7.
12. Rose PS, et al. Risk of fracture after single fraction image-guided intensity-modulated radiation therapy to spinal metastases. J Clin Oncol. 2009;27(30):5075–9.
13. Virk MS, et al. Frequency of symptomatic vertebral body compression fractures requiring intervention following single-fraction stereotactic radiosurgery for spinal metastases. Neurosurg Focus. 2017;42(1):E8.

14. Sahgal A, et al. Stereotactic body radiotherapy versus conventional external beam radiotherapy in patients with painful spinal metastases: an open-label, multicentre, randomised, controlled, phase 2/3 trial. Lancet Oncol. 2021;22(7):1023–33.
15. Yarnold JR. 8 Gy single fraction radiotherapy for the treatment of metastatic skeletal pain: randomised comparison with a multifraction schedule over 12 months of patient follow-up. Radiother Oncol. 1999;52(1):111–21.
16. Zeng KL, et al. Mature local control and reirradiation rates comparing spine stereotactic body radiation therapy with conventional palliative external beam radiation therapy. Int J Radiat Oncol Biol Phys. 2022;114(2):293–300.
17. Katagiri H, et al. Clinical results of nonsurgical treatment for spinal metastases. Int J Radiat Oncol Biol Phys. 1998;42(5):1127–32.
18. Medin PM, et al. Spinal cord tolerance to reirradiation with single-fraction radiosurgery: a swine model. Int J Radiat Oncol Biol Phys. 2012;83(3):1031–7.
19. Fred GL, Wong CS. Time-dependent neurosphere-forming ability of adult rat spinal cord after irradiation. Radiat Res. 2007;168(4):453–61.
20. Ang KK, et al. The tolerance of primate spinal cord to re-irradiation. Int J Radiat Oncol Biol Phys. 1993;25(3):459–64.
21. Laufer I, et al. Local disease control for spinal metastases following "separation surgery" and adjuvant hypofractionated or high-dose single-fraction stereotactic radiosurgery: outcome analysis in 186 patients. J Neurosurg Spine. 2013;18(3):207–14.
22. Moore A, et al. 40 gray in 5 fractions for salvage reirradiation of spine lesions previously treated with stereotactic body radiotherapy. Neurosurgery. 2024;95(2):380–91.
23. Thibault I, et al. Salvage Stereotactic Body Radiotherapy (SBRT) following in-field failure of initial SBRT for spinal metastases. Int J Radiat Oncol Biol Phys. 2015;93(2):353–60.
24. Lucido JJ, et al. Local control after re-irradiation of spinal metastases with stereotactic body radiation therapy. In: ASTRO 2023. San Diego: Int J Radiat Oncol Biol Phys; 2023. p. e132.
25. Serrand J, Ayadi M, Tanguy R, Sunyach MP. Spinal re-irradiation by Stereotactic Body Radiotherapy (SBRT): safety and efficiency. In: Radiosurgery Society SRS/SBRT scientific meeting 2016; 2016.
26. Ito K, et al. Postoperative re-irradiation using stereotactic body radiotherapy for metastatic epidural spinal cord compression. J Neurosurg Spine. 2018;29(3):332–8.
27. Hashmi A, et al. Re-irradiation stereotactic body radiotherapy for spinal metastases: a multi-institutional outcome analysis. J Neurosurg Spine. 2016;25(5):646–53.
28. Sasamura K, et al. Outcomes after reirradiation of spinal metastasis with stereotactic body radiation therapy (SBRT): a retrospective single institutional study. J Radiat Res. 2020;61(6):929–34.
29. Ito K, Ogawa H, Nakajima Y. Efficacy and toxicity of re-irradiation spine stereotactic body radiotherapy with respect to irradiation dose history. Jpn J Clin Oncol. 2021;51(2):264–70.
30. Patel PP, et al. Oncologic outcomes and safety after spinal re-irradiation with stereotactic body radiation therapy. In: ASTRO 2023. San Diego: Int J Radiat Oncol Biol Phys; 2023.
31. Detsky J, et al. Re-irradiation with spine stereotactic body radiotherapy in a heavily pre-treated cohort. Int J Radiat Oncol Biol Phys. 2019;105(1):E122.
32. Boyce-Fappiano D, et al. Reirradiation of the spine with stereotactic radiosurgery: efficacy and toxicity. Pract Radiat Oncol. 2017;7(6):e409–17.
33. Bate BG, et al. Stereotactic radiosurgery for spinal metastases with or without separation surgery. J Neurosurg Spine. 2015;22(4):409–15.
34. Sellin JN, et al. Factors affecting survival in 37 consecutive patients undergoing de novo stereotactic radiosurgery for contiguous sites of vertebral body metastasis from renal cell carcinoma. J Neurosurg Spine. 2015;22(1):52–9.
35. Ghia AJ, et al. Single-fraction versus multifraction spinal stereotactic radiosurgery for spinal metastases from renal cell carcinoma: secondary analysis of phase I/II trials. J Neurosurg Spine. 2016;24(5):829–36.

36. Bernard V, et al. Heterogeneity in treatment response of spine metastases to spine stereotactic radiosurgery within "radiosensitive" subtypes. Int J Radiat Oncol Biol Phys. 2017;99(5):1207–15.
37. Park HJ, et al. Stereotactic Body Radiotherapy (SBRT) for spinal metastases: who will benefit the most from SBRT? Technol Cancer Res Treat. 2015;14(2):159–67.
38. Anand AK, et al. Hypofractionated stereotactic body radiotherapy in spinal metastasis - with or without epidural extension. Clin Oncol (R Coll Radiol). 2015;27(6):345–52.
39. Bishop AJ, et al. Outcomes for spine stereotactic body radiation therapy and an analysis of predictors of local recurrence. Int J Radiat Oncol Biol Phys. 2015;92(5):1016–26.
40. Guckenberger M, et al. Safety and efficacy of stereotactic body radiotherapy as primary treatment for vertebral metastases: a multi-institutional analysis. Radiat Oncol. 2014;9:**226**.
41. Thibault I, et al. Spine stereotactic body radiotherapy for renal cell cancer spinal metastases: analysis of outcomes and risk of vertebral compression fracture. J Neurosurg Spine. 2014;21(5):711–8.
42. Sohn S, et al. Stereotactic radiosurgery compared with external radiation therapy as a primary treatment in spine metastasis from renal cell carcinoma: a multicenter, matched-pair study. J Neuro-Oncol. 2014;119(1):121–8.
43. Folkert MR, et al. Outcomes and toxicity for hypofractionated and single-fraction image-guided stereotactic radiosurgery for sarcomas metastasizing to the spine. Int J Radiat Oncol Biol Phys. 2014;88(5):1085–91.
44. Al-Omair A, et al. Surgical resection of epidural disease improves local control following postoperative spine stereotactic body radiotherapy. Neuro-Oncology. 2013;15(10):1413–9.
45. Chang UK, Kim MS, Han CJ, Lee DH. Clinical result of stereotactic radiosurgery for spinal metastasis from hepatocellular carcinoma: comparison with conventional radiation therapy. J Neuro-Oncol. 2014;119(1):141–8.
46. Bahig H, et al. A study of Pseudoprogression after spine stereotactic body radiation therapy. Int J Radiat Oncol Biol Phys. 2016;96(4):848–56.
47. Guckenberger M, et al. Dose-intensified hypofractionated stereotactic body radiation therapy for painful spinal metastases: results of a phase 2 study. Cancer. 2018;124(9):2001–9.
48. Rothrock RJ, et al. Hypofractionated spinal stereotactic body radiation therapy for high-grade epidural disease. J Neurosurg Spine. 2020;33:1–8.
49. Zeng KL, et al. Dose-escalated 2-fraction spine stereotactic body radiation therapy: 28 Gy versus 24 Gy in 2 daily fractions. Int J Radiat Oncol Biol Phys. 2023;115(3):686–95.

Chapter 10
Treatment Planning for Spine SBRT

Masoud Zarepisheh, Lei Zhang, and Linda Hong

Introduction

Stereotactic body radiation therapy (SBRT) is increasingly utilized as a safe and effective treatment modality for spine tumors [8, 23, 35]. This high-precision radiotherapy technique delivers ablative doses of radiation in one or a few fractions to the target while minimizing dose to surrounding healthy tissues. There is growing evidence to support the role of SBRT as an alternative for conventional external beam radiotherapy or surgical decompression, in de novo disease as well as re-irradiation setting to provide durable local control or pain relief [31].

SBRT became feasible thanks to the technological advancements in imaging, treatment planning, patient immobilization, and image guidance for treatment delivery. Advanced imaging techniques such as high-resolution computed tomography (CT) and magnetic resonance imaging (MRI) have been implemented to visualize and delineate the tumor and organs-at-risk. The development of modern planning and delivery techniques such as intensity-modulated radiation therapy (IMRT) and volumetric modulated arc therapy (VMAT) have enabled plan optimization to generate complex dose distributions that target the disease with biologically more potent high doses while minimizing dose to nearby critical structures. Online 3D image guidance and real-time tumor tracking techniques that modern linear accelerators are equipped with ensure confidence in the accuracy of treatment delivery which is critical in the high dose and often high risk SBRT treatments [2, 11, 18, 20].

At Memorial Sloan Kettering Cancer Center (MSKCC), spine SBRT was first implemented in the clinic in the early 2000s. The technique, safety and efficacy have been well documented [17, 21, 22, 44, 51]. The clinical workflow has been

M. Zarepisheh (✉) · L. Zhang · L. Hong
Department of Medical Physics, Memorial Sloan Kettering Cancer Center, New York, NY, USA
e-mail: zarepism@mskcc.org; zhangl7@mskcc.org; hongl@mskcc.org

Y. Yamada et al. (eds.), *Multidisciplinary Spine Tumor Management*,
https://doi.org/10.1007/978-3-032-07519-2_10

evolving to adopt new and more advanced techniques as they become available, and to implement standardized approaches to improve consistency and quality of the treatment [32]. In recent years, we have also developed automated and clinically optimal treatment planning tools at our institution [19, 48, 49], internally known as Expedited Constrained Hierarchical Optimization (ECHO), which has been instrumental in improving the clinical efficiency of our spine SBRT program and its expansion across our network. ECHO employs advanced optimization tools, such as hierarchical constrained optimization, convex approximations, and Lagrangian methods, to improve the speed, quality, and applicability of SBRT treatment planning. These tools are able to generate reliable and consistent high-quality plans and have greatly improved and expedited the treatment planning processes. This has benefited a large number of patients with spine tumors, including many patients in severe pain and in urgent need of treatment who might have otherwise required longer hospital stays or undergone unnecessary procedures to control the progression of their disease.

In this chapter, we provide a review of the physical and clinical aspects of spine SBRT treatment planning and delivery with an emphasis on our institution's approach, as well as a detailed description of the MSK ECHO program.

Imaging, Simulation, and Immobilization

Spine SBRT features a tight planning margin, a high fractional dose, complex dose distribution with steep dose gradient due to close proximity of the target to critical and sensitive organs, including the spinal cord and cauda equina, as well as gastrointestinal structures such as esophagus and bowels, depending on the location of vertebrae being treated. Such intricate treatment demands high precision in localizing the target and organs-at-risk (OAR) to ensure the safety and dosimetric accuracy. Proper positioning of the patient and effective immobilization are crucial in limiting inter-fractional setup variation as well as intra-fractional motion.

Patient Immobilization

Patients should be simulated in a stable and consistently reproducible position. Rigid or near-rigid immobilization devices are utilized to provide adequate support to various parts of the anatomy and to minimize motion. The simulation position and immobilization system should be comfortable for the patient to tolerate during the relatively long treatment time. This is particularly important given that often many of the patients are in pain due to the disease in the spine. In addition, it is crucial to ensure that the simulation position is compatible with the planning technique and beam arrangement and has clearance at the treatment machine without interfering with the ancillary systems.

At our institution, spine SBRT patients are typically simulated in a supine position with both arms down at the sides or on the chest for comfort. The patient is positioned on rigid or near-rigid immobilization devices. Historically, two types of immobilization devices developed at MSKCC were used in spine SBRT: the Memorial stereotactic body frame and the Memorial body cradle, which provide reliable and accurate patient setup under 3D image guidance [46, 47]. In recent years, we have transitioned to using commercial solutions designed for spine SBRT that incorporate similar features and additional flexibility [32]. Dedicated spine SBRT simulation protocols are customized based on the treatment location (level of vertebrae) and use various components of immobilization devices. For cervical and upper thoracic spine treatment, a custom head and neck mold is created together with a thermoplastic open-face mask and shoulder drape. A couch-end extension, which allows an extra degree of flexibility in adjusting the pitch and roll, is very helpful for upper cervical spine setup. Custom vacuum cushions such as Vac-Lok (CIVCO Radiotherapy, IA) or Alpha Cradle are used to support the patient's trunk and arms for treatments of the thoracic and lumbar-sacral spine. Side paddles with indexing bars are used to provide additional immobilization to the pelvis and ensure the spinal column is in a straight and reproducible position. Attention must be paid to positioning the patient's arms and elbows to ensure they are well supported by the vacuum cushion and elevated to be anterior to the spinal column, such that they do not interfere with placing treatment beams at wide oblique angles. When treating the lumbar spine and sacrum, the patient's forearms and hands are positioned high on the chest and away from the treatment area. Lower extremities are supported with cushions to ensure patient comfort.

Each component of the entire immobilization system is attached or indexed to an couch top overlay, which is indexable to the treatment couch to ensure consistency in the setup. Figure 10.1 illustrates examples of immobilization for the cervical and upper thoracic spine (left) and for the lower thoracic spine (right).

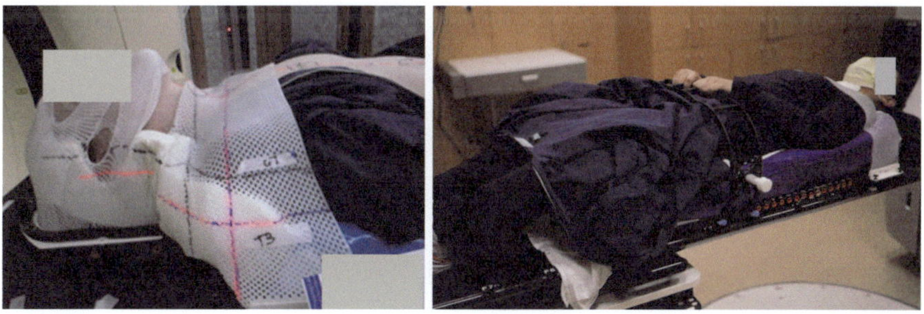

Fig. 10.1 Examples of patient immobilization for spine SBRT at MSKCC for cervical and upper thoracic spine (left) and for lower thoracic spine (right) using the CDR system (CDR Systems Inc., Canada). For the cervical and upper thoracic spine, a custom cranial and shoulder mold, along with a face and shoulder mask, is used. For the lower thoracic spine, a shoulder mask, custom vacuum bag, and pelvic paddles are used. The individual components of the immobilization devices are indexed to an overlay that is, in turn, indexed to the treatment couch

CT Scanning Protocol

The simulation CT scans over the entire vertebral column in the cranial-caudal direction with 1–2 mm slice thickness. The reconstruction field of view (FOV) should encompass the patient's full anatomy at the treatment level and any immobilization devices that need to be considered during dose calculation. Metal artifact reduction algorithm is applied when implanted hardware is present in or near the treatment area. Small bowel contrast may be used for lumbar spine and sacrum cases where the tumor comes close to the small bowel. For certain cases with paraspinal tumor extension, particularly cervical spine tumors that may encase vasculature, IV contrast can be helpful for tumor delineation.

Spinal Cord Delineation with CT Myelogram or CT/MRI Fusion

There are typically two methods for visualizing the spinal cord. Prior to simulation, patients can undergo myelography, where a contrast material is injected into the thecal sac. This allows for direct visualization of the spinal cord, thecal sac, and any epidural disease (Fig. 10.2). CT myelography remains an important tool, especially in post-operative patients with spinal hardware.

Alternatively, high-quality spine MRI offers a non-invasive option for visualizing the spinal cord, cauda equina, thecal sac, and epidural disease when myelography is contraindicated or unavailable. A dedicated MRI protocol for spine SBRT uses high-resolution 3D axial scans with 1–2 mm slice thickness and usually includes T1-weighted and T2-weighted images, as well as post-contrast sequences. A 2D sagittal scan is also included for localization and vertebrae counting. Unlike diagnostic spine MRI, axial scans in such protocol should be acquired orthogonal to the couch to match the CT simulation scanning axis. The FOV for the axial scans

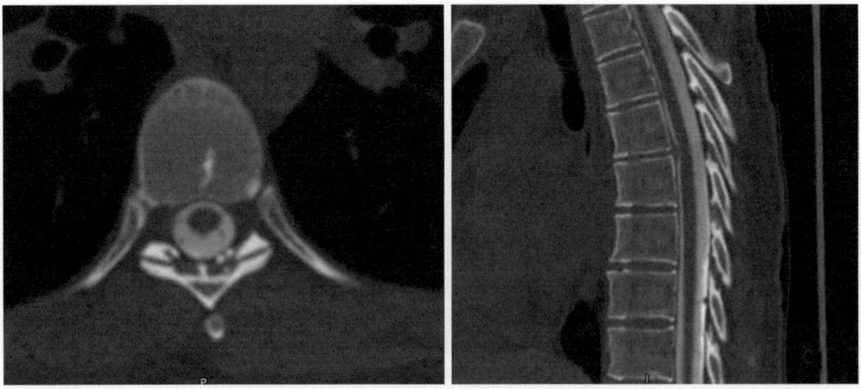

Fig. 10.2 Example of CT myelogram

typically extends to include atleast one vertebral body above and one below the target area. However, MRI may not be suitable for patients with certain types of implanted devices or when metal hardware is present in the treatment area that often causes severe susceptibility artifacts. Figure 10.3 illustrates examples of the Focal Spine MR images used at Memorial Sloan Kettering Cancer Center for spine SBRT.

To facilitate contouring, CT/MRI fusions are created between each MR sequence and the planning CT through image registration with a focus primarily on the targeted vertebral bodies. T2-weighted images are typically used for visualizing the spinal cord and cauda equina nerve roots. To account for registration uncertainty as well as intrinsic image distortion associated with the MR images, a 3D expansion of 1–2 mm is added to the true cord or cauda equina defined on T2 MRI to create the planning risk volume (PRV), which is then used for planning.

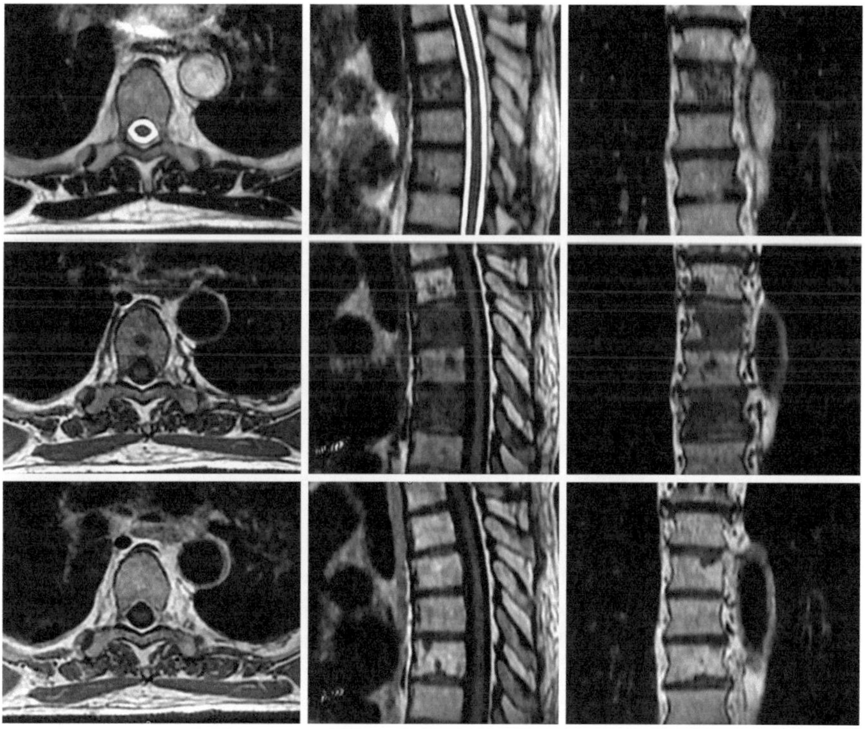

Fig. 10.3 The Focal Spine MRI protocol used for spine SBRT at Memorial Sloan Kettering Cancer Center. The top panel showcases a T2-weighted 3D axial scan; the middle panel displays a T1-weighted 3D axial scan; and the bottom panel exhibits a T1-weighted post-contrast 3D axial scan

Target Delineation

Target volumes are contoured based on both CT and MR images and in accordance with the International Spine Radiosurgery Consortium consensus guidelines [8]. Briefly, the gross tumor volume (GTV) is defined based on both CT and spine MRI to encompass the total extent of gross disease in the vertebra and any epidural and paraspinal involvement. The clinical target volume (CTV) should include any involved compartments of the vertebra and an adjacent normal bony expansion to account for subclinical tumor spread. The planning target volume (PTV) is typically a 2 mm 3-dimensional expansion from the CTV, excluding the thecal sac. Similar contouring guidelines are followed for targets in the sacrum [12].

Planning Techniques, Clinical Criteria, Plan Evaluation

IMRT and Arc Therapy

Spine SBRT treatment planning utilizes intensity modulated radiation therapy (IMRT) with coplanar beams to achieve highly conformal dose coverage around the target and rapid dose fall-off to the spinal cord and other nearby OARs. Typically seven to nine fields are used, primarily from posterior angles to avoid traversing through significant volumes of normal tissue, as well as mobile or highly deformable organs and those filled with air pockets. The posterior anatomy also tends to be more stable and less prone to setup or motion-related uncertainties. Beams from wide oblique angles should also avoid entering through arms and shoulders [19, 32].

The treatment fields are usually spread out at 20–25 degrees apart to improve dose conformity and to reduce skin dose. For treatment in the cervical spine, selected anterior oblique beam angles can be used while avoiding direct entrance through the oral cavity. Complementary collimator angles alternate between fields, with 0 and 90 degrees being commonly used in our clinic to achieve the desired modulation and reduce interleaf transmission. Both 6 MV and 10 MV photons are commonly used in spine SBRT. Higher energy photons are not recommended due to increased dosimetric penumbra, higher transmission through the multileaf collimator (MLC), and neutron production. Spine SBRT is feasible with standard MLC on modern linear accelerators (linac), although high-def MLC may offer additional dosimetric advantage which can be more beneficial in re-irradiation setting and cases with extensive epidural disease. Dose calculation should be performed with a fine dose grid size (1–2 mm) and heterogeneity correction, using an advanced photon dose calculation algorithm such as convolution/superposition based as well as Monte Carlo in accordance with the recommendations from the AAPM Task Group 101 report [2].

Many modern linear accelerators allow the delivery of arc therapy, which offers a faster delivery compared to static gantry IMRT. Typically, two to four coplanar arcs are used. A similar approach to IMRT can be applied when selecting the arc range and collimator angles. When anterior angles are needed, using full arcs with avoidance sectors for areas such as shoulders and oral cavity could further reduce delivery time while minimizing uncertainties related to mobile body parts and unnecessary entrance dose to certain organs or normal tissue. Examples of beam arrangements and dose distributions from IMRT and Volumetric Modulated Arc Therapy (VMAT) plans generated from the Varian Eclipse (Varian Medical Systems, Palo Alto, CA) treatment planning system are shown in Fig. 10.4.

Spine SBRT plans are characterized by extremely heterogeneous dose distribution across the treatment area that often requires significant plan modulation. The large fractional dose, together with the high modulation factor, results in treatment plans with a large number of monitor units per field, thus significantly longer treatment times than conventional treatment. In recent years, flattening-filter-free (FFF) photon beams became available on modern linac, offering a dose rate 2–4 times higher than that of the traditional flattened beams. The use of FFF in spine SBRT has expedited the radiation delivery, making the treatment more tolerable, especially for patients suffering from severe pain due to spinal disease. It also helps to reduce dosimetric uncertainties due to intra-fractional motion that is often associated with prolonged treatment times.

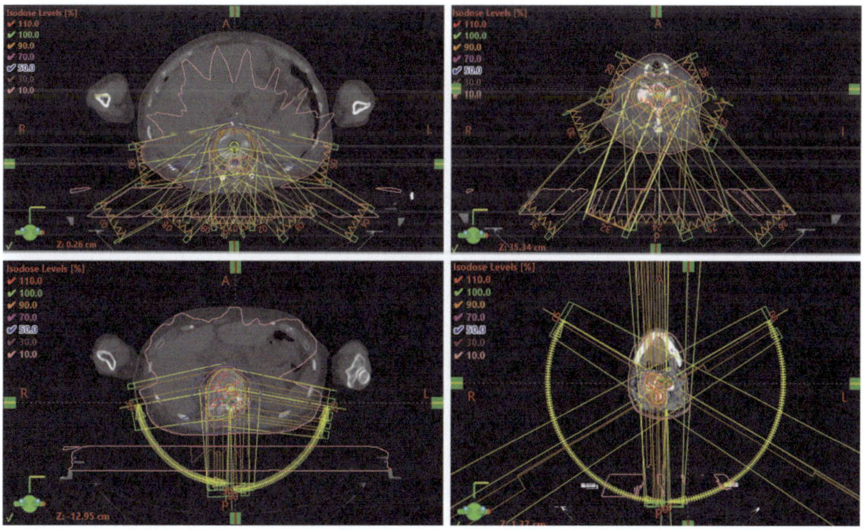

Fig. 10.4 Illustrations of spine SBRT plans with IMRT and VMAT generated using the Varian Eclipse external beam treatment planning system. Top panel: examples of static gantry IMRT using 9 fields, with all posterior beams for thoracic spine (left) and added anterior oblique beams for cervical spine (right); bottom left: VMAT with four posterior partial arcs for thoracic spine; bottom right: VMAT with an extended arc span anteriorly and shoulder avoidance for cervical spine

Clinical Criteria

Prescriptions for Spine SBRT typically vary from 1 to 5 fractions, depending upon many factors such as tumor histology, the number of vertebrae included in the PTV, abutment of critical organs to the target, history of prior radiation, etc. Given the hypofractionated nature and the close proximity to critical structures, clearly defined dosimetric guidelines for treatment planning are imperative to ensure the quality and safety of spine SBRT.

Clinical criteria, i.e., planning objectives, should include goals for target coverage, and constraints on OAR—most importantly the spinal cord, cauda equina, as well as mucosal structures nearby. All clinical criteria should be specified based on the prescribed dose and fractionation. In terms of target coverage, volume receiving 100% and 95% of the prescribed dose, i.e., V100% and V95% for the PTV, are used together with near-minimum dose criteria for the CTV and GTV to assess coverage adequacy [28, 32, 45].

A central aspect of spine SBRT is the protection of the spinal cord. Both maximum point dose and dose to small volumes (D0.35cc) are often used to optimize and evaluate dose to the spinal cord. Additionally, a transection constraint is also used to ensure that no high dose is axially traversing the spinal cord on any slice throughout the entire treatment volume, especially when treating multiple vertebral bodies. Depending on the location of the target, many other organs could become relevant or even dose-limiting. Point dose and appropriate volumetric dose constraints should be provided for each relevant OAR. Figure 10.5 illustrates the target coverage and cord transection constraint for a thoracic spine SBRT treatment plan with a prescription of 30 Gy in 3 fractions.

SBRT has been found to be safe as salvage treatment for previously irradiated spine metastases and provides excellent disease control and palliation, thanks to the sharp dose gradient that allows the delivery of biologically more potent doses to the target area while sparing the spinal cord [7, 10, 24]. Currently, guidelines and detailed data on cumulative dose tolerance are limited [34]. Therefore, tissue dose constraints for re-treatment are often guided by institutional experience and existing literature, and the dose delivered in a single course should be considered, as well as cumulative doses from prior treatment and current treatment. When designing treatment plans for patients with prior radiation treatment, the extent of overlap with the prior treatment fields should be carefully examined and ideally determined based on image registration with the prior planning CT. The regions of structures that have received prior RT should be clearly delineated and optimized following perspective re-irradiation constraints. Special considerations should be given to the uncertainties associated with the individual contours, image registration, setup and patient motion. Tools and functionalities in the treatment planning system or standalone software that allow dose accumulation and assessment of organ dose on a voxel level are highly desired to accurately assess the relevance, extent and dose distribution of the prior treatment plan on the current planning anatomy and aid the design of a treatment plan for re-irradiation. Such development is already on the horizon

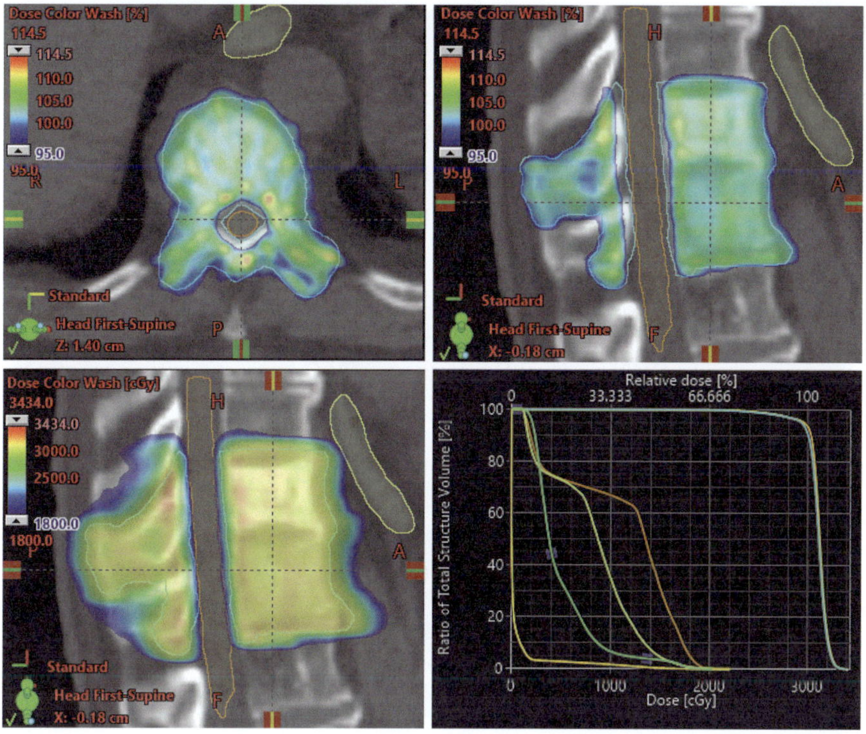

Fig. 10.5 (Top panel): Example of treatment plan (axial and sagittal view) for T10-T11 with a circumferential target. Prescription dose: 30 Gy in 3 fractions. PTV is contoured in cyan, the MRI-defined spinal cord PRV is in brown, and the esophagus contour is in light green. The plan was generated using our in-house auto-planning algorithm (ECHO) with 9-field static gantry IMRT. The color wash illustrates target coverage with a 95% Rx dose. (Bottom left): color wash showing the spinal cord transection constraint (18 Gy for 3 fractions) that does not traverse the cord on any axial slice. (Bottom right): dose-volume-histogram (DVH) for (from left to right) skin, stomach, esophagus, spinal cord PRV, PTV, and CTV

and will likely become an essential component of the clinical workflow in re-irradiation settings [29, 43]. As overdosing certain critical organs could face serious consequences in spine SBRT, it is also important to have a peer-review mechanism where individual clinical cases can be consulted among credentialed members of the team when a challenging scenario arises, or specific clinical criteria cannot be met.

Common prescriptions and corresponding dosimetric constraints used at MSKCC for spine SBRT in de novo and re-irradiation settings are listed in Tables 10.1 and 10.2, respectively [21, 32].

Table 10.1 Dosimetric guidelines and common prescriptions used at MSKCC for de novo spine SBRT

		1-Fraction	3-Fraction	5-Fraction
	Prescription Dose	24 Gy × 1	9–10 Gy × 3	6–8 Gy × 5
Target coverage	PTV Coverage	PTV $V_{100\%} \geq 90\%$ and PTV $V_{95\%} \geq 95\%$ (Ideal) PTV $V_{100\%} \geq 80\%$ and PTV $V_{95\%} \geq 90\%$ (Acceptable)		
	Minimum CTV Coverage[a] (Ideal)	$DC_{0.035cc} \geq 15$ Gy	$DC_{0.035cc} \geq 21$ Gy	$DC_{0.035cc} \geq 25$ Gy
	Minimum GTV Coverage[a] (Acceptable)	$DC_{0.035cc} \geq 15$ Gy	$DC_{0.035cc} \geq 21$ Gy	$DC_{0.035cc} \geq 25$ Gy
Neurologic constraints	Spinal Cord (Cord PRV if MRI Fusion)	$D_{max} < 14$ Gy or 12 Gy[b] $D_{0.35cc} < 10$ Gy	$D_{max} < 26$ Gy or 24 Gy[b] $D_{0.35cc} < 18$ Gy, $D_{0.1cc} < 19.1$ Gy	$D_{max} < 30$ Gy $D_{0.35cc} < 23$ Gy
	Spinal Cord Transection Constraint	10 Gy	18 Gy	23 Gy
	Cauda Equina	$D_{max} < 18$ Gy $D_{5cc} < 14$ Gy	$D_{max} < 26$ Gy $D_{5cc} < 22$ Gy	$D_{max} < 35$ Gy $D_{5cc} < 30$ Gy
	Brachial Plexus	$D_{max} < 24$ Gy[c]	$D_{max} < 27$ Gy[c]	$D_{max} < 35$ Gy[c]
	Lumbosacral Plexus	$D_{max} < 24$ Gy[c]	$D_{max} < 27$ Gy[c]	$D_{max} < 35$ Gy[c]
Mucosal constraints	Esophagus[d]	Level I: $V_{14Gy} < 2.5$ cc Level II: $V_{18\,Gy} < 2.5$ cc	Level I: $D_{0.035cc} < 27.6$ Gy $D_{5cc} < 16.8$ Gy Level II: $D_{0.035cc} < 30$ Gy $D_{5cc} < 22$ Gy	Level I: $D_{0.035cc} < 32.2$ Gy $D_{5cc} < 19$ Gy Level II: $D_{0.035cc} < 50$ Gy $D_{5cc} < 27.5$ Gy
	Stomach	$D_{max} < 15$ Gy $D_{5cc} < 12$ Gy	$D_{max} < 27$ Gy or 30 Gy[e] $D_{5cc} < 21$ Gy	$D_{max} < 30$ Gy or 33 Gy[e] $D_{5cc} < 25$ Gy
	Small Bowel	$D_{max} < 16$ Gy $D_{5cc} < 12$ Gy	$D_{max} < 27$ Gy or 30 Gy[e] $D_{5cc} < 21$ Gy	$D_{max} < 30$ Gy or 33 Gy[e] $D_{5cc} < 25$ Gy $V_{20Gy} < 100$ cc

[a]Use near-minimum absorbed dose metric $DC_{0.035cc}$, i.e., max dose to the coolest 0.035 cc
[b]Use the lower value if PTV is circumferential
[c]Applies only to portion 3 mm away from the PTV. The portion inside the PTV is limited to 110% of Rx
[d]Attempt level I constraints first. Use level II constraints if level I compromises coverage
[e]User the higher value if overlapping with PTV

Automated Planning

Traditional manual planning can be intricate, time-consuming, and labor-intensive, resulting in notable discrepancies in plan quality both within and between hospitals. This makes the plan quality significantly reliant on the expertise of the planners. To streamline this process, recent research has focused on developing advanced

Table 10.2 Dosimetric guidelines used at MSKCC for spine SBRT with prior radiation[a]

		1-Fraction	3-Fraction	5-Fraction
Neurologic constraints	Spinal Cord (Cord PRV if MRI Fusion)[b]	$D_{max} < 12$ Gy or 10.2 Gy[c] $D_{0.35cc} < 9$ Gy	$D_{max} < 14.5$ Gy or 13.9 Gy[c] $D_{0.35cc} < 10$ Gy	$D_{max} < 18$ Gy or 17 Gy[c] $D_{0.35cc} < 14$ Gy
	Cauda Equina[b]	$D_{max} < 14$ Gy $D_{5cc} < 11$ Gy	$D_{max} < 15$ Gy $D_{5cc} < 13$ Gy	$D_{max} < 20$ Gy $D_{5cc} < 17$ Gy
	Brachial Plexus	No hot spot	$D_{max} < 17.7$ Gy[d]	$D_{max} < 22$ Gy[d]
	Lumbosacral Plexus	No hot spot	$D_{max} < 17.7$ Gy[d]	$D_{max} < 22$ Gy[d]
Mucosal constraints	Esophagus[e]	No hot spot	$D_{0.035cc} < 20.4$ Gy Cumulative $D_{0.035cc} < 100$ Gy in 2 Gy equivalents ($\alpha/\beta = 3$)	$D_{0.035cc} < 25$ Gy Cumulative $D_{0.035cc} < 100$ Gy in 2 Gy equivalents ($\alpha/\beta = 3$)
	Stomach/Small Bowel[e]	No hot spot	Cumulative $D_{5cc} < 85$ Gy in 2 Gy equivalents ($\alpha/\beta = 3$) Cumulative $D_{max} < 65$ Gy in 2 Gy equivalents ($\alpha/\beta = 3$)	Cumulative $D_{5cc} < 85$ Gy in 2 Gy equivalents ($\alpha/\beta = 3$) Cumulative $D_{max} < 65$ Gy in 2 Gy equivalents ($\alpha/\beta = 3$)

[a]Only apply to patients with one course of prior radiation that was treated at least 3 months before
[b]To use the spinal cord or cauda equina re-irradiation constraints, the Rx of prior conventional treatment should not exceed 30 Gy in 10 fractions or 50 Gy in 25 fractions; or the spinal cord D_{max} from prior SBRT should not exceed 14 Gy in 1 fraction, 21 Gy in 3 fractions, or 26 Gy in 5 fractions, the cauda D_{max} from prior SBRT should not exceed 18 Gy in 1 fraction, 26 Gy in 3 fractions, or 30 Gy in 5 fractions
[c]Use the lower value if PTV is circumferential
[d]Apply only to the portion 3 mm away from the PTV. The portion inside the PTV is limited to 110% of Rx
[e]The cumulative constraints are total equivalent doses in 2 Gy fractions over the prior and current course of radiation

techniques that overcome the limitations of manual planning. These techniques include: (1) knowledge-based planning (KBP) [1, 6, 40, 41, 50], (2) multiple criteria optimization (MCO) [9, 30], and (3) constrained hierarchical optimization (also referred to as prioritized optimization or lexicographic optimization) [4, 48, 49].

KBP, marketed as RapidPlan™ by Varian, primarily extracts information from the data of previously treated patients to assist treatment planning for new patients. Early KBP methods, which form the groundwork of the current RapidPlan, created models to learn the relationship between a patient's geometry (defined by factors like distance and overlap between PTV and OARs) and the achievable optimal DVH. KBP predicts the achievable DVH for new patients and uses this to expedite plan creation. With recent advancements in artificial intelligence and deep learning, KBP models are now designed to learn the relationship between patients' geometries (represented by CT images and contours) and the optimal 3D dose distribution. The significant advantage of KBP is that it is fully automated and fast once trained, making it particularly suitable for applications like online adaptive radiotherapy.

Nevertheless, constructing a new KBP model based on previously treated patients can be challenging and labor-intensive. Additionally, alterations in clinical criteria may render an existing KBP model obsolete, necessitating re-training. KBP is also unable to cater to patients with specific requirements, such as those who have previously undergone radiation, a limitation that is practically important, with many spine patients having received previous radiation (about 30% in our institution).

MCO, commercialized as MCO™ by RaySearch, generates a set of Pareto optimal plans considering key clinical objectives that require trade-offs. Users navigate through these Pareto plans to select the one that best suits their preferences. Unlike KBP, MCO does not rely on prior knowledge, can accommodate patients with specific requirements, and adapt to changes in clinical criteria. However, it is not fully automated, as it still necessitates user intervention for the selection of the optimal plan, which may lead to variations in plan quality depending on user experiences.

The principal concept in constrained hierarchical optimization involves defining non-negotiable clinical criteria as hard constraints and ranking desirable clinical objectives, optimizing them sequentially. This traditional optimization method has been applied to address complex multicriteria optimization issues in radiotherapy. Recently, MSK incorporated a variant of this technique, known as ECHO (Expedited Constrained Hierarchical Optimization), into its clinical practice. ECHO is not reliant on learning techniques and can handle complex geometries not seen in previous datasets. Moreover, ECHO is fully automated. It has been implemented at MSK as an in-house system, incorporated into Eclipse using API scripting, and is utilized in daily clinical routines [14, 19, 33, 49]. The reader is referred to section "Automated Planning Using MSK-ECHO" for a detailed explanation of ECHO. Table 10.3 offers a comparison of these automation planning techniques, highlighting their respective advantages and disadvantages.

Table 10.3 A Comparative overview of three advanced treatment planning techniques: knowledge-based planning (KBP), multiple criteria optimization (MCO), and constrained hierarchical optimization

	Fast (suitable for online adaptive planning)	Adapts to changes in clinical criteria	Handles special requirements (e.g., preRT)	Fully automated
Knowledge-based planning (Varian RapidPlan™)	√	×	×	√
Multicriteria optimization (RaySearch MCO™)	×	√	√	×
Expedited constrained hierarchical optimization (MSK-ECHO)	×	√	√	√

Quality Assurance and Treatment Delivery

Quality Assurance

Given the highly precise and potent nature of spine SBRT, the importance of conducting thorough Quality Assurance (QA) cannot be overstated. Our institution has vigorous QA protocols regarding the treatment machine, dose calculation, and treatment delivery processes. These QA procedures comply with the guidelines of AAPM Task Group 40 report [27], Task Group 142 report [25] and Task Group 101. All spine SBRT treatments are planned and delivered on dedicated linear accelerators that meet stringent SBRT and IGRT standards.

Patient-specific pre-treatment dose measurements are typically performed using an electronic portal imaging device (EPID) for all single-fraction SBRT patients. Other types of dosimeters, such as MapCHECK and SRS MapCHECK (Sun Nuclear Corp., FL), my QASRS (IBA Dosimetry, Germany) are also used in our clinic. For hypofractionated treatments, pre-treatment dose measurement is substituted by a comprehensive QA program that includes MLC QA, pre-treatment plan integrity check, and an in-house automatic script for post-treatment QA that analyzes machine trajectory log files after each fraction [26, 38], and measurement is only performed on case-by-case basis when indicated. Each treatment on the Varian TrueBeam™ treatment machine generates a set of trajectory log files that record accumulated MU, MLC positions, and gantry angle every 10 ms during delivery. Any discrepancies between planned and actual leaf positions are examined via an automated computer program. If any leaf surpasses a discrepancy of 0.5 mm for over 15% of the total beam-on time, the program flags this occurrence and sends an alert to a physicist for further investigation before the next treatment appointment. The overnight QA check program also monitors the integrity of the treatment planning system database, including machine beam data, ECHO program parameters, etc.

In recent years, to enhance efficiency and safety in initial chart check for complex treatments, our clinic adopted an automated plan check tool (PCT), which is a script implemented in the Varian Eclipse treatment planning system [3]. Briefly, the PCT performs checks on 6 stages of a treatment plan: Manual Review Items (Stage 1), Electronic Prescription (Stage 2), Contours (Stage 3), Naming Conventions and Demographics (Stage 4), Beams, Optimization, and Calculation (Stage 5), and QA/Approvals/Aria (Stage 6). It offers configurable checks specific to different disease sites. Figure 10.6 provides a snapshot of the PCT output for an ECHO spine SBRT plan. For example, the PCT verifies the plan complexity by calculating and comparing the duty cycle with the typical range based on our clinical experience [19]. When a plan is flagged with unusually high duty cycle, it will prompt the physics team to look into the cause of high MUs (such as multiple vertebrae large PTV volume or re-treatment resulting in steeper dose gradient due to stricter OAR constraints) and, if necessary, request dose measurement prior to first treatment to verify the deliverability of the plan and accuracy of the dose calculation. This way,

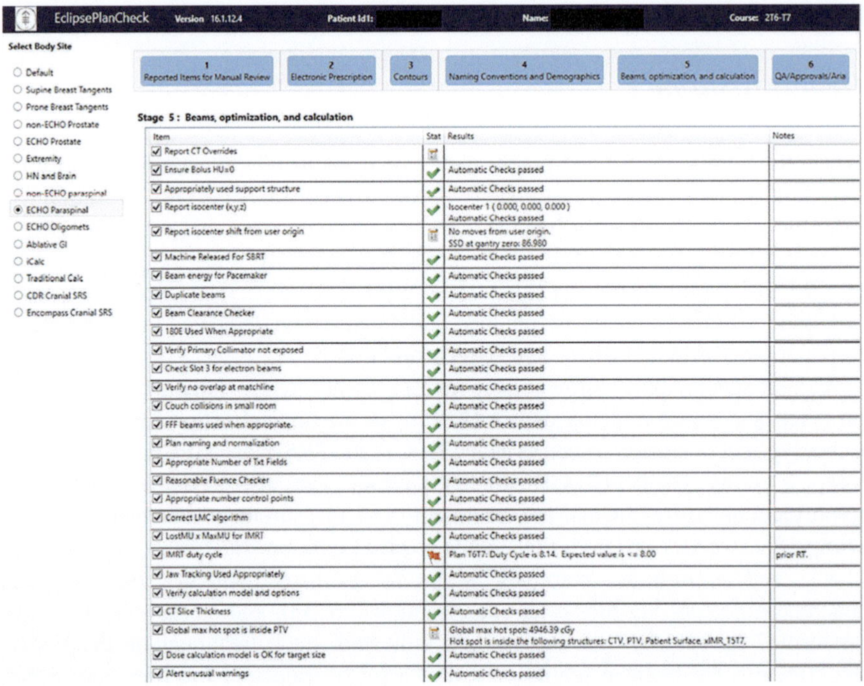

Fig. 10.6 Display of Plan Check Tool (PCT) output for a spine patient treated with ECHO. The PCT systematically reviews six stages of the treatment plan. In Stage 5, it scrutinizes the parameters related to beams, optimization, and calculation. In this instance, the duty cycle was flagged for review, prompting the planner to provide an explanation involving prior radiation therapy

it could catch plans that are overly modulated and may experience delivery and dosimetric challenges. Other parameters such as beam model and independent dose calculation status are also verified by PCT.

Patient Setup and Treatment Delivery

The safety and dosimetric accuracy of spine SBRT rely on consistent reproducibility of patient position at each treatment. Image guidance plays an essential role in patient setup to align the anatomy in accordance with the planning CT. Modern linear accelerators are equipped with an on-board kV imager (OBI) that allows planar radiographs as well as cone-beam CT (CBCT) and online 3D matching. In general, the patient is first positioned in the immobilization device on the treatment couch such that the treatment target is aligned to the radiation isocenter using the room lasers based on the skin markings. An orthogonal kV image pair is acquired for the initial bony alignment and to verify that the correct level of the spine is being targeted. A CBCT is subsequently acquired, which should capture patient's full anatomy in the treatment area, especially along the paths where the radiation beams enter. The entire target area of the spine and any spinal hardware (if present) should be aligned according to the planning CT in all 3 views. The alignment of the spinal canal in the treatment area should be carefully examined through each slice. The position of all other nearby OAR, especially mobile organs, as well as any avoidance structures taken into planning, such as arms and shoulders, should also be verified. A robotic treatment couch with 6 degrees of freedom can be very helpful in fine-tuning the positioning and alignment, especially for the cervical spine and when the target is located in the curved spine area.

Compared to conventional treatment, spine SBRT often requires significantly longer time at the treatment machine from setup to radiation delivery; deviation of the target position from the initial setup position could occur during treatment. A study of over 1000 treatment sessions from 194 patients treated at MSKCC reported that, although rare, shifts greater than 2 mm in any direction could occur in immobilized patients during spine SBRT [42]. Because of the large dose gradient around the spinal cord, a small shift could result in a significant dose uncertainty in the epidural space, concerning both spinal cord safety and dose coverage to epidural disease. As such, continuous intra-fractional motion monitoring is crucial to detect patient motion and ensure alignment of the target throughout treatment delivery, thus minimizing dose uncertainties to the target and critical organs. A shift in any direction that exceeds clinical criteria would require immediate interruption of the radiation delivery. The alignment of the anatomy should be reassessed using CBCT and couch corrections applied before resuming treatment. Periodic kV imaging using the OBI offers a direct way to verify bony anatomy but requires frequent interruptions to the treatment beam and additional time for gantry rotation. Certain brand linacs offer automatically triggered imaging at predefined locations or time intervals using the OBI without interfering with the MV beam. This is implemented as the Intrafractional Motion Review (IMR) on Varian TrueBeam (Siemens Healthineers USA), where a predefined contour—usually the targeted vertebral body or the spinal hardware—from the planning CT is overlaid on the triggered kV image to provide a visual assessment of target alignment. Quantitative methods using triggered kV imaging [15] or combined kV and MV imaging are being investigated in the clinic [5]. Other standalone in-room X-ray imaging systems such as ExacTrac (BrainLab Inc., Germany) are also widely used for image-guided setup and on-treatment motion monitoring in spine SBRT.

Automated Planning Using MSK-ECHO

ECHO Workflow

ECHO stands for Expedited Constrained Hierarchical Optimization and is the automated optimization algorithm developed at Memorial Sloan Kettering Cancer Center. It is integrated with Eclipse using API scripting; however, it operates

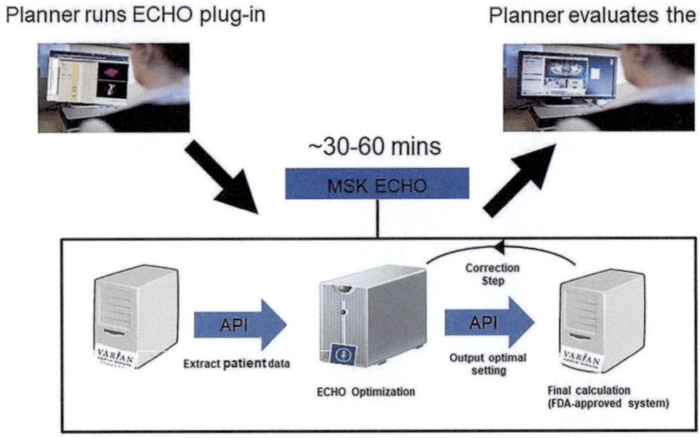

Fig. 10.7 The ECHO Clinical Workflow: (1) The process begins with the planner creating a template plan and initiating the ECHO plug-in. (2) Next, essential data for optimization is extracted from the Treatment Planning System (TPS). (3) Following this, the optimization problems are solved using commercial optimization engines on an institutional server. (4) The optimal results, including fluence maps for IMRT and control points for VMAT, are then reintegrated into the TPS for the final dose calculation. (5) To rectify any discrepancies between the optimized dose and the final dose, a corrective step is implemented. (6) Upon completion, the user is notified via email to review the finalized plan within the TPS

independently of the Eclipse optimization engine and has its own distinct optimization engine. Figure 10.7 illustrates the ECHO workflow. First, the user creates a template plan with a preferred set of beams (for IMRT) or arcs (for VMAT). Then, the user runs the ECHO plug-in provided in Eclipse and selects the anatomical structures to include in the optimization (i.e., PTV, OARs). API scripting is employed to extract all the necessary data for optimization (e.g., beam/contour data, influence matrix) from the TPS and save it on an institutional server for running the optimization problems. The resulting constrained optimization problems are solved using commercial optimization engines Artelys KNITRO™ (Artelys Corp., Chicago, IL) and AMPL™ (AMPL Optimization Inc., Evanston, IL) and MOSEK™ (MOSEK ApS, Copenhagen, Denmark). The output of the optimization problems (optimal fluence map for IMRT and optimal control points for VMAT) is imported back into the TPS for final dose calculation. ECHO then calculates the discrepancies between the optimized dose and the final dose and feeds them back into the optimization to correct the discrepancies. The new optimal machine parameters are imported back into the TPS for final dose calculation, and the user is notified by email that the plan is ready for review. The email also includes plan quality reports in the form of two PDF file attachments (Fig. 10.8). The entire aforementioned workflow is automated using API scripting.

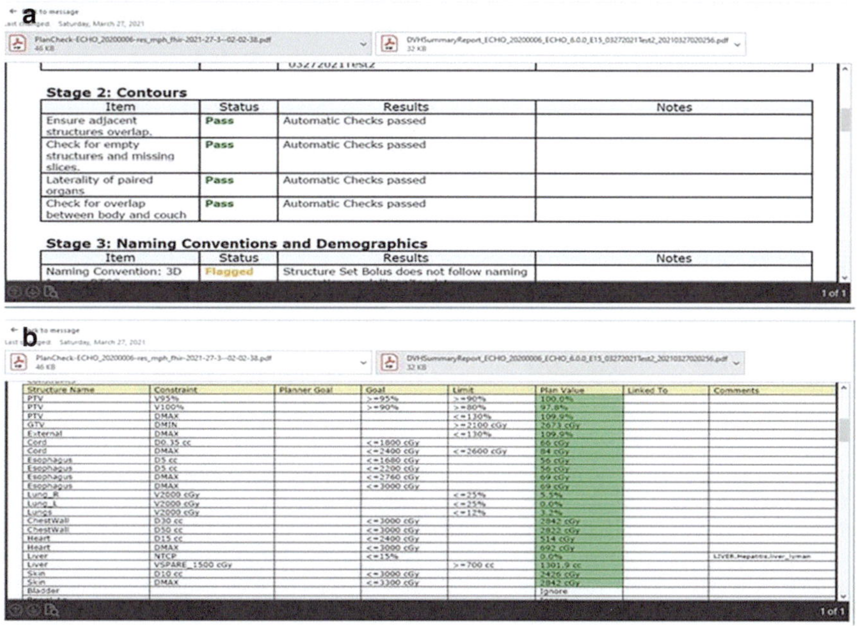

Fig. 10.8 Upon completion of the plan within the Treatment Planning System (TPS), an automated email is dispatched to the user. This email includes two essential PDF attachments: a detailed report outlining the quality and safety parameters of the plan generated by our in-house plan check tool (PCT) (**a**), and a comprehensive summary of Dose-Volume Histogram (DVH) metrics related to plan quality (**b**)

2-Step Constrained Hierarchical Optimization

ECHO solves two constrained optimization problems. Figure 10.9 displays the results of both steps using a simple example. In Step 1, PTV coverage is maximized while imposing all mean/max/DVH hard constraints on PTV and OARs. Step 2 aims to further reduce OAR doses, beyond their specified hard constraints, in the vicinity of Step 1 results. ECHO's IMRT and VMAT implementations exhibit slight differences in how their Step-2 problems search the vicinity of the Step-1 result.

Technical Challenges

The Eclipse optimization engine does not provide support for constrained optimization, making it unsuitable for ECHO. ECHO is a comprehensive optimization engine that accommodates a variety of objective functions and constraints (e.g., mean, max, DVH, gEUD) for both IMRT and VMAT. Developing ECHO involved addressing numerous technical challenges, including computational difficulties

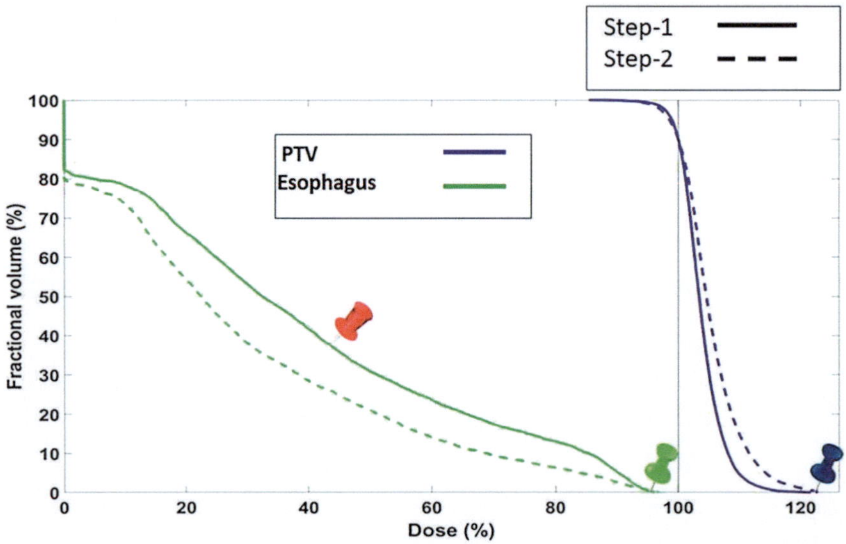

Fig. 10.9 A simple example illustrating ECHO's two-step optimization technique: The pins represent the DVH/max hard constraints. Step 1 aims for the best PTV coverage/homogeneity while enforcing the hard constraints (solid line). Step 2 further reduces the OAR doses, beyond the specified hard constraints, while slightly relaxing the PTV coverage achieved in Step 1 (dashed line)

arising from solving large-scale constrained optimization problems, non-convexity resulting from DVH criteria and VMAT optimization, and discrepancies between optimized and final doses. Table 10.4 outlines some of these technical challenges along with a brief description of the tools employed to address them and the corresponding publications. As indicated in the table, some techniques are still under development.

Adding a New Disease Site or New Prescription

To incorporate a new disease site or a different prescription/fractionation scheme in ECHO, we generate new template files (in the form of text/xml files). These files primarily consist of clinical criteria (max/mean/DVH) for PTV and OARs, which are based on the established departmental guidelines (Tables 10.1 and 10.2). Additionally, a few parameters, including the type of gEUD functions utilized for each structure and the rind structures created to control dose fall-off, require some fine-tuning. These parameters are adjusted using a small number of patients as a training dataset (typically 6–20) and can often be applied to various prescription and fractionation schemes. If the clinical criteria change, we can readily modify the template files without re-tuning the parameters.

Table 10.4 A summary of the technical challenges raised during the development of ECHO, mathematical solutions, and corresponding publications

Implementation Status	Challenge	Solution	Publication
Clinically Implemented	Multicriteria problem and trade-offs between PTV coverage and OAR sparing	Hierarchical constrained nonlinear optimization	[19, 48, 49]
	Dose discrepancies between the optimized dose and the final dose	Correction Method	[49]
	Non-convex DVH criteria	Mixed Integer Programming, Convex Relaxation	[33]
	Non-convex VMAT optimization	Sequential Convex Programming	[13, 14]
Research/ Development	Proton: Beam Angle Selection	Bayesian Optimization	[37]
	Proton: Uncertainty Management	Robust Optimization (P-Norm Function)	[36]
	Proton: Computational Complexity	Distributed Optimization (ADMM)	[16]
	Reducing IMRT plan complexity	Wavelet-induced smoothness	[39]

To ensure that employing automated planning with ECHO does not compromise plan quality, for each site or new prescription, we conduct retrospective analyses on the performance of ECHO using randomly selected patients (typically 20–40) as a test dataset. We then compare the plans generated by ECHO and the manual plans used to treat the patients using established dosimetric plan quality metrics. Additionally, 2–3 expert physicists are involved in thoroughly evaluating the plan quality by examining the 3D dose distribution, DVH, and other factors.

ECHO Performance

Since its inception in 2017, ECHO has been employed in the treatment of over 8000 patients up to 2023. Figure 10.10a illustrates the monthly output of ECHO plans, averaging 180 plans per month, and highlights the chronological addition of disease sites to the ECHO system (Table 10.5). As demonstrated in Fig. 10.10b, the bulk of the plans generated pertain to spine and oligometastasis (non-spine metastasis) cases. Notably, as depicted in Fig. 10.10c, around 30% of spine ECHO plans had received radiation treatment previously, necessitating lower dose parameters for the previously irradiated structures. Within the ECHO system, users have the option to manually designate the maximum/mean dose constraints for such structures, which are subsequently enforced as strict limits. Figure 10.10d provides a depiction of the various prescription dosages and fractionation schemes used in the creation of ECHO spine plans.

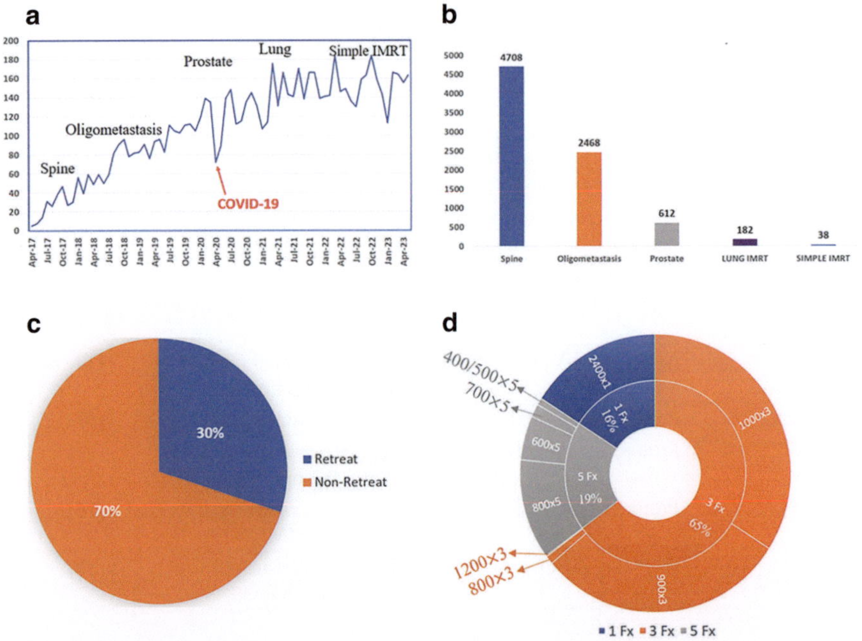

Fig. 10.10 ECHO plans statistics. (**a**) Monthly generation of ECHO plans. (**b**) Distribution of ECHO plans across various disease sites. (**c**) Proportion of spine/oligometastasis plans with and without prior radiation treatment. (**d**) Various prescription doses and fractions utilized in ECHO plans for treating spine/oligometastasis patients

Table 10.5 The quantity of patients in the training and test datasets for spine and non-spine metastasis (oligometastasis) cases, as well as ECHO-eligible prescription/fractionation schemes

Disease site	# of Training patients	# of training patients	ECHO eligible Rx
Spine/ oligometastasis SBRT	6 spine single fraction 24Gy × 1	75 spine (25 for 24Gy × 1, 25 for 9Gy × 3 without pre-RT and 25 patients 9Gy × 3 with pre-RT)	All SBRT for spine and metastatic tumor sites, with or without pre-RT. (dose/fx from 5 to 24Gy, #fx from 1 to 6).

If the plan generated by ECHO is not satisfactory, the user may re-run ECHO after making appropriate modifications (e.g., changing beams, arcs, optimization structures, max/mean/DVH criteria). Figure 10.11-left shows that the first ECHO plan is found to be satisfactory about 77% of the time. Figure 10.11-right illustrates various reasons for plans after the first run not being satisfactory. In 47% of re-run cases, the issue was related to user input (e.g., incorrect contours, beam arrangement changes), 17% of the time for re-run, it was related to MD changes (e.g., adjusting clinical criteria), and in 36% of re-run cases, it was related to the ECHO

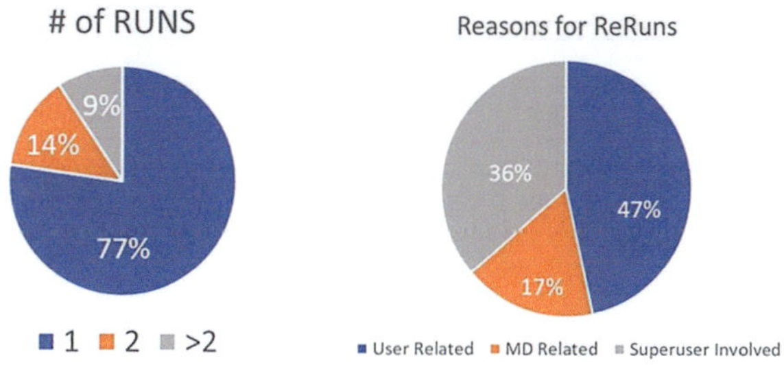

Fig. 10.11 (Left): The number of ECHO runs required to produce a satisfactory plan. (Right): The underlying reasons for multiple ECHO runs in the planning process

optimization engine (e.g., discrepancies between optimized and final dose), requiring the intervention of a designated user, referred to internally as super-user.

ECHO Benefits

Employing automated planning enhances plan quality while also reducing variability. Figure 10.12 retrospectively compares automated ECHO plans with manually generated plans used for treatment in 75 spine patients across three prescription/fractionation schemes. The results demonstrate that ECHO plans offer improved and more consistent PTV coverage as well as OAR sparing [49].

ECHO has effectively reduced the total treatment planning time (from simulation to delivery) by 1 day, decreasing it from 5 days to 4 days. ECHO has also enabled same-day treatment for oligometastasis patients and ultra-expedited treatment (within 3 days) for spine patients in our institution.

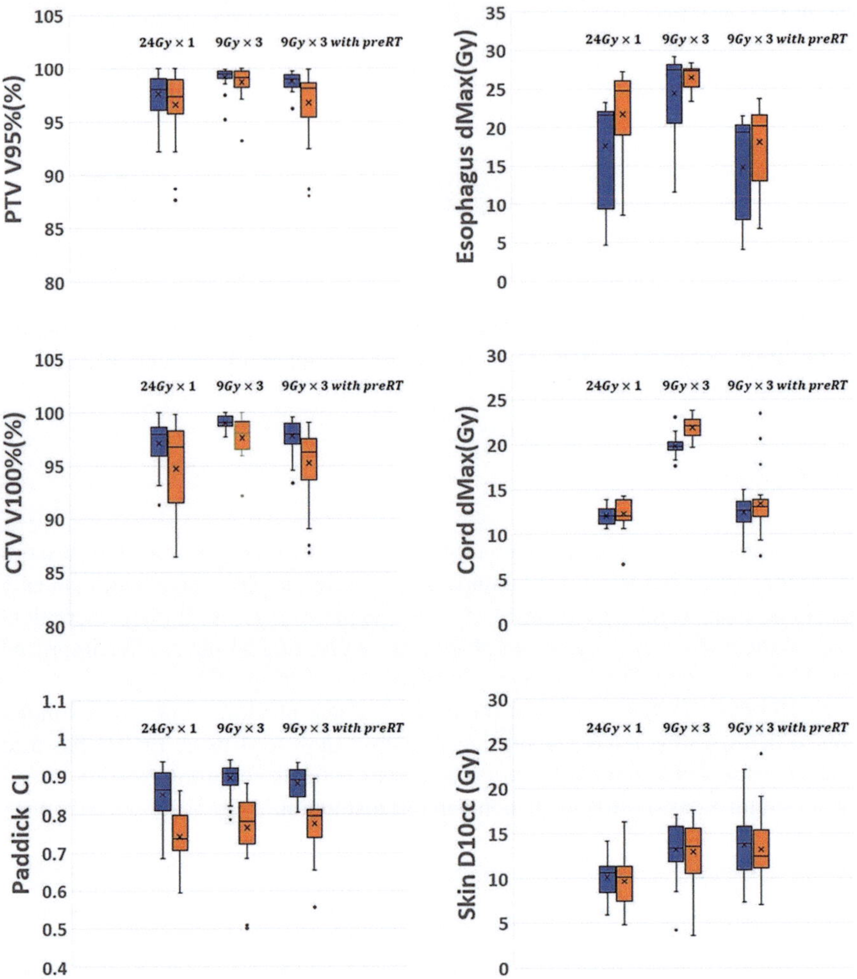

Fig. 10.12 Comparison of automated ECHO plans (blue bars, left) and manually created plans (orange bars, right) for 75 SBRT spine plans with three distinct prescription/fractionation schemes (25 plans per scheme). For the coverage and conformity comparisons in the left plots, higher values are better, while lower values are better for OAR sparing comparisons in the right plots

Summary

SBRT is becoming an essential component in the multidisciplinary management of spine tumors. Technological advancements in imaging, patient setup, planning and treatment delivery all play important roles in ensuring the safety and quality of spine SBRT treatment. In this chapter, we reviewed the treatment planning process for spine SBRT and shared our clinical experience on patient positioning, imaging, planning techniques, and quality assurance aspects. The automated planning algorithm ECHO developed at MSKCC has been a great success, and has largely simplified and expedited the treatment planning process with consistently high-quality plans for spine SBRT and beyond.

There remain challenges and prospects in spine SBRT. A better understanding of normal tissue tolerance in the re-irradiation setting, a robust deformable image registration algorithm, and advanced dose accumulation software will likely lead to further improvement in clinical practice. Research is needed in new treatment modalities such as proton therapy as well as flash radiotherapy, which may hold new promise of further sparing in the critical organs and allowing dose escalation, especially for radioresistant tumors.

Acknowledgments This work was partially supported by MSK Cancer Center Support Grant/Core Grant from the NIH (P30 CA008748).

References

1. Appenzoller LM, Michalski JM, Thorstad WL, Mutic S, Moore KL. Predicting dose-volume histograms for organs-at-risk in IMRT planning. Med Phys Wiley. 2012;39(12):7446–61.
2. Benedict SH, Yenice KM, Followill D, Galvin JM, Hinson W, Kavanagh B, et al. Stereotactic body radiation therapy: the report of AAPM Task Group 101. Med Phys Wiley Online Library. 2010;37(8):4078–101.
3. Berry SL, Zhou Y, Pham H, Elguindi S, Mechalakos JG, Hunt M. Efficiency and safety increases after the implementation of a multi-institutional automated plan check tool at our institution. J Appl Clin Med Phys Wiley. 2020;21(4):51–8.
4. Breedveld S, Storchi PRM, Heijmen BJM. The equivalence of multi-criteria methods for radiotherapy plan optimization. Phys Med Biol IOP Publishing. 2009;54(23):7199–209.
5. Cai W, Fan Q, Li F, He X, Zhang P, Cervino L, et al. Markerless motion tracking with simultaneous MV and kV imaging in spine SBRT treatment-a feasibility study. Phys Med Biol IOP Publishing. 2023;68(3):035012.
6. Chanyavanich V, Das SK, Lee WR, Lo JY. Knowledge-based IMRT treatment planning for prostate cancer. Med Phys Wiley. 2011;38(5):2515–22.
7. Choi CYH, Adler JR, Gibbs IC, Chang SD, Jackson PS, Minn AY, et al. Stereotactic radiosurgery for treatment of spinal metastases recurring in close proximity to previously irradiated spinal cord. Int J Radiat Oncol Biol Phys Elsevier BV. 2010;78(2):499–506.
8. Cox BW, Spratt DE, Lovelock M, Bilsky MH, Lis E, Ryu S, et al. International Spine Radiosurgery Consortium consensus guidelines for target volume definition in spinal stereotactic radiosurgery. Int J Radiat Oncol Biol Phys Elsevier. 2012;83(5):e597–605.
9. Craft D, Bortfeld T. How many plans are needed in an IMRT multi-objective plan database? Phys Med Biol IOP Publishing. 2008;53(11):2785–96.
10. Damast S, Wright J, Bilsky M, Hsu M, Zhang Z, Lovelock M, et al. Impact of dose on local failure rates after image-guided reirradiation of recurrent paraspinal metastases. Int J Radiat Oncol Biol Phys Elsevier BV. 2011;81(3):819–26.
11. De Los SJ, Popple R, Agazaryan N, Bayouth JE, Bissonnette J-P, Bucci MK, et al. Image guided radiation therapy (IGRT) technologies for radiation therapy localization and delivery. Int J Radiat Oncol Biol Phys Elsevier BV. 2013;87(1):33–45.
12. Dunne EM, Sahgal A, Lo SS, Bergman A, Kosztyla R, Dea N, et al. International consensus recommendations for target volume delineation specific to sacral metastases and spinal stereotactic body radiation therapy (SBRT). Radiother Oncol Elsevier BV. 2020;145:21–9.
13. Dursun P, Hong L, Jhanwar G, Huang Q, Zhou Y, Yang J, et al. Automated VMAT treatment planning using sequential convex programming: algorithm development and clinical implementation. Phys Med Biol [Internet]. 2023; https://doi.org/10.1088/1361-6560/ace09e.

14. Dursun P, Zarepisheh M, Jhanwar G, Deasy JO. Solving the volumetric modulated arc therapy (VMAT) problem using a sequential convex programming method. Phys Med Biol [Internet]. 2021;66(8) https://doi.org/10.1088/1361-6560/abee58.
15. Fan Q, Pham H, Li X, Zhang P, Zhang L, et al. Toward quantitative intrafractional monitoring in paraspinal SBRT using a proprietary software application: clinical implementation and patient results, Phys. Med. Biol. 2024, 69 045015.
16. Fu A, Taasti VT, Zarepisheh M. Distributed and scalable optimization for robust proton treatment planning. Med Phys. 2023;50(1):633–42.
17. Greco C, Zelefsky MJ, Lovelock M, Fuks Z, Hunt M, Rosenzweig K, et al. Predictors of local control after single-dose stereotactic image-guided intensity-modulated radiotherapy for extracranial metastases. Int J Radiat Oncol Biol Phys Elsevier. 2011;79(4):1151–7.
18. Hong L. WE-E-BRCD-01: SBRT treatment planning: practical considerations. Med Phys amos3.aapm.org. 2012;39(6Part27):3955.
19. Hong L, Zhou Y, Yang J, Mechalakos JG, Hunt MA, Mageras GS, et al. Clinical experience of automated SBRT Paraspinal and other metastatic tumor planning with constrained hierarchical optimization. Adv Radiat Oncol Elsevier. 2020;5(5):1042–50.
20. Hong LX, Shankar V, Shen J, Kuo H-C, Mynampati D, Yaparpalvi R, et al. Spine stereotactic body radiation therapy plans: achieving dose coverage, conformity, and dose falloff. Med Dosim Elsevier. 2015 Autumn;40(3):181–5.
21. Jackson CB, Boe LA, Zhang L, Apte A, Ruppert LM, Haseltine JM, et al. Radiation Myelitis Risk After Hypofractionated Spine Stereotactic Body Radiation Therapy. JAMA Oncology. 2025;11(2):128. https://doi.org/10.1001/jamaoncol.2024.5387.
22. Jackson CB, Boe LA, Zhang L, Apte A, Jackson A, Ruppert LM, et al. (2025) Histologic Classifier of Radiosensitivity to Spine Stereotactic Body Radiation Therapy International Journal of Radiation Oncology*Biology*Physics. 2025;123(3):829–38. https://doi.org/10.1016/j.ijrobp.2025.05.078.
23. Katsoulakis E, Kumar K, Laufer I, Yamada Y. Stereotactic body radiotherapy in the treatment of spinal metastases. Semin Radiat Oncol Elsevier. 2017;27(3):209–17.
24. Katsoulakis E, Riaz N, Cox B, Mechalakos J, Zatcky J, Bilsky M, et al. Delivering a third course of radiation to spine metastases using image-guided, intensity-modulated radiation therapy. J Neurosurg Spine J Neurosurg Publishing Group (JNSPG). 2013;18(1):63–8.
25. Klein EE, Hanley J, Bayouth J, Yin F-F, Simon W, Dresser S, et al. Task Group 142 report: quality assurance of medical accelerators. Med Phys Wiley. 2009;36(9):4197–212.
26. Kumar R, Amols HI, Lovelock M, Sharma SD, Datta D. Quick, efficient and effective patient-specific intensity-modulated radiation therapy quality assurance using log file and electronic portal imaging device. J Cancer Res Ther journals.lww.com. 2017;13(2):297–303.
27. Kutcher GJ, Coia L, Gillin M, Hanson WF, Leibel S, Morton RJ, et al. Comprehensive QA for radiation oncology: report of AAPM Radiation Therapy Committee Task Group 40. Med Phys w2fisicaunammx. 1994;21(4):581–618.
28. Lovelock DM, Zhang Z, Jackson A, Keam J, Bekelman J, Bilsky M, et al. Correlation of local failure with measures of dose insufficiency in the high-dose single-fraction treatment of bony metastases. Int J Radiat Oncol Biol Phys Elsevier BV. 2010;77(4):1282–7.
29. Mechalakos J, Zhang L, Shah N, Hu Y, Zhang P, Ballangrud A, Kuo L, Deasy J, Cervino L. Accounting for dose accumulation uncertainty in spine reirradiation. THE 2021 AAPM Annual Meeting Program, 2021. p. e117–3408.
30. Monz M, Küfer KH, Bortfeld TR, Thieke C. Pareto navigation: algorithmic foundation of interactive multi-criteria IMRT planning. Phys Med Biol IOP Publishing. 2008;53(4):985–98.
31. Moussazadeh N, Lis E, Katsoulakis E, Kahn S, Svoboda M, DiStefano NM, et al. Five-year outcomes of high-dose single-fraction spinal stereotactic radiosurgery. Int J Radiat Oncol Biol Phys Elsevier BV. 2015;93(2):361–7.
32. Mueller B, Zhang L, Yerramill D, and Yamada Y, Spine SBRT, Chapter 2 in Radiation Oncology Clinical Fundamentals, Eds. John J. Cuaron, and Lior Z. Braunstein, Springer Nature, 2025
33. Mukherjee S, Hong L, Deasy JO, Zarepisheh M. Integrating soft and hard dose-volume constraints into hierarchical constrained IMRT optimization. Med Phys Wiley. 2020;47(2):414–21.

34. Nieder C, Langendijk JA, Guckenberger M, Grosu AL. Second re-irradiation: a narrative review of the available clinical data. Acta Oncol. 2018;57(3):305–10.
35. Ryu S, Pugh SL, Gerszten PC, Yin F-F, Timmerman RD, Hitchcock YJ, et al. RTOG 0631 phase II/III study of image-guided stereotactic radiosurgery for localized (1-3) spine metastases: phase II results. Int J Radiat Oncol Biol Phys Elsevier BV. 2011;81(2):S131–2.
36. Taasti VT, Hong L, Deasy JO, Zarepisheh M. Automated proton treatment planning with robust optimization using constrained hierarchical optimization. Med Phys. 2020a;47(7):2779–90.
37. Taasti VT, Hong L, Shim JSA, Deasy JO, Zarepisheh M. Automating proton treatment planning with beam angle selection using Bayesian optimization. Med Phys. 2020b;47(8):3286–96.
38. Tang G, Chan M, Wang A, Yang J, Zhang P, Mageras G. SU-D-105-04: automated QA analysis of VMAT delivery errors using trajectory log files. Med Phys Wiley. 2013;40(6Part3):100–1.
39. Tefagh M, Zarepisheh M. Built-in wavelet-induced smoothness to reduce plan complexity in intensity modulated radiation therapy (IMRT). Phys Med Biol [Internet]. 2023;68(6) https://doi.org/10.1088/1361-6560/acbefe.
40. Wang H, Dong P, Liu H, Xing L. Development of an autonomous treatment planning strategy for radiation therapy with effective use of population-based prior data. Med Phys Wiley. 2017;44(2):389–96.
41. Wu B, Ricchetti F, Sanguineti G, Kazhdan M, Simari P, Jacques R, et al. Data-driven approach to generating achievable dose-volume histogram objectives in intensity-modulated radiotherapy planning. Int J Radiat Oncol Biol Phys Elsevier BV. 2011;79(4):1241–7.
42. Wu J, Wu J, Ballangrud Å, Mechalakos J, Yamada J, Lovelock DM. Frequency of large intrafractional target motions during spine stereotactic body radiation therapy. Pract Radiat Oncol Elsevier BV. 2020;10(1):e45–9.
43. Hu Y, Kuo L, Mechalakos J, Zhang L, Shah N, Ballangrud A, Li A, Deasy J, Cervino L, Zhang P. RAdiotherapy Dose Accumulation Routine (RADAR) - a fast dose accumulation tool for planning with previous treatments. THE 2021 AAPM Annual Meeting Program. 2021. p. e117–3408.
44. Yamada Y, Bilsky MH, Lovelock DM, Venkatraman ES, Toner S, Johnson J, et al. High-dose, single-fraction image-guided intensity-modulated radiotherapy for metastatic spinal lesions. Int J Radiat Oncol Biol Phys Elsevier BV. 2008;71(2):484–90.
45. Yamada Y, Katsoulakis E, Laufer I, Lovelock M, Barzilai O, McLaughlin LA, et al. The impact of histology and delivered dose on local control of spinal metastases treated with stereotactic radiosurgery. Neurosurg Focus J Neurosurg Publishing Group (JNSPG). 2017;42(1):E6.
46. Yamada Y, Lovelock DM, Yenice KM, Bilsky MH, Hunt MA, Zatcky J, et al. Multifractionated image-guided and stereotactic intensity-modulated radiotherapy of paraspinal tumors: a preliminary report. Int J Radiat Oncol Biol Phys Elsevier BV. 2005;62(1):53–61.
47. Yenice KM, Lovelock DM, Hunt MA, Lutz WR, Fournier-Bidoz N, Hua C-H, et al. CT image-guided intensity-modulated therapy for paraspinal tumors using stereotactic immobilization. Int J Radiat Oncol Biol Phys Elsevier BV. 2003;55(3):583–93.
48. Zarepisheh M, Hong L, Zhou Y, Huang Q, Yang J, Jhanwar G, et al. Automated and clinically optimal treatment planning for cancer radiotherapy. INFORMS J Appl Anal pubsonlineinformsorg. 2022;52(1):69–89.
49. Zarepisheh M, Hong L, Zhou Y, Oh JH, Mechalakos JG, Hunt MA, et al. Automated intensity modulated treatment planning: the expedited constrained hierarchical optimization (ECHO) system. Med Phys Wiley Online Library. 2019;46(7):2944–54.
50. Zarepisheh M, Long T, Li N, Tian Z, Romeijn HE, Jia X, et al. A DVH-guided IMRT optimization algorithm for automatic treatment planning and adaptive radiotherapy replanning. Med Phys Wiley. 2014;41(6):061711.
51. Zelefsky MJ, Yamada Y, Greco C, Lis E, Schöder H, Lobaugh S, et al. Phase 3 multi-center, prospective, randomized trial comparing single-dose 24 Gy radiation therapy to a 3-fraction SBRT regimen in the treatment of Oligometastatic cancer. Int J Radiat Oncol Biol Phys Elsevier. 2021;110(3):672–9.

Chapter 11
Spine Radiation Toxicity and Management

Boris Mueller

Introduction

Despite the success of spine SBRT in achieving local control and pain relief in patients with spine metastases, SBRT can cause toxicity, including pain flare, myelopathy, vertebral compression fracture, myositis, GI/esophageal toxicity, and plexopathy. Understanding and recognizing the toxicity of spine SBRT is critical for radiation oncologists so that the patients can be effectively managed when they develop side effects.

Pain Flare

The most common acute side effect of spine SBRT is pain flare, which typically manifests within the initial 24–48 hours after SBRT [1, 2]. The pathophysiology of a pain flare is felt to be secondary to increased edema from treatment-induced inflammation [3, 4]. Pain flare occurs in approximately 25% of patients, with reports ranging from 23% to 68% [1, 5]. Risk factors were evaluated as part of secondary analysis of Phase 1/2 trials [195 evaluable patients] and the only independent predictor of pain flare was the radiation fraction number. For treatment regimens of 1, 3, and 5 fractions, pain flare occurred in 34%, 20%, and 8%, respectively [5].

The Cleveland Clinic evaluated 348 spine patients who had undergone SRS and noted a pain flare incidence of 14.4% [6]. Pain flare was defined as an increase in pain within 7 days of treatment, which resolved with steroids. Predictors for the

B. Mueller (✉)
MSKCC, Radiation Oncology, New York, NY, USA
e-mail: muellerb@mskcc.org

Y. Yamada et al. (eds.), *Multidisciplinary Spine Tumor Management*,
https://doi.org/10.1007/978-3-032-07519-2_11

development of pain flare included higher KPS, female gender, higher prescription dose, and cervical/thoracic tumor location.

A published recursive partitioning analysis of over 400 patients identified 125 total pain flares (20%) and five variables met significance ($P < 0.02$) for model inclusion: renal primary, soft tissue involvement, Bilsky >0, spinal instability neoplastic score >6, and gross tumor volume >8 cc [7]. Patients with zero risk factors had pain flare rates of 7%, one risk factor had pain flare rates of 14% and two or more risk factors had a pain flare rate of 28%.

Minimizing the Risk of Pain Flare

More fractionated radiation regimens appear to minimize the risk of a pain flare as noted above. Prophylactic steroids can also reduce the risk of developing a pain flare. A commonly used regimen is a 6-day course of methylprednisolone [Medrol Dosepak]. The University of Toronto has published on the use of prophylactic oral dexamethasone (4 mg) 1 hour before and for 4 days following SBRT [2]. Prophylactic treatment with 4 mg of 8 mg reduced the incidence of pain flare from 68% to 19% with improved worst pain scores and improved general activity outcome.

Management of Pain Flare

Active pain flares can be managed with a short course (3–5 days) of corticosteroids [1, 2].

NSAIDs and Cox-2 inhibitors may also be beneficial in reducing inflammation and discomfort.

Myelopathy

The most severe side effect associated with spine SBRT is radiation myelopathy due to its debilitating consequences [8–11]. In the medical literature the general incidence of radiation myelopathy in the de novo setting is reported at <5% [12]. However the incidence of radiation myelopathy after SBRT is considered to be <1% [11] [in the de novo or re-irradiation setting] when closely following existing guidelines, using modern delivery techniques, and using established safe dose schedules [4, 11]. Dose constraints are suggested by an international survey for SBRT for spinal metastases [13] and are shown in Table 11.1. MSK Guidelines for neurologic tissues are shown in Table 11.2 for de novo spine cases and Table 11.3 for re-irradiation spine cases.

Table 11.1 Common spinal cord constraints applied to either true cord or surrogate of the true cord (cord PRV or thecal sac) according to no prior and common prior radiation dose exposure

Prior conventional RT dose	1 Fraction	2 Fractions	3 Fractions	4 Fractions	5 Fractions
No prior RT & no cord compromise	10–14Gy D_{max} 10Gy to <10%cord	17Gy D_{max}	18–21Gy D_{max}	23–26Gy D_{max}	25–30Gy D_{max}
No prior RT but cord compromise	8–14Gy D_{max} 10Gy to <10% cord	17Gy D_{max}	18–21Gy D_{max}	23–26Gy D_{max}	25–28Gy D_{max}
800 cGy in 1 fraction	9Gy D_{max}	12.2Gy D_{max}	14–21Gy D_{max}	16.2Gy D_{max}	17.5–27.5 D_{max}
2000 cGy in 5 fractions	9–12Gy D_{max}	12.2Gy D_{max}	14–21Gy D_{max}	16.2Gy D_{max}	15–27.5Gy D_{max}
3000 cGy in 5 fractions	9–12Gy D_{max}	12.2Gy D_{max}	14–21Gy D_{max}	16.2Gy–24Gy D_{max}	17.5–26Gy D_{max}
4000 cGy in 20 fractions	9–12Gy D_{max}	12.2Gy D_{max}	14–21Gy D_{max}	16.2Gy D_{max}	12–25Gy D_{max}
4500 cGy in 5 fractions	9–12Gy D_{max}	12.2Gy D_{max}	14–21Gy D_{max}	16.2Gy D_{max}	12–18Gy D_{max}

Table 11.2 MSK Dosimetric Guidelines for Neurologic Tissues for De Novo Spine Cases

	1-Fraction	3 Fractions	5-Fractions
Prescription dose	24 Gy × 1	9–10 Gy × 3	8 Gy × 5
Spinal cord (PRV if MRI fusion)	D_{max} < 14 Gy or 12 Gy $D_{0.35cc}$ < 10 Gy	D_{max} < 26 Gy or 24 Gy $D_{0.35cc}$ < 18 Gy	D_{max} < 30 Gy $D_{0.35cc}$ < 23 Gy
Spinal cord transection constraint	10 Gy	18 Gy	23 Gy
Cauda equina	D_{max} < 18 Gy D_{5cc} < 14 Gy	D_{max} < 26 Gy D_{5cc} < 22 Gy	D_{max} < 35 Gy D_{5cc} < 30 Gy

Table 11.3 MSK Dosimetric Guidelines for Neurologic Tissues for Re-irradiation Spine Cases

	1-Fraction	3-Fractions	5-Fractions
Spinal cord (PRV if MRI fusion)	D_{max} < 12 Gy or 10.2 Gy $D_{0.35cc}$ < 9 Gy	D_{max} < 14.5 Gy or 13.9 Gy $D_{0.35cc}$ < 10 Gy	D_{max} < 18 Gy or 17 Gy $D_{0.35cc}$ < 14 Gy
Cauda equina	D_{max} < 14 Gy D_{5cc} < 11 Gy	D_{max} < 15 Gy D_{5cc} < 13 Gy	D_{max} < 20 Gy D_{5cc} < 17 Gy

Minimizing the Risk of Myelopathy

Minimizing risk of radiation myelopathy for spine SBRT patients begins at the time of simulation with the use of near-rigid immobilization [14]. Identifying and contouring the spinal cord correctly is also critical [13, 15]. An MRI fused to the planning CT, or the use of a CT-myelogram, is essential for defining the spinal cord and delineating organs-at-risk. A planning organ-at-risk volume (PRV) of 1.5 mm for the spinal cord is advised, especially when using MRI fusion.

During radiation planning, it is important to adhere to dose constraints for spinal cord and cauda equina tissue [16]. During radiation delivery, verifying spine position using inter- and intrafraction on-board imaging is important for optimal accuracy [17].

Management of Myelopathy

Corticosteroids are the first line and primary treatment for radiation myelopathy. Since patients will often require a prolonged course of steroids, a steroid taper should also be initiated when possible in order to minimize the impact of corticosteroid-induced myopathy [18]. Extrapolating from patients who had developed brain necrosis from radiosurgery, there may also be a benefit to the use of Vitamin E and pentoxifylline in patients who present with radiation myelopathy [19]. Another small study of patients with radiation-induced nervous system injury [included 1 patient with radiation myelopathy] showed a benefit with full anticoagulation using heparin and warfarin over 3–6 months [19].

There are also several small studies that suggest a benefit to the use of hyperbaric oxygen in the setting of radiation myelopathy [20, 21]. One case report of a patient with cervical spine myelopathy revealed resolution of spinal cord swelling and subtotal resolution of 2 intramedullary enhancing areas just two months after completion of HBO. The patient reported clinical improvement of symptoms during and at the end of HBO. Objective clinical features and the neurologic examination also became progressively better [20].

Bevacizumab may also be beneficial in the management of CNS necrosis and may have promise in radiation myelopathy. In a small, randomized study of 14 patients with cerebral radiation necrosis, bevacizumab improved neurological symptoms and radiological outcomes [22]. A larger study randomized 112 nasopharyngeal carcinoma patients who developed radiation necrosis to treatment with either bevacizumab or corticosteroids. Patients who received bevacizumab had better symptom and radiological responses versus patients who received corticosteroids [23].

Several case reports describing the use of bevacizumab specifically for RM also show a benefit and the ability to reverse neurological symptoms and preserve neurologic function [24–26].

Vertebral Compression Fracture

Vertebral compression fracture [VCF] is a relatively common complication after spine SBRT. VCF rates after SBRT vary significantly in the medical literature, ranging from 5% to 42% [27]. A large review of 11 spine SABR studies reported a mean crude VCF event rate of 13.9% [27]. Fractures occurred a median of 1.6–3.3 months after treatment for 10 of the studies, whereas a longer median time of 25 months occurred in 1 study [27]. MSKCC reported the incidence of VCF of 38% after single fraction spine SBRT in a series of 61 patients, prescribed to 18 to 24 Gy [28].

A prospective study of 145 patients with 279 de novo spinal metastases treated with 24 Gy in 2 fractions reported VCF rates of 8.5% at 1 year and 13.8% at 2 years [29]. In a more recent publication, the University of Toronto published on VCF incidence in spine SBRT patients living more than 3 years. The incidence of VCF was 2.2% at 1 year, 7.4% at 2 years, 10.4% at 3 years and 14.4% at 5 years [30].

Several variables are predictive of VCF development, including: (1) age > 55 years, (2) radiation dose >20Gy, (3) baseline VCF, (4) lytic disease, (5) >40% VB tumor involvement and (6) spinal deformity [27, 31].

Minimizing the Risk of VCF

Spine SBRT candidates should be assessed for spinal stability with a validated scoring system prior to radiation therapy. MSK practitioners use the SINS scoring system (see Tables 11.4 and 11.5) [32] to help determine if a patient is at high risk for fracture and which patients should undergo surgical fixation prior to radiation therapy [33].

Sahgal and colleagues have described a pathway for surgical evaluation prior to SBRT, as shown in Fig. 11.1.

In choosing radiation fractionation regimens, practitioners should be mindful that single fraction treatment with doses ≥20Gy may significantly increase the risk of VCF versus more fractionated regimens [28]. The benefit of a higher local control rate with single fraction treatment needs to be weighed against the higher fracture risk. More fractionated regimens of 12Gy × 2 or 9Gy × 3 still provide excellent local control with significantly lower risk of VCF [29, 34].

Table 11.4 Spinal instability neoplastic score (SINS) system

Component	Score
Location	
Junctional (O-C2; C7-T2; T11-L1; L5-S1)	3
Mobile spine (C3-6; L2-4)	2
Semirigid (T3-10)	1
Rigid (S2-S5)	0
Mechanical pain	
Yes	3
No	2
Pain free lesion	1
Bone lesion	
Lytic	2
Mixed (lytic/blastic)	1
Blastic	0
Radiographic spinal alignment	
Subluxation/translation present	4
Deformity (kyphosis/scoliosis)	2
Normal	0
Vertebral body collapse	
>50% collapse	3
<50% collapse	2
No collapse with >50% body involved	1
None of the above	0
Posterolateral involvement	
Bilateral	3
Unilateral	1
None of the above	0

Table 11.5 Total SINS: determination of stability SCORE (Total = 0–18)

0–6	7–12	13–18
Stable spine	Potentially unstable	Unstable spine

Management of VCF

Patients experiencing painful pathologic fractures may achieve symptomatic relief through non-surgical interventions like vertebroplasty or kyphoplasty [35]. More severe fractures associated with pain may require surgical intervention [27]. At present, there is no clear role for prophylactic stabilization in patients with a stable spine and risk factors for VCF.

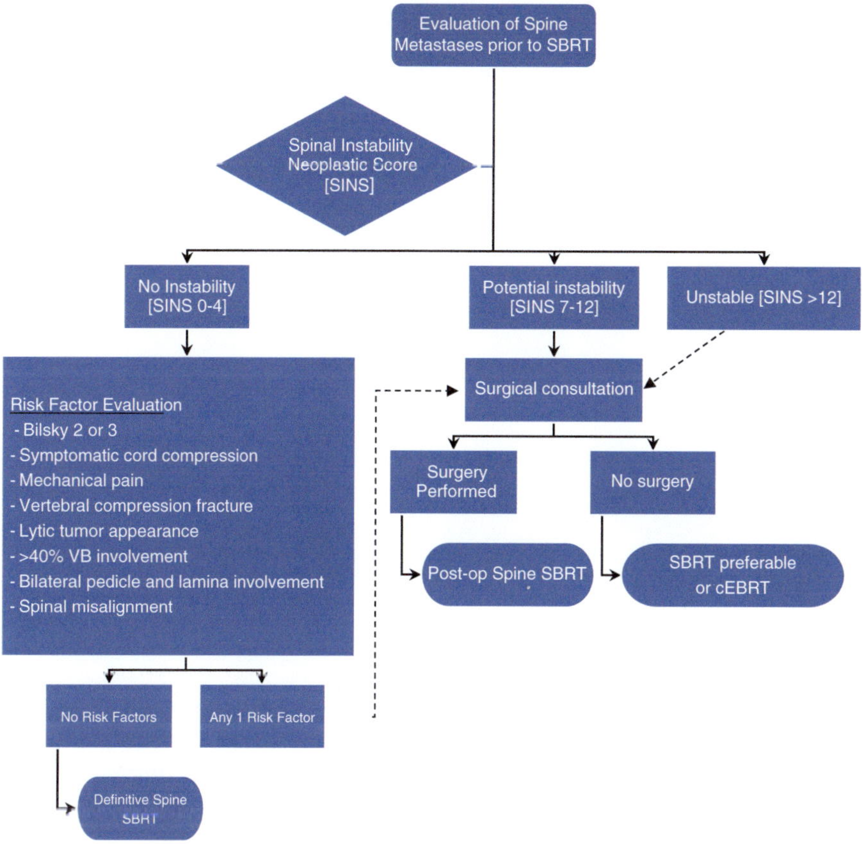

Fig. 11.1 Algorithm for surgical evaluation prior to spine SBRT or EBRT

Myositis

Radiation myositis after spine radiosurgery is a rare but important delayed complication that can cause debilitating pain and motor dysfunction. In a large retrospective series of over 600 patients undergoing single-fraction and multi-fraction SRS, myositis occurred in only 1.9% of patients, with a median time to development of clinical symptoms occurring at 1.4 months and a median time to imaging of 4.7 months [36]. Single-fraction spine SBRT had an increased risk of developing myositis. There was otherwise no correlation with myosotis and anti-VEGF therapy [36].

Figure 11.2 depicts an example of radiation myositis, which developed 6 months after spine SBRT to the L3 vertebral body level [36]. Image A shows an axial T2-weighted MRI of the L3 vertebral body and paraspinal muscles prior to radiation therapy. Image B shows an MRI 6 months after radiation therapy at the onset of myositis symptoms, showing T2 hyperintensity of the left psoas muscle and erector

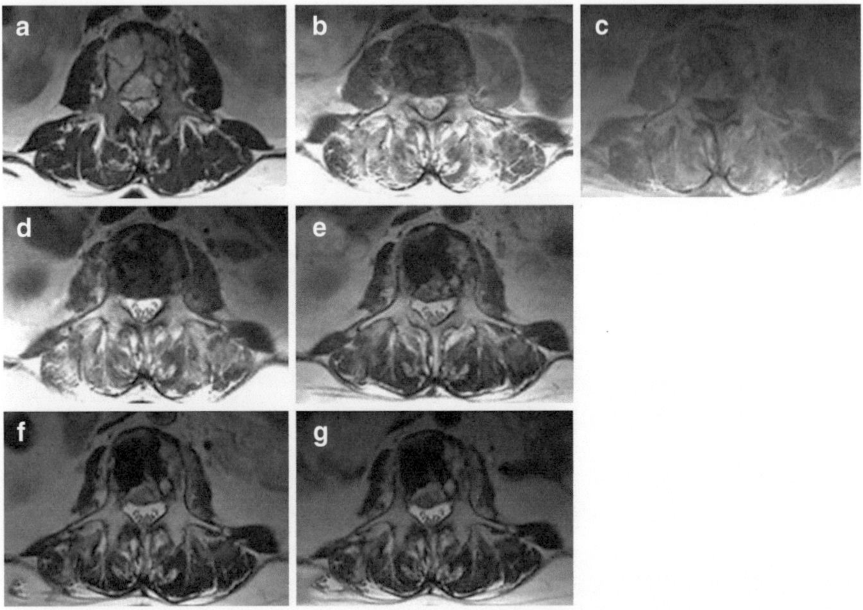

Fig. 11.2 Radiation myositis after spine SBRT. (Image obtained from Lockney et al. [36])

spinae muscles. Image C shows a lack of contrast enhancement on a T1-weighted postcontrast scan 6 months after radiation therapy. Image D shows an axial T2-weighted MR image eight months after radiation therapy at the time of the clinical resolution of myositis symptoms. Images E–G show T2-weighted MR images at 1.2 years (E), 1.6 years (F), and 2.5 years (G) after radiation therapy, showing volume loss of the left psoas with vague residual T2 hyperintensity.

It is noteworthy that myositis after spine SBRT can also present as radiation recall myositis. Radiation recall myositis is defined as acute inflammation in previously irradiated tissues, which is felt to be induced by subsequent systemic therapy [chemotherapy such as gemcitabine, targeted therapy, and antibiotics] [37].

Minimizing the Risk of Radiation Myositis

No clear guidelines exist for mitigating the risk of myositis secondary to paucity of data in the medical literature. However, single-fraction schedules may be associated with an increased risk of myositis versus multi-fraction regimens [36].

Management of Radiation Myositis

Radiation myositis is typically treated with a several-week course of steroids, NSAIDS and pain medication [36].

Esophageal Toxicity

Severe esophageal toxicities after spine SBRT are rare complications that can occur in either the acute or the late setting. Manifestations include radiation esophagitis (see Fig. 11.3) [38], intractable pain, ulcer, fistula formation and in rare cases death.

In a systematic review of 12 postoperative spine radiosurgery series, only 1 of 445 patients developed Grade 4 esophageal toxicity with associated fistula formation requiring surgical repair [39].

A single institution series from Stanford University evaluated patients with lung or spine tumors within close proximity to the esophagus treated with a single or multifraction SBRT regimens (range: 16–50 Gy in 1–5 fractions) [40]. Only 2 of 31 patients developed grade 4–5 esophageal toxicity [40]. It is noteworthy that both patients had received chemotherapy prior to SBRT, which may have triggered radiation recall reactions.

The largest single institution series in the medical literature is from MSK, which included 182 spine SBRT patients [41]. This study reported a 6.8% rate of acute late grade 3+ esophageal toxicity at a median FU of 12 months. Risk factors correlating with increased toxicity included: volume of tissue receiving ≤12 Gy (V12Gy) = 3.78 cc (relative risk [RR] 3.7, $P = 0.05$), V15Gy = 1.87 cc (RR 18, $P = 0.0013$), V20Gy = 0.11 cc (RR 6, $P = 0.01$), and Dmax V22Gy – 0.0 cc (RR 13, $P = 0.0013$). A logistical regression model was developed based on the median split

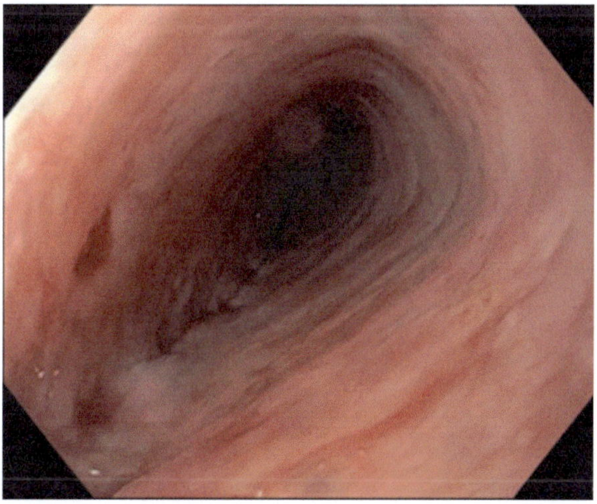

Fig. 11.3 Radiation esophagitis after spine radiation. (Image obtained from Ajayi et al. [38])

Table 11.6 MSK Dosimetric Guidelines for Esophageal Tissue for De Novo Spine Cases

	1-Fraction	3-Fractions	5-Fractions
Prescription dose	24 Gy × 1	9–10 Gy × 3	8 Gy × 5
Esophagus	Level I: $V_{14Gy} < 2.5$ cc Level II: $V_{18\,Gy} < 2.5$ cc	Level I: $D_{0.035cc} < 27.6$ Gy $D_{5cc} < 16.8$ Gy Level II: $D_{0.035cc} < 30$ Gy $D_{5cc} < 22$ Gy	Level I: $D_{0.035cc} < 32.2$ Gy $D_{5cc} < 19$ Gy Level II: $D_{0.035cc} < 50$ Gy $D_{5cc} < 27.5$ Gy

Attempt level I constraints first. Use level II constraints if level I compromises coverage

of D 2.5 cc = 14.02 (RR 6, $P = 0.01$), suggesting that limiting D 2.5 cc < 14 Gy yields <5% risk of grade 3+ toxicity with a steep increase in toxicity thereafter.

The MSK series also found that all the grade 4+ toxicities ($n = 7$) were associated with chemotherapy administered prior to SBRT (e.g., doxorubicin or gemcitabine, which are associated with radiation recall reactions) or when there was iatrogenic manipulation of the irradiated esophagus.

The Cleveland Clinic's experience of esophageal toxicity after liver and lung SBRT within proximity to the esophagus was similarly limited by a low event rate of 3.7% (2 patients). In this study, the median SBRT dose was 50Gy in 10 fractions with various dose regimens (range: 37.5–60 Gy in 3–10 fractions) [42]. Both of these patients had Dmax >51 Gy and V48 Gy >1 cc and received VEGF-modulating agents in close temporal proximity to SBRT.

Minimizing the Risk of Esophageal Toxicity

During radiation planning, it is important to adhere to dose constraints for esophageal tissue.

The MSK dose constraints for esophageal tissue are shown in Tables 11.6 and 11.7.

Esophageal biopsy or any surgical manipulation of the esophagus after SBRT should be avoided. Avoiding the administration of antiangiogenic therapies immediately prior to, during, and immediately after spine SBRT can also reduce the risk of esophageal side effects. We also emphasize the significance of being vigilant towards systemic therapies [i.e., Doxorubicin and Gemcitabine], which can potentially lead to a radiation recall reaction.

Table 11.7 MSK Dosimetric Guidelines for Esophageal Tissue for Re-irradiation Spine Cases

	1-Fraction	3-Fractions	5-Fractions
Prescription dose	24Gy × 1	9–10Gy × 3	8Gy × 5
Esophagus	No Hot Spot	$D_{0.035cc}$ < 20.4 Gy Cumulative $D_{0.035cc}$ < 100 Gy in 2 Gy equivalents ($\alpha/\beta = 3$)	$D_{0.035cc}$ < 25 Gy Cumulative $D_{0.035cc}$ < 100 Gy in 2 Gy equivalents ($\alpha/\beta = 3$)

Management of Esophageal Toxicity

Acute radiation esophagitis is typically managed with pain medication, IV hydration and nutritional supplements. Sucralfate suspension has been studied in the prevention of acute esophagitis in a prospective trial [43]. Several randomized studies have also evaluated Amifostine (a radioprotector) with mixed results regarding its ability to reduce esophagitis [44].

It is recommended that SBRT be delivered with caution after recent administration of antiangiogenic drugs or systemic therapy associated with recall reactions. Surgical manipulation of the esophagus should also be avoided after radiation therapy [3].

Radiofrequency ablation is an option for the management of late hemorrhagic radiation esophagitis. A case report of a patient who developed hemorrhagic esophagitis 2 years after chemoradiation was successfully treated with RFA treatment of the lower esophagus and GE junction 2 years after chemoradiation [45].

Esophageal stricture is an additional late complication of radiation therapy. The Mayo Clinic published a case report where a patient was successfully managed with serial balloon dilatation and hyperbaric oxygen therapy [38].

Plexopathy

Spine radiation can cause injury to the brachial plexus [C5-T1 nerve roots], the lumbosacral plexus [L4-S1 nerve roots] and other nerve roots in rare cases. Symptoms include neurogenic pain, numbness, paresthesia, dysesthesia, lymphedema, motor weakness and in some cases paralysis [46, 47].

Radiation-induced plexopathy [RIP] can manifest as soon as 1 month after treatment, but symptoms more commonly develop within a timeframe of 1–5 years. In cases of brachial plexopathy, clinical signs may take several decades to appear after radiation exposure. While some patients may experience some improvement or stabilization, gradual worsening is the usual course, and the chances of natural recovery are generally low [48].

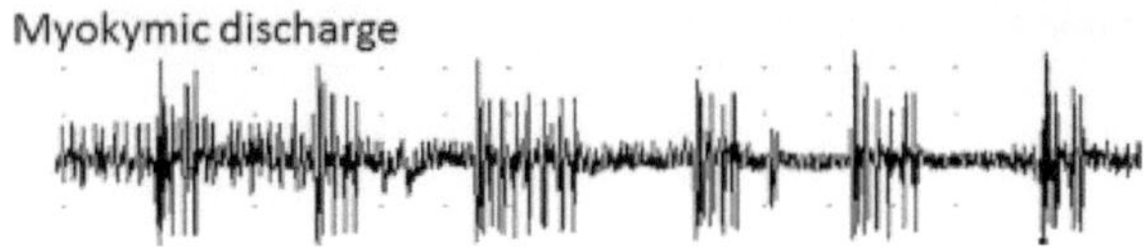

Fig. 11.4 Myokymic discharge. (Adapted from Stalberg et al. [51])

Electromyographic (EMG) and evoked potentials testing are helpful in characterizing plexopathies. Such testing can determine the severity of the deficits and define their level and extension. Electrodiagnostic abnormalities related to radiation injury are typically unilateral [46]. Electrodiagnostic studies of radiation-induced plexus injury reveal axonal loss indicators, such as reduced SNAP and CMAP amplitudes, neurogenic motor unit potentials, and occasional fibrillation potentials [49]. A hallmark of radiation-related injury seen on EMG is the presence of myokymia [49], defined by spontaneous bursts of consecutive myokymic discharges with slow, irregular firing frequencies [50, 51]. An example of a myokymic discharge is shown in Fig. 11.4 [51].

Unfortunately, there is limited information in the medical literature on radiation-induced plexopathy for patients who have undergone spine SBRT [3]. In an MSKCC series of over 90 patients who underwent single-fraction spine SBRT to a dose of 18 to 24Gy, there were no reported cases of plexopathy [28, 52]. Another MSK series examined 447 patients treated with 557 courses of single fraction spine SBRT with 18–26Gy in the de novo setting [53]. Within this study, 13 patients (2.9%) reported a total of 14 cases of plexopathy, occurring at a median of 10 months after SBRT. It is noteworthy that the treatment location was either the cervical or lumbosacral spine in each reported case.

In a more recent retrospective review of 52 patients undergoing spine SBRT [median dose 24Gy over 2 fractions] for cervical and sacral metastases, there was 1 case of brachial plexopathy and 1 case of lumbosacral plexopathy [54]. In a subsequent publication, the same group evaluated spine SBRT patients who lived more than 3 years and found the 3-year and 5-year rates of plexopathy to be 2.2% and 5.1%, respectively [30].

Minimizing Risk of Plexopathy

To mitigate the risk of brachial and lumbosacral plexopathy, it is imperative to accurately contour the brachial plexus [55] and lumbosacral plexus anatomy [56] when treating spinal segments in their corresponding regions. It is also critical to follow dose constraints for the nerve plexus. The MSK dose constraints for the brachial plexus and lumbosacral plexus are shown in Tables 11.8 and 11.9.

Table 11.8 MSK Dosimetric Guidelines for Brachial & Lumbosacral Plexus for De Novo Spine Cases

	1-Fraction	3-Fractions	5-Fractions
Prescription dose	24 Gy × 1	9–10 Gy × 3	8 Gy × 5
Brachial plexus	D_{max} < 24 Gy	D_{max} < 27 Gy	D_{max} < 35 Gy
Lumbosacral plexus	No Hot Spot	D_{max} < 27 Gy	D_{max} < 35 Gy

Table 11.9 MSK Dosimetric Guidelines for Brachial & Lumbosacral Plexus for Re-irradiation Spine Cases

	1-Fraction	3-Fractions	5-Fractions
Spinal cord (PRV if MRI fusion)*	D_{max} < 12 Gy or 10.2 Gy $D_{0.35cc}$ < 9 Gy	D_{max} < 14.5 Gy or 13.9 Gy $D_{0.35cc}$ < 10 Gy	D_{max} < 18 Gy or 17 Gy $D_{0.35cc}$ < 14 Gy
Cauda equina*	D_{max} < 14 Gy D_{5cc} < 11 Gy	D_{max} < 15 Gy D_{5cc} < 13 Gy	D_{max} < 20 Gy D_{5cc} < 17 Gy
Brachial plexus	No Hot Spot	D_{max} < 17.7 Gy	D_{max} < 22 Gy
Lumbosacral plexus	No Hot Spot	D_{max} < 17.7 Gy	D_{max} < 22 Gy

Management of Radiation-Induced Plexopathy

Both the diagnosis and treatment of radiation plexopathy are challenging since there is no proven therapy that reverses or prevents its progression [57]. The primary focus is pain management, which includes the use of narcotics, continuous infusion pumps, local, and regional blocks, sympathectomy, or rhizotomy. Dysesthesias may improve with nerve stimulation, gabapentin, carbamazepine, topiramate, valproic acid, tricyclic antidepressants, and phenytoin. Regional nerve blocks, sympathetic ganglion blocks and epidural anesthetics can also provide pain relief [58].

Physical and occupational therapy can also aid in regaining patient independence and help prevent muscle atrophy [50, 57, 59].

Conclusion

Stereotactic body radiation therapy (SBRT) is a powerful and effective tool for achieving tumor control and alleviating pain for spinal cancer. However, its success is tempered by potential toxicities, such as pain flare, myelopathy, vertebral compression fracture, myositis, gastrointestinal/esophageal toxicity, and plexopathy. The importance of understanding and managing these toxicities cannot be overstated, as it directly impacts patient outcomes. Critical to this management is the accurate identification and treatment of nearby organs at risk, as well as the employment of appropriate clinical strategies to minimize side effects. Future research, particularly well-designed randomized controlled trials, is essential to refine dosing and fractionation protocols for spine SBRT. This will enable us to maximize the therapeutic benefits while simultaneously reducing both acute and long-term toxicities, thereby enhancing the overall quality of life for patients undergoing this treatment.

References

1. Chiang A, et al. Pain Flare is a common adverse event in steroid-naive patients after spine stereotactic body radiation therapy: a prospective clinical trial. Int J Radiat Oncol Biol Phys. 2013;86(4):638–42.
2. Khan L, et al. Prophylactic dexamethasone effectively reduces the incidence of pain flare following spine stereotactic body radiotherapy (SBRT): a prospective observational study. Support Care Cancer. 2015;23(10):2937–43.
3. Schaub SK, et al. Strategies to mitigate toxicities from stereotactic body radiation therapy for spine metastases. Neurosurgery. 2019;85(6):729–40.
4. Glicksman RM, et al. Stereotactic ablative radiotherapy for the management of spinal metastases: a review. JAMA Oncol. 2020;6(4):567–77.
5. Pan HY, et al. Incidence and predictive factors of pain flare after spine stereotactic body radiation therapy: secondary analysis of phase 1/2 trials. Int J Radiat Oncol Biol Phys. 2014;90(4):870–6.
6. Balagamwala EH, et al. Pain flare after stereotactic radiosurgery for spine metastases. J Radiosurg SBRT. 2018;5(2):99–105.
7. Kowalchuk RO, et al. Development and internal validation of a recursive partitioning analysis-based model predictive of pain flare incidence after spine stereotactic body radiation therapy. Pract Radiat Oncol. 2022;12(4):e269–77.
8. Folkert MR, et al. Outcomes and toxicity for hypofractionated and single-fraction image-guided stereotactic radiosurgery for sarcomas metastasizing to the spine. Int J Radiat Oncol Biol Phys. 2014;88(5):1085–91.
9. Myrehaug S, et al. Reirradiation spine stereotactic body radiation therapy for spinal metastases: systematic review. J Neurosurg Spine. 2017;27(4):428–35.
10. Guckenberger M, et al. Safety and efficacy of stereotactic body radiotherapy as primary treatment for vertebral metastases: a multi-institutional analysis. Radiat Oncol. 2014;9:226.
11. Hall WA, et al. Stereotactic body radiosurgery for spinal metastatic disease: an evidence-based review. Int J Surg Oncol. 2011;2011:979214.
12. Sahgal A, et al. Probabilities of radiation myelopathy specific to stereotactic body radiation therapy to guide safe practice. Int J Radiat Oncol Biol Phys. 2013;85(2):341–7.
13. Redmond KJ, et al. Consensus contouring guidelines for postoperative stereotactic body radiation therapy for metastatic solid tumor malignancies to the spine. Int J Radiat Oncol Biol Phys. 2017;97(1):64–74.
14. Jabbari S, et al. Stereotactic body radiotherapy for spinal metastases: practice guidelines, outcomes, and risks. Cancer J. 2016;22(4):280–9.
15. Cox BW, et al. International Spine Radiosurgery Consortium consensus guidelines for target volume definition in spinal stereotactic radiosurgery. Int J Radiat Oncol Biol Phys. 2012;83(5):e597–605.
16. Sahgal A, et al. Spinal cord dose tolerance to stereotactic body radiation therapy. Int J Radiat Oncol Biol Phys. 2021;110(1):124–36.

17. Hazelaar C, et al. Verifying tumor position during stereotactic body radiation therapy delivery using (limited-arc) cone beam computed tomography imaging. Radiother Oncol. 2017;123(3):355–62.
18. Ong WL, et al. Radiation myelopathy following stereotactic body radiation therapy for spine metastases. J Neuro-Oncol. 2022;159(1):23–31.
19. Williamson R, et al. Adverse radiation effects after radiosurgery may benefit from oral vitamin E and pentoxifylline therapy: a pilot study. Stereotact Funct Neurosurg. 2008;86(6):359–66.
20. Calabro F, Jinkins JR. MRI of radiation myelitis: a report of a case treated with hyperbaric oxygen. Eur Radiol. 2000;10(7):1079–84.
21. Smith JA, Fenderson JL. Diving into radiation necrosis: hyperbaric oxygen therapy in cerebral radiation necrosis. JCO Oncol Pract. 2020;16(8):519–21.
22. Levin VA, et al. Randomized double-blind placebo-controlled trial of bevacizumab therapy for radiation necrosis of the central nervous system. Int J Radiat Oncol Biol Phys. 2011;79(5):1487–95.
23. Xu Y, et al. Bevacizumab monotherapy reduces radiation-induced brain necrosis in nasopharyngeal carcinoma patients: a randomized controlled trial. Int J Radiat Oncol Biol Phys. 2018;101(5):1087–95.
24. Shah N, Ranjan S. Successful treatment of quadriparesis from radiation myelopathy with bevacizumab in a patient with metastatic breast cancer. BMJ Case Rep. 2022;15(2):e246470.
25. Canedo G, et al. Treatment of radiation-induced myelopathy with bevacizumab. Clin Transl Oncol. 2020;22(6):957–60.
26. Psimaras D, et al. Bevacizumab in late-onset radiation-induced myelopathy. Neurology. 2016;86(5):454–7.
27. Faruqi S, et al. Vertebral compression fracture after spine stereotactic body radiation therapy: a review of the pathophysiology and risk factors. Neurosurgery. 2018;83(3):314–22.
28. Yamada Y, et al. High-dose, single-fraction image-guided intensity-modulated radiotherapy for metastatic spinal lesions. Int J Radiat Oncol Biol Phys. 2008;71(2):484–90.
29. Tseng CL, et al. Imaging-based outcomes for 24 Gy in 2 daily fractions for patients with de Novo spinal metastases treated with spine Stereotactic Body Radiation Therapy (SBRT). Int J Radiat Oncol Biol Phys. 2018;102(3):499–507.
30. Zeng KL, et al. Prognostic factors associated with surviving less than 3 months vs greater than 3 years specific to spine stereotactic body radiotherapy and late adverse events. Neurosurgery. 2021;88(5):971–9.
31. Sahgal A, et al. Vertebral compression fracture after spine stereotactic body radiotherapy: a multi-institutional analysis with a focus on radiation dose and the spinal instability neoplastic score. J Clin Oncol. 2013;31(27):3426–31.
32. Fisher CG, et al. A novel classification system for spinal instability in neoplastic disease: an evidence-based approach and expert consensus from the Spine Oncology Study Group. Spine (Phila Pa 1976). 2010;35(22):E1221–9.
33. Fourney DR, et al. Spinal instability neoplastic score: an analysis of reliability and validity from the spine oncology study group. J Clin Oncol. 2011;29(22):3072–7.
34. Wang XS, et al. Stereotactic body radiation therapy for management of spinal metastases in patients without spinal cord compression: a phase 1-2 trial. Lancet Oncol. 2012;13(4):395–402.
35. Chi JH, Gokaslan ZL. Vertebroplasty and kyphoplasty for spinal metastases. Curr Opin Support Palliat Care. 2008;2(1):9–13.
36. Lockney DT, et al. Myositis following spine radiosurgery for metastatic disease: a case series. J Neurosurg Spine. 2018;28(4):416–21.
37. Borroni G, et al. Radiation recall dermatitis, panniculitis, and myositis following cyclophosphamide therapy: histopathologic findings of a patient affected by multiple myeloma. Am J Dermatopathol. 2004;26(3):213–6.
38. Ajayi OD, et al. Esophageal stricture following radiation, concurrent immunochemotherapy, treated with hyperbaric oxygen and dilation. Mayo Clin Proc Innov Qual Outcomes. 2019;3(2):241–5.

39. Faruqi S, et al. Stereotactic radiosurgery for postoperative spine malignancy: a systematic review and International Stereotactic Radiosurgery Society practice guidelines. Pract Radiat Oncol. 2022;12(2):e65–78.
40. Abelson JA, et al. Esophageal tolerance to high-dose stereotactic ablative radiotherapy. Dis Esophagus. 2012;25(7):623–9.
41. Cox BW, et al. Esophageal toxicity from high-dose, single-fraction paraspinal stereotactic radiosurgery. Int J Radiat Oncol Biol Phys. 2012;83(5):e661–7.
42. Stephans KL, et al. Esophageal dose tolerance to hypofractionated stereotactic body radiation therapy: risk factors for late toxicity. Int J Radiat Oncol Biol Phys. 2014;90(1):197–202.
43. McGinnis WL, et al. Placebo-controlled trial of sucralfate for inhibiting radiation-induced esophagitis. J Clin Oncol. 1997;15(3):1239–43.
44. Bradley J, Movsas B. Radiation esophagitis: predictive factors and preventive strategies. Semin Radiat Oncol. 2004;14(4):280–6.
45. Marin FS, et al. Successful treatment of hemorrhagic radiation esophagitis with radiofrequency ablation. Endoscopy. 2022;54(S 02):E830–1.
46. Ko K, et al. Clinical, electrophysiological findings in adult patients with non-traumatic Plexopathies. Ann Rehabil Med. 2011;35(6):807–15.
47. Killer HE, Hess K. Natural history of radiation-induced brachial plexopathy compared with surgically treated patients. J Neurol. 1990;237(4):247–50.
48. Dhawan PS. Electrodiagnostic assessment of Plexopathies. Neurol Clin. 2021;39(4):997–1014.
49. Harper CM Jr, et al. Distinction between neoplastic and radiation-induced brachial plexopathy, with emphasis on the role of EMG. Neurology. 1989;39(4):502–6.
50. Almeida LR, et al. Radiation-induced lumbosacral plexopathy. Cureus. 2023;15(3):e36842.
51. Stalberg E, et al. Standards for quantification of EMG and neurography. Clin Neurophysiol. 2019;130(9):1688–729.
52. Moussazadeh N, et al. Five-year outcomes of high-dose single-fraction spinal stereotactic radiosurgery. Int J Radiat Oncol Biol Phys. 2015;93(2):361–7.
53. Stubblefield MD, et al. Peripheral nervous system injury after high-dose single-fraction image-guided stereotactic radiosurgery for spine tumors. Neurosurg Focus. 2017;42(3):E12.
54. Zeng KL, et al. Stereotactic body radiotherapy for spinal metastases at the extreme ends of the spine: imaging-based outcomes for cervical and sacral metastases. Neurosurgery. 2019;85(5):605–12.
55. Truong MT, et al. Brachial plexus contouring with CT and MR imaging in radiation therapy planning for head and neck cancer. Radiographics. 2010;30(4):1095–103.
56. Yi SK, et al. Development of a standardized method for contouring the lumbosacral plexus: a preliminary dosimetric analysis of this organ at risk among 15 patients treated with intensity-modulated radiotherapy for lower gastrointestinal cancers and the incidence of radiation-induced lumbosacral plexopathy. Int J Radiat Oncol Biol Phys. 2012;84(2):376–82.
57. Dyck PJ, Thaisetthawatkul P. Lumbosacral plexopathy. Continuum (Minneap Minn). 2014;20(5 Peripheral Nervous System Disorders):1343–58.
58. Jaeckle KA. Neurological manifestations of neoplastic and radiation-induced plexopathies. In: Seminars in neurology. Copyright© 2004 by Thieme Medical Publishers, Inc; 2004.
59. Jaeckle KA, Young DF, Foley KM. The natural history of lumbosacral plexopathy in cancer. Neurology. 1985;35(1):8–15.

Chapter 12
Toxicities of Overlapping Spine Radiotherapy and Systemic Therapy

Justin Haseltine

Introduction

Radiotherapy with concurrent systemic therapy is commonly used in the definitive treatment of several non-metastatic cancer types. However, in cancer metastases, overlapping RT and systemic therapy can increase toxicity without a clear improvement in outcomes. The amount and quality of data on toxicity with concurrent RT and systemic therapies are highly variable, but general treatment approaches and recommendations can be informed by available data. In this chapter, we will review interactions between various systemic therapies and RT for cancer metastases to the spine, as well as recommendations for avoiding synergistic toxicity.

Cytotoxic Chemotherapy

Cytotoxic chemotherapies include agents such as alkylating agents (e.g. cyclophosphamide, ifosfamide, dacarbazine, temozolomide, mitomycin, cisplatin, carboplatin, oxaliplatin), antimetabolites (e.g. methotrexate, pemetrexed, fluorouracil, capecitabine, cytarabine, gemcitabine, azacitidine), anti-microtubule agents (e.g. vincristine, vinblastine, vinorelbine, paclitaxel, docetaxel), topoisomerase inhibitors (e.g. irinotecan, topotecan, etoposide), and cytotoxic antibiotics (e.g. doxorubicin, daunorubicin, actinomycin, bleomycin).

As a general recommendation, clinicians should consider holding cytotoxic chemotherapies for at least 1 week or 1–2 half-lives (whichever is longer) before and

J. Haseltine (✉)
Memorial Sloan Kettering Cancer Center, Department of Radiation Oncology, New York, NY, USA
e-mail: haseltij@mskcc.org

Y. Yamada et al. (eds.), *Multidisciplinary Spine Tumor Management*,
https://doi.org/10.1007/978-3-032-07519-2_12

after spine RT. With doxorubicin or in cases where the chemotherapy has known toxicities affecting organs that are in or near the radiation field and expected to receive a meaningful RT dose, consider holding the chemotherapy for at least 2 weeks or at least 2 half-lives.

Doxorubicin

Increased toxicity with concurrent RT and doxorubicin has been reported since at least the 1970s, including synergistic cardiotoxicity [1], increased esophagitis [2] and dermatitis [2, 3]. A prospective trial from Finland published in 1992 included 200 stage II breast cancer patients treated post-operatively from 1981 to 1984 with randomization to arms including adjuvant breast RT and adjuvant doxorubicin-based chemotherapy administered every 4 weeks, with breast RT given to 45 Gy in 15 fractions between the third and fourth chemo cycles [4]. This schedule, by definition, allowed only a few days of chemotherapy washout before and after RT. Rates of symptomatic radiation pneumonitis were significantly increased from 4% with RT alone to 23–33% with concurrent RT and chemotherapy.

A prospective, non-randomized study from The Netherlands published in 2003 included breast cancer patients who received adjuvant treatment from 1996 to 1999 with RT alone ($n = 42$) or doxorubicin-based chemo and concurrent RT ($n = 61$) [5]. RT was to 50 Gy in 25 fractions and included a boost of 14–20 Gy in 7–10 fractions for patients who underwent breast conservation. Doxorubicin-based chemo was administered every 21 days for 4 cycles and 80% of patients started breast RT after 1–2 cycles of chemotherapy. Concurrent doxorubicin and RT, compared with RT alone, was associated with significantly increased rates of severe skin toxicity (70% vs 26%), moderate to severe esophagitis (36% vs 5%) and moderate to severe anorexia (51% vs 4%). Rates of pneumonitis were 5% or less in both groups.

Another study published in 2003 included 35 patients with retroperitoneal sarcoma who underwent concurrent doxorubicin and escalating RT doses up to 50.4 Gy in 28 fractions [6]. Four patients required hospitalization during or shortly after concurrent therapy. Patients who received 50.4 Gy had 18% acute grade 3/4 nausea.

More recently, a non-randomized phase II trial of 27 patients with locally advanced thyroid cancer included treatment with RT with or without doxorubicin [7]. There were significantly increased rates of acute grade 2+ dermatitis (90% vs 50%), mucositis (74% vs 25%), and dysphagia (63% vs 13%) with concurrent therapy, but few late toxicities were noted in either group.

Actinomycin

Concurrent actinomycin and RT has been reported to produce additive toxicity since at least the 1950s, including dermatitis and mucositis [8, 9]. Other reports raised concerns about actinomycin lowering the threshold at which radiation hepatitis, nephritis and pneumonitis occur [10].

Animal model experiments have corroborated the clinical findings of additive toxicity of actinomycin and RT. Dermatitis was increased in studies using rat and mouse models [11, 12]. Other studies demonstrated increased intestinal toxicity of concurrent treatment in mouse models [13, 14] and a canine model [15]. The study by Phillips et al. also demonstrated increased toxicity in the lung and esophagus.

Pneumonitis was highlighted as a toxicity of great clinical relevance in this setting in a 1991 case report of death from pulmonary failure in a pediatric Ewing's sarcoma patient who received whole lung RT to 12 Gy with combination chemotherapy including actinomycin. Whole lung RT to 12 Gy would not otherwise be expected to cause high-grade pneumonitis. Actinomycin was felt to be the most likely culprit drug given data showing that it had the greatest dose effect factor for increased pulmonary toxicity [14].

5-Fluorouracil

The use of 5-Fluorouracil (5FU) with concurrent RT has been studied extensively in the definitive treatment of non-metastatic cancers, often in combination with other chemotherapeutic agents. There is less data available on outcomes and toxicity when 5FU is used in combination with RT in the metastatic setting. Data on the concurrent use of 5FU and RT in the definitive setting demonstrates that mucosal toxicity is of particular concern [16]. Mucosal toxicity, especially esophagitis, is very important in spine RT given the proximity of the esophagus to the vertebral body.

Gemcitabine

Concurrent gemcitabine and RT has been associated with pneumonitis and mucositis in the definitive treatment of non-metastatic cancers. An initial phase II study of concurrent gemcitabine and RT in locally advanced non-small cell lung cancer (NSCLC) used a high dose of gemcitabine (1000 mg/m^2 weekly) with conventionally fractionated RT to 60 Gy [17]. Of 8 patients treated, 3 patients had grade 5 toxicity (2 pulmonary, 1 hemorrhage), 3 patients had severe acute pneumonitis or esophagitis, and 2 patients had other significant side effects. Subsequent trials in NSCLC reduced the dose of gemcitabine, which improved toxicity, but still included clinically meaningful rates of esophagitis and pneumonitis. For example, a trial of 21 patients gave gemcitabine at 125–190 mg/m^2 weekly and reported acute grade 3/4 esophagitis of 30% [17]. Another study of 17 patients gave gemcitabine at 10–50 mg/m^2 twice weekly and reported acute grade 3 pneumonitis of 25% and acute grade 3/4 esophagitis of 18% [18].

In pancreatic cancer, a study of 51 patients with locally advanced, unresectable disease were treated with concurrent gemcitabine (250–500 mg/m^2 weekly) and RT (30–33 Gy in 10–11 fractions) [19]. Severe acute toxicity was reported in 24% of patients, including admission for supportive care >5 days ($n = 8$), more than 3 gemcitabine dose deletions ($n = 5$), and gastrointestinal bleed with evidence of ulceration ($n = 3$).

Irinotecan

Irinotecan has been administered concurrently with RT in the treatment of locally advanced NSCLC and upper gastrointestinal (GI) cancers. The main toxicities of concern that are associated with concurrent administration are esophagitis and pneumonitis.

A phase I/II study published in 1999 reported on 26 patients with NSCLC treated with conventionally fractionated RT to 60 Gy in 30 fractions and concurrent irinotecan at increasing dose levels [20]. Three of five patients treated at the highest irinotecan dose level developed Grade 3 or 4 esophagitis and pneumonitis. Additionally, one patient treated at an intermediate dose level experienced grade 5 pneumonitis. A similar phase I trial including 13 patients with NSCLC and similar RT and irinotecan dosing, again found grade 3 or 4 esophagitis in 2 of 3 patients at the highest irinotecan dose level [21]. The worst toxicity at the intermediate dose level was grade 2 esophagitis in 1 patient. The lowest dose level, with 7 patients enrolled, was notable for 1 patient who experienced grade 5 esophagitis; there was no esophagitis in the other patients at this dose level. A phase I study of patients with upper GI cancers included 15 patients treated to up to 50.4 Gy in 28 fractions with concurrent irinotecan and reported grade 3/4 toxicities, including nausea, vomiting, dehydration and anorexia. There were no grade 5 toxicities.

A study of stereotactic body radiotherapy (SBRT) with concurrent irinotecan in patients with oligometastatic colorectal cancer to liver or lung included 44 patients with 51 lesions ($n = 39$ liver, $n = 12$ lung) [22]. There were no acute toxicities (within 3 months of SBRT) greater than grade 2 (and no grade 2 esophagitis or pneumonitis). Late toxicities included 1 case of grade 2 pneumonitis and 1 case of grade 3 liver enzyme elevation in the setting of liver progression.

Taxanes

Concurrent administration of taxanes with RT has been associated with mucositis and pneumonitis in patients treated definitively for non-metastatic cancers. An abstract on 28 patients treated for esophageal cancer with concurrent docetaxel (10–15 mg/m^2 weekly) and RT (ranging 30.6–65 Gy, conventionally fractionated) reported grade 3 esophagitis in 35% of patients and grade 3 pneumonitis in 10% [23].

A phase III randomized trial of 356 patients undergoing weekly docetaxel (15 mg/m^2) and conventionally fractionated RT for definitive treatment of locally advanced head and neck squamous cell carcinoma found significantly higher rates of grade 3 mucositis (50% vs 22%) and dysphagia (50% vs 33%) with concurrent docetaxel [24]. There were also increased rates of aspiration pneumonia (6.7% vs 1.7%, $p = 0.032$) and grade 3 dermatitis (15% vs 8.5%, $p = 0.070$).

Targeted Therapy

Targeted therapies include monoclonal antibodies such as anti-vascular endothelial growth factor (VEGF) (bevacizumab) and small molecule drugs such as epidermal growth factor receptor (EGFR) inhibitors (e.g., erlotinib, gefitinib, osimertinib), BRAF inhibitors (e.g., vemurafenib, dabrafenib) and multikinase inhibitors (e.g., sunitinib, sorafenib, cabozantinib).

As a general recommendation, clinicians should consider holding small molecule drugs for 2 days before and after spine RT, or 1–2 half-lives, whichever is longer. Consider holding bevacizumab for 1–2 weeks or more as clinically allowed. In our practice, efforts are made to hold bevacizumab when possible; however, the clinical urgency of spine treatment often takes precedence, and we have not observed excess toxicity among patients treated to the spine around the time of bevacizumab administration.

Recent review papers have summarized data on combining targeted therapy and immunotherapy with metastasis-directed RT [25] and SBRT [26].

Bevacizumab

Bevacizumab can be associated with an increased risk of bowel toxicity, fistula formation, and hemorrhage when administered around the time of intra-abdominal or lung RT.

A report in 2013 showed increased severe bowel toxicity in patients who received a VEGF inhibitor and abdominal SBRT [27]. The overall population included 66 patients who underwent abdominal SBRT (with or without use of VEGF inhibitor), 7 of whom (9% of overall cohort) experienced a grade 3–5 bowel event. Among the

26 patients who received a VEGF inhibitor within 3 months of abdominal SBRT, the 6-month estimate of a serious bowel injury was 38%. No serious bowel injury occurred in patients who did not have VEGF inhibitor treatment.

Subsequent reports in patients with primary and metastatic tumors of the lung who underwent SBRT for tumors abutting the proximal bronchial tree showed unacceptably high rates of grade 5 toxicity involving 4 patients, 2 of whom had exposure to bevacizumab [28]. A later report from the same group showed that bevacizumab exposure among patients with more fractionated radiation schedules of 15 fractions was still associated with severe toxicities, including grade 4 tracheal necrosis and grade 3 tracheoesophageal fistula [29].

Conventionally fractionated radiation combined with bevacizumab has also been shown to increase bowel toxicity. In a study of 302 patients with cervical cancer, the 3-year cumulative incidence of fistula was significantly elevated in patients exposed to bevacizumab (27% vs 3%) [30]. They found a longer interval between RT and bevacizumab of 10 months or more to be associated with a reduced incidence of fistula.

EGFR Inhibitors

Treatment with RT and concurrent EGFR inhibitors is associated with esophagitis and pneumonitis in the treatment of non-metastatic esophageal and lung cancers. Patients treated to esophageal primary with conventionally fractionated RT doses of 46–70 Gy and concurrent erlotinib [31] or gefitinib [32] have experienced grade 3 esophagitis rates of 20–30%. Grade 3/4 pneumonitis was reported in 5–10%, and grade 3 dermatitis in 5–10%.

In a prospective phase II trial testing the addition of erlotinib to thoracic RT (66 Gy in 33 fractions) for locally advanced NSCLC, grade 3+ dyspnea was not increased with the addition of erlotinib (14% without vs 10% with) [33]. However, the rate of any grade 3+ event was nearly doubled in the erlotinib arm (50% vs 27%), appearing to be mostly driven by dermatitis/desquamation, fatigue, and anorexia. A subsequent report of 11 patients with NSCLC treated with thoracic RT and concurrent osimertinib reported a 45% rate of grade 3+ pneumonitis, including one death [34].

A prospective phase II study of 24 patients with NSCLC and progression on platinum-based chemotherapy administered treatment with concurrent erlotinib and SBRT to extracranial sites of disease [35]. The toxicities considered attributable to SBRT included 1 grade 5 event, 1 grade 4 event, and 2 grade 3 events. There were 3 grade 4 events attributed to erlotinib.

A retrospective study of 158 patients undergoing SBRT with targeted therapy evaluated whether there was a difference in outcomes among patients who had a pause in targeted therapy during SBRT versus those who continued targeted therapy uninterrupted [36]. 68 patients were on an EGFR inhibitor. Rates of any grade toxicity were significantly increased when the EGFR inhibitor was continued during

SBRT; however, rates of grade 3+ toxicity were low (acute grade 3+ in 1.6%, late grade 3+ in 4.9%) and were not different among patients who continued or paused the EGFR inhibitor.

BRAF Inhibitors

Dermatitis is the most commonly reported adverse event when BRAF inhibitors are used with concurrent RT, though other toxicities have also been reported. The first known case report of significant dermatitis in this setting was also associated with grade 5 hepatic hemorrhage, although direct causality is unclear [37]. A retrospective report of 70 patients treated with concurrent BRAF inhibitor and RT found grade 2+ dermatitis in 36% of cases [38]. Follicular cystic proliferation occurred in 13% of patients. No hepatotoxicity was reported.

The Eastern Cooperative Oncology Group (ECOG) published consensus guidelines in 2016 regarding the use of BRAF inhibitors and RT. [39] They noted that in addition to dermatological toxicities, some visceral toxicities have been reported, including deaths possibly related to combination treatment in the previously noted hepatotoxicity as well as bowel perforation and pulmonary hemorrhage (although rates of pneumonitis overall do not appear elevated). ECOG recommends holding BRAF inhibitors for at least 3 days before and after fractionated RT and at least 1 day before and after stereotactic RT.

Multikinase Inhibitors

Multikinase inhibitors administered with concurrent spine SBRT have been reported to be generally well tolerated. A retrospective study of 100 patients with metastatic renal cell carcinoma undergoing spine SBRT described different treatment conditions, including concurrent drug therapy (defined as drug administration on the day of spine SBRT) [40]. The use of concurrent first-line drug therapy was associated with better local control than in treatment-naïve patients. Importantly, concurrent therapy was well tolerated with no grade 3 or greater events reported.

Immunotherapy

Immune checkpoint inhibitors (ICI) promote an anti-tumor immune response by removing inhibitory signaling. ICIs include anti-CTLA4 (e.g., ipilimumab), anti-PD-1 (e.g., nivolumab, pembrolizumab), and anti-PD-L1 (e.g., durvalumab, atezolizumab).

As a general recommendation, ICIs can be continued during radiation therapy. If a patient has previously experienced an ICI-related toxicity in an organ at risk from planned spine RT (e.g., pneumonitis), then clinicians may wish to administer RT halfway between ICI cycles or possibly delay an ICI cycle at their discretion.

Recent review papers have summarized data on combining targeted therapy and immunotherapy with metastasis-directed RT [25] and SBRT [26].

Anti-CTLA4

Multiple prospective trials have evaluated concurrent administration of ipilimumab and RT with low rates of significant toxicity. A phase II trial of ipilimumab with SBRT in patients with non-melanoma metastatic cancer to liver, lung, or adrenal gland evaluated 106 patients [41]. SBRT was to 50 Gy in 4 fractions or 60 Gy in 10 fractions and was administered during the first dose (concurrent) or 1 week after the second dose (sequential) of ipilimumab. There were no grade 4/5 treatment-related toxicities. There were 4 grade 3 respiratory events in the lung-lesion treatment group, including 1 pneumonitis. There were no differences in toxicity between concurrent and sequential dosing.

The above trial was preceded by a phase I trial that included 35 patients and used the same RT and ipilimumab dosing [42]. Similarly, there were no grade 4/5 treatment-related toxicities and no patient experienced greater than grade 1 pneumonitis.

A phase I dose escalation trial including 13 patients with metastatic melanoma administered SBRT in 3 fractions (every other day) with increasing total doses of 24 Gy, 30 Gy, and 36 Gy [43]. SBRT was given between the second and third cycles of ipilimumab. There were 3 grade 3/4 toxicities, all attributed to ipilimumab (1 diarrhea, 2 colitis).

Anti-PD-1 or Anti-PD-L1

Several prospective clinical trials have demonstrated that concurrent administration of RT with anti-PD-1 or anti-PD-L1 therapies is generally safe. In a phase I study, 79 patients with metastatic solid tumors were treated with SBRT and pembrolizumab (initiated within 7 days after completion of SBRT) [44]. There were 6 patients with severe treatment-related toxicity, including 3 grade 3 pneumonitis, 2 grade 3 colitis, and 1 grade 3 hepatic toxicity. Among patients with at least 3-month follow-up, the rate of dose-limiting toxicity was 9.7%.

A randomized, phase II study treated patients with metastatic NSCLC with pembrolizumab alone ($n = 40$) or pembrolizumab within 7 days after SBRT to 24 Gy in 3 fractions ($n = 36$) [45]. Fatigue and pneumonia occurred more commonly with SBRT (51% vs 27% ($p = 0.05$) and 26% vs 8% ($p = 0.06$), respectively). Grade 3–5 toxicity was reported in 12 patients and was not significantly different between treatment arms.

A randomized, phase II trial including 62 patients with metastatic head and neck squamous cell carcinoma treated patients with either nivolumab alone or nivolumab with SBRT (27 Gy in 3 fractions) administered to a metastatic lesion between the first and second dose of nivolumab [46]. There was no significant difference between trial arms in overall adverse events (70% nivo alone vs 87% nivo/SBRT, $p = 0.12$) or in grade 3–5 events (13% nivo alone vs 10% nivo/SBRT, $p = 0.70$).

A phase II, single-arm study of nivolumab with SBRT administered within 7 days of the first nivolumab dose included 69 patients with metastatic renal cell carcinoma [47]. SBRT was given to 30 Gy in 3 fractions. There were no treatment-related deaths, and grade 3/4 treatment-related toxicity occurred in 18 patients. Of note, all toxicities occurred outside the irradiated field, and there were no differences in toxicity between arms.

A phase II, single-arm study of 31 patients with metastatic castrate-resistant prostate cancer administered treatment with avelumab and SBRT [48]. SBRT was given with 20 Gy in 1 fraction to 1 or 2 sites before the first and second doses of avelumab. There were no treatment-related deaths. Grade 3/4 adverse events occurred in 5 patients, including 1 pneumonitis.

Antibody-Drug Conjugates

Antibody-drug conjugates (ADCs) are a relatively newer class of anti-cancer therapy. They work by linking a drug, often a cytotoxic chemotherapy, with an antibody to molecules present on cancer cellular membranes, which serves to concentrate the treatment at sites of cancer. Trastuzumab-emtansine (T-DM1) is one example of an ADC and is used in some patients with HER2-amplified breast cancer. In our practice, we try to administer spine RT midway between ADC cycles.

T-DM1

Most data on the use of T-DM1 with RT is in the setting of RT to the breast/chest wall or brain. A recent systematic review and meta-analysis reported on the safety of RT and T-DM1 [49]. Rates of brain radionecrosis were elevated with grade 3+ events in 17% of patients. Grade 3+ pneumonitis (<1%) and skin toxicity (1%) were low.

Table 12.1 Summary of concurrent RT and systemic therapy recommendations

Cytotoxic chemotherapy	Consider holding at least 1 week or 1–2 half-lives (whichever is longer) before and after RT
Doxorubicin	Consider holding at least 2 weeks before and after RT
Targeted therapy	Consider holding 2 days before, during, and 2 days after RT
Bevacizumab	Consider holding 1–2 weeks, or more as clinically allowed
Immunotherapy	Continue during RT, consider administering RT between cycles
Antibody-drug conjugates	Continue during RT, consider administering RT between cycles
Hormone therapy	Continue during RT

Other Systemic Therapies

Other systemic therapies used in cancer management may include hormone therapies (e.g., androgen deprivation therapy in prostate cancer, endocrine therapy in breast cancer), radionuclide therapies (e.g., radium-223, lutetium-177 conjugates), and cellular therapies (e.g., chimeric antigen receptor T-cells).

Hormone therapies are routinely combined with RT across the cancer care continuum and are considered safe to continue with concurrent RT. Radionuclide therapies have little data in the setting of concurrent external beam RT. In our practice, we consider the radiation dose to normal tissue from radionuclide therapies to be negligible and do not account for such dose or alter standard normal tissue constraints when planning RT. Cellular therapies are most used in blood cancers. There is little data on the combination of RT and cellular therapies. Given the generally radiosensitive nature of blood cancers, conventionally fractionated palliative dosing of RT is often appropriate (Table 12.1).

References

1. Merrill J, Greco FA, Zimbler H, Brereton HD, Lamberg JD, Pomeroy TC. Adriamycin and radiation: synegistic cardiotoxicity. Ann Intern Med. 1975;82(1):122–3.
2. Greco FA, Brereton HD, Kent H, Zimbler H, Merrill J, Johnson RE. Adriamycin and enhanced radiation reaction in normal esophagus and skin. Ann Intern Med. 1976;85(3):294–8.
3. Aristizabal SA, Miller RC, Schlichtemeier AL, Jones SE, Boone ML. Adriamycin-irradiation cutaneous complications. Int J Radiat Oncol Biol Phys. 1977;2(3–4):325–31.
4. Blomqvist C, Tiusanen K, Elomaa I, Rissanen P, Hietanen T, Heinonen E, et al. The combination of radiotherapy, adjuvant chemotherapy (cyclophosphamide-doxorubicin-ftorafur) and tamoxifen in stage II breast cancer. Long-term follow-up results of a randomised trial. Br J Cancer. 1992;66(6):1171–6.
5. Fiets WE, van Helvoirt RP, Nortier JWR, van der Tweel I, Struikmans H. Acute toxicity of concurrent adjuvant radiotherapy and chemotherapy (CMF or AC) in breast cancer patients. A prospective, comparative, non-randomised study. Eur J Cancer. 2003;39(8):1081–8.
6. Pisters PWT, Ballo MT, Fenstermacher MJ, Feig BW, Hunt KK, Raymond KA, et al. Phase I trial of preoperative concurrent doxorubicin and radiation therapy, surgical resection, and

intraoperative electron-beam radiation therapy for patients with localized retroperitoneal sarcoma. J Clin Oncol. 2003;21(16):3092–7.
7. Romesser PB, Sherman EJ, Whiting K, Ho ML, Shaha AR, Sabra MM, et al. Intensity-modulated radiation therapy and doxorubicin in thyroid cancer: a prospective phase 2 trial. Cancer. 2021;127(22):4161–70.
8. D'angio GJ, Farber S, Maddock CL. Potentiation of x-ray effects by actinomycin D. Radiology. 1959;73:175–7.
9. D'angio GJ. Clinical and biologic studies of actinomycin D and roentgen irradiation. Am J Roentgenol Radium Therapy, Nucl Med. 1962;87:106–9.
10. Pearson D, Deakin DP, Hendry JH, Moore JV. The interaction of actinomycin D and radiation. Int J Radiat Oncol Biol Phys. 1978;4(1–2):71–3.
11. Liebner EJ. Actinomycin D and radiation therapy. Am J Roentgenol Radium Therapy, Nucl Med. 1962;87:94–105.
12. Redpath JL, Colman M. The effect of adriamycin and actinomycin D on radiation-induced skin reactions in mouse feet. Int J Radiat Oncol Biol Phys. 1979;5(4):483–6.
13. Concannon JP, Dalbow MH, Hagemann RF, Frich JC, Hodgson SE, Weil CS, et al. Radiation and actinomycin D mortality studies in C57BL 6 mice. II. Combined treatment and gastrointestinal lethality. Cancer. 1973;32(3):553–61.
14. Phillips TL, Wharam MD, Margolis LW. Modification of radiation injury to normal tissues by chemotherapeutic agents. Cancer. 1975;35(6):1678–84.
15. Concannon JP, Summers RE, King J, Tcherkow G, Cole C, Rogow E. Enhancement of x-ray effects on the small intestinal epithelium of dogs by actinomycin D. Am J Roentgenol Radium Therapy, Nucl Med. 1969;105(1):126–36.
16. Rich TA, Shepard RC, Mosley ST. Four decades of continuing innovation with fluorouracil: current and future approaches to fluorouracil chemoradiation therapy. J Clin Oncol. 2004;22(11):2214–32.
17. Mornex F, Girard N. Gemcitabine and radiation therapy in non-small cell lung cancer: state of the art. Ann Oncol. 2006;17(12):1743–7.
18. Blackstock AW, Lesser GJ, Fletcher-Steede J, Case LD, Tucker RW, Russo SM, et al. Phase I study of twice-weekly gemcitabine and concurrent thoracic radiation for patients with locally advanced non-small-cell lung cancer. Int J Radiat Oncol Biol Phys. 2001;51(5):1281–9.
19. Crane C, Janjan N, Evans D, Wolff R, Ballo M, Milas L, et al. Toxicity and efficacy of concurrent gemcitabine and radiotherapy for locally advanced pancreatic cancer. Int J Gastrointest Cancer. 2001;29(1):9–18.
20. Takeda K, Negoro S, Kudoh S, Okishio K, Masuda N, Takada M, et al. Phase I/II study of weekly irinotecan and concurrent radiation therapy for locally advanced non-small cell lung cancer. Br J Cancer. 1999;79(9–10):1462–7.
21. Choy H, Chakravarthy A, Devore RF, Jagasia M, Hande KR, Roberts JR, et al. Weekly irinotecan and concurrent radiation therapy for stage III unresectable NSCLC. Oncology (Williston Park). 2000;14(7 Suppl 5):43–6.
22. Vaugier L, Mirabel X, Martel-Lafay I, Racadot S, Carrie C, Vendrely V, et al. Radiosensitizing chemotherapy (Irinotecan) with stereotactic body radiation therapy for the treatment of inoperable liver and/or lung metastases of colorectal cancer. Cancers (Basel). 2021;13(2):248.
23. Satoh Y, Shirai K, Kitamoto Y, Higuchi K, Tamaki Y, Hokamura S. Efficacy and toxicity of weekly low dose docetaxel with concurrent radiotherapy in patients with esophageal cancer - interim analysis of phase I/II study. Int J Radiat Oncol Biol Phys. 2008;72(1):S271–2.
24. Patil VM, Noronha V, Menon N, Singh A, Ghosh-Laskar S, Budrukkar A, et al. Results of phase III randomized trial for use of Docetaxel as a Radiosensitizer in patients with head and neck cancer, unsuitable for Cisplatin-based chemoradiation. J Clin Oncol. 2023;41(13):2350–61.
25. Guimond E, Tsai CJ, Hosni A, O'Kane G, Yang J, Barry A. Safety and tolerability of metastasis-directed radiation therapy in the era of evolving systemic, immune, and targeted therapies. Adv Radiat Oncol. 2022;7(6):101022.

26. Kroeze SGC, Pavic M, Stellamans K, Lievens Y, Becherini C, Scorsetti M, et al. Metastases-directed stereotactic body radiotherapy in combination with targeted therapy or immunotherapy: systematic review and consensus recommendations by the EORTC-ESTRO OligoCare consortium. Lancet Oncol. 2023;24(3):e121–32.
27. Barney BM, Markovic SN, Laack NN, Miller RC, Sarkaria JN, Macdonald OK, et al. Increased bowel toxicity in patients treated with a vascular endothelial growth factor inhibitor (VEGFI) after stereotactic body radiation therapy (SBRT). Int J Radiat Oncol Biol Phys. 2013;87(1):73–80.
28. Haseltine JM, Rimner A, Gelblum DY, Modh A, Rosenzweig KE, Jackson A, et al. Fatal complications after stereotactic body radiation therapy for central lung tumors abutting the proximal bronchial tree. Pract Radiat Oncol. 2016;6(2):e27–33.
29. Wang C, Rimner A, Gelblum DY, Flynn J, Jackson A, Yorke E, et al. Analysis of toxic effects with antiangiogenic agents plus stereotactic body radiation in ultracentral lung tumors. JAMA Oncol. 2019;5(5):737–9.
30. Kim N, Choi SH, Chang JS, Kim YT, Kim SW, Kim GM, et al. Use of bevacizumab before or after radiotherapy increases the risk of fistula formation in patients with cervical cancer. Int J Gynecol Cancer. 2021;31(1):59–65.
31. Zhai Y, Hui Z, Wang J, Zou S, Liang J, Wang X, et al. Concurrent erlotinib and radiotherapy for chemoradiotherapy-intolerant esophageal squamous cell carcinoma patients: results of a pilot study. Dis Esophagus. 2013;26(5):503–9.
32. Xu Y, Zheng Y, Sun X, Yu X, Gu J, Wu W, et al. Concurrent radiotherapy with gefitinib in elderly patients with esophageal squamous cell carcinoma: preliminary results of a phase II study. Oncotarget. 2015;6(35):38429–39.
33. Martínez E, Martínez M, Rico M, Hernández B, Casas F, Viñolas N, et al. Feasibility, tolerability, and efficacy of the concurrent addition of erlotinib to thoracic radiotherapy in locally advanced unresectable non-small-cell lung cancer: a phase II trial. Onco Targets Ther. 2016;9:1057–66.
34. Jia W, Guo H, Jing W, Jing X, Li J, Wang M, et al. An especially high rate of radiation pneumonitis observed in patients treated with thoracic radiotherapy and simultaneous osimertinib. Radiother Oncol. 2020;152:96–100.
35. Iyengar P, Kavanagh BD, Wardak Z, Smith I, Ahn C, Gerber DE, et al. Phase II trial of stereotactic body radiation therapy combined with erlotinib for patients with limited but progressive metastatic non-small-cell lung cancer. J Clin Oncol. 2014;32(34):3824–30.
36. Kroeze SGC, Fritz C, Schaule J, Blanck O, Kahl KH, Kaul D, et al. Continued versus interrupted targeted therapy during metastasis-directed stereotactic radiotherapy: a retrospective multi-center safety and efficacy analysis. Cancers (Basel). 2021;13(19):4780.
37. Anker CJ, Ribas A, Grossmann AH, Chen X, Narra KK, Akerley W, et al. Severe liver and skin toxicity after radiation and vemurafenib in metastatic melanoma. J Clin Oncol. 2013;31(17):e283–7.
38. Hecht M, Zimmer L, Loquai C, Weishaupt C, Gutzmer R, Schuster B, et al. Radiosensitization by BRAF inhibitor therapy-mechanism and frequency of toxicity in melanoma patients. Ann Oncol. 2015;26(6):1238–44.
39. Anker CJ, Grossmann KF, Atkins MB, Suneja G, Tarhini AA, Kirkwood JM. Avoiding severe toxicity from combined BRAF inhibitor and radiation treatment: consensus guidelines from the Eastern Cooperative Oncology Group (ECOG). Int J Radiat Oncol Biol Phys. 2016;95(2):632–46.
40. Miller JA, Balagamwala EH, Angelov L, Suh JH, Rini B, Garcia JA, et al. Spine stereotactic radiosurgery with concurrent tyrosine kinase inhibitors for metastatic renal cell carcinoma. J Neurosurg Spine. 2016;25(6):766–74.
41. Welsh JW, Tang C, de Groot P, Naing A, Hess KR, Heymach JV, et al. Phase II trial of Ipilimumab with stereotactic radiation therapy for metastatic disease: outcomes, toxicities, and low-dose radiation-related Abscopal responses. Cancer Immunol Res. 2019;7(12):1903–9.

42. Tang C, Welsh JW, de Groot P, Massarelli E, Chang JY, Hess KR, et al. Ipilimumab with stereotactic ablative radiation therapy: phase I results and immunologic correlates from peripheral T cells. Clin Cancer Res. 2017;23(6):1388–96.
43. Sundahl N, De Wolf K, Kruse V, Meireson A, Reynders D, Goetghebeur E, et al. Phase 1 dose escalation trial of Ipilimumab and stereotactic body radiation therapy in metastatic melanoma. Int J Radiat Oncol Biol Phys. 2018;100(4):906–15.
44. Luke JJ, Lemons JM, Karrison TG, Pitroda SP, Melotek JM, Zha Y, et al. Safety and clinical activity of Pembrolizumab and multisite stereotactic body radiotherapy in patients with advanced solid tumors. J Clin Oncol. 2018;36(16):1611–8.
45. Theelen WSME, Peulen HMU, Lalezari F, van der Noort V, de Vries JF, Aerts JGJV, et al. Effect of Pembrolizumab after stereotactic body radiotherapy vs Pembrolizumab alone on tumor response in patients with advanced non-small cell lung cancer: results of the PEMBRO-RT phase 2 randomized clinical trial. JAMA Oncol. 2019;5(9):1276–82.
46. McBride S, Sherman E, Tsai CJ, Baxi S, Aghalar J, Eng J, et al. Randomized phase II trial of Nivolumab with stereotactic body radiotherapy versus Nivolumab alone in metastatic head and neck squamous cell carcinoma. J Clin Oncol. 2021;39(1):30–7.
47. Masini C, Iotti C, De Giorgi U, Bellia RS, Buti S, Salaroli F, et al. Nivolumab in combination with stereotactic body radiotherapy in pretreated patients with metastatic renal cell carcinoma. Results of the phase II NIVES study. Eur Urol. 2022;81(3):274–82.
48. Kwan EM, Spain L, Anton A, Gan CL, Garrett L, Chang D, et al. Avelumab combined with stereotactic ablative body radiotherapy in metastatic Castration-resistant prostate cancer: the phase 2 ICE-PAC clinical trial. Eur Urol. 2022;81(3):253–62.
49. Salvestrini V, Kim K, Caini S, Alkner S, Ekholm M, Skyttä T, et al. Safety profile of trastuzumab-emtansine (T-DM1) with concurrent radiation therapy: a systematic review and meta-analysis. Radiother Oncol. 2023;186:109805.

Chapter 13
Genomic Biomarkers to Guide the Management of Spine Metastases

Gustav Cederquist and Adam Schmitt

Abbreviations

cfDNA	Cell-free DNA
ctDNA	Circulating tumor DNA
DDR	DNA damage response pathway
DNA	Deoxyribonucleic acid
DSB	Double-strand DNA break
EBV	Epstein Barr Virus
HR	Hormone Receptor
MAPK	Mitogen-activated protein kinase signaling pathway
NOMS	Neurologic, oncologic, mechanical, systemic framework
PI3K	Phosphoinositide 3-kinase signaling pathway
RAS	Rat sarcoma virus pathway
SBRT	Stereotactic body radiotherapy
SNP	Single-nucleotide polymorphism
SRS	Stereotactic radiosurgery
TKI	Tyrosine kinase inhibitor
WNT	Wingless/integrated signaling pathway

Introduction

15–40% of cancer patients will develop spine metastases [1–3]. Among these patients, the incidence of epidural spinal cord compression is estimated to be 5–10% [1, 4]. Advances in systemic therapy over the past few decades have significantly

G. Cederquist · A. Schmitt (✉)
Department of Radiation Oncology, Memorial Sloan Kettering Cancer Center, New York, NY, USA
e-mail: cederqug@mskcc.org; schmitta@mskcc.org

Y. Yamada et al. (eds.), *Multidisciplinary Spine Tumor Management*,
https://doi.org/10.1007/978-3-032-07519-2_13

improved the overall prognosis and survival for many subgroups of cancer patients. As patients live longer with spine metastases, the risk of progression to pain or functional neurologic deficit increases [5]. Therefore, achieving durable local tumor control in the spine, while minimizing treatment-related morbidity, is becoming increasingly important.

The management of metastatic spine disease has evolved into an integrated multidisciplinary specialty [6]. The transformative pillars underlying metastatic spine oncology are (1) stereotactic radiosurgery (SRS) which allows for the precise delivery of ablative doses of ionizing radiation to vertebral and epidural targets; (2) minimally invasive surgical approaches resulting in reduced treatment related morbidity and improved outcomes; and (3) targeted systemic therapies and immunotherapies which have substantially improved the overall prognosis of patients with metastatic disease. The integration of these therapeutic advances into a unified management approach is supported by the neurologic, oncologic, mechanical, systemic (NOMS) framework [7]. The NOMS framework extracts critical clinical factors from these 4 domains to arrive at a coherent and consistent treatment decision.

In addition to providing a coherent treatment paradigm, the NOMS framework is flexible and allows for the continued integration of new knowledge and treatment approaches. The NOMS framework achieves this by asking the clinician to evaluate its four domains within the context of current clinical practice, rather than scoring static clinical factors. For example, whereas HER2 amplified breast cancers were initially associated with poor overall prognosis, the development of HER2 targeted agents has substantially improved outcomes [8, 9]. The NOMS framework can accommodate this new knowledge without changing its core structure.

Advances in genomic sequencing technology have unlocked new biology and therapeutic inroads for the treatment of metastatic disease. The widespread use of tumor sequencing has revolutionized cancer care [10]. The use of genomic biomarkers in spine oncology is only in its infancy, and an important question moving forward is how best to incorporate tumor genetic profile into the NOMS framework. Here, we will discuss how genomic data has been and can be utilized in the treatment of spinal metastases. Broadly, tumor mutational profiles can be used as biomarkers of (1) overall prognosis and risk stratification, (2) therapeutic sensitivity to radiotherapy, and (3) direct targets of systemic therapy. We envision that the development of liquid biopsy technologies, especially circulating tumor DNA (ctDNA) and cell-free DNA (cfDNA), will greatly enhance the ability to assess tumor genetic profiles, extent of metastatic disease, treatment response, and normal tissue toxicity.

The Biology of Metastatic Spread to the Spine

Observations by Oscar Batson in 1940 noted that prostate cancer tends to spread to the lumbar spine, sacrum, and iliac wings through a communicating venous plexus [11]. This seminal observation linked metastatic spread to the spine through hematogenous anatomical routes. This notion was further corroborated by an extensive autopsy study of 1885 prostate cancer patients, which identified the lumbar spine to be frequently involved in cases of single organ metastatic involvement, suggesting the venous connection between the prostate gland and lumbar spine is a conduit for metastatic spread [12]. However, while hematogenous routes clearly influence patterns of metastatic spread to the spine, this is not the entire story.

Prior to Batson's work, Stephen Paget reported on necropsy studies of 735 breast cancer patients in the year 1889. Like Batson, Paget observed that the patterns of metastatic tumor spread were not random. For example, breast cancer cells had a predilection for the liver and bone. Paget also noted, however, that the pattern of metastatic seeding could not be described solely by the hematogenous connections between organs [13]. These observations led to the well-known "seed and soil" hypothesis that posits that metastatic colonization requires a receptive host organ; non-receptive host organs limit metastatic spread, resulting in the observed non-random, organotropic pattern of metastatic spread. More recent analyses of the patterns of metastatic spread have identified apparent metastatic subtypes even within the same tumor histology. For example, radio-recurrent prostate cancer relapses in discrete anatomical patterns that include local-regional, lymphotropic, osteotropic, and multi-organ/visceral, each with a different prognosis [14]. Similarly, a subset of metastatic breast cancer patients will present with bone-only disease, which carries a more favorable prognosis than those with visceral-only disease [15]. Finally, while soft tissue sarcomas tend to metastasize to the lung, 17% of patients with myxoid liposarcoma will develop bone metastasis. Among these patients, bone is typically the first site of metastatic involvement, suggesting a distinct underlying biological program [16].

What accounts for the osteotropic nature of certain tumors? One hypothesis is that metastatic tumors may evolve specific driver mutations that confer tropism to the bone. Barzilai and colleagues examined the tumor genetic profile of spine tumor samples using a targeted next-generation sequencing panel, MSK-IMPACT [17]. Interestingly, greater than 95% concordance in driver mutations was observed between spine metastasis samples and with either the primary tumor or an additional metastatic site [18]. The high concordance argues against the hypothesis that specific osteotropic tumor mutations evolve during the course of tumor progression. This appears to be true more broadly; large-scale sequencing of matched primary and metastatic samples reveals little heterogeneity at the single gene level [19, 20].

On the other hand, a recent study by Nguyen et al. used MSK-IMPACT to profile over 25,000 metastatic tumor samples and evaluated for genetic changes that correlate with organ-specific metastasis [21]. The study was able to identify certain genetic alterations enriched in patients with bone metastasis. For example, among breast cancer patients, hormone receptor (HR) positive/HER2-amplification negative samples were associated with bone metastasis compared with HR negative/HER2-amplification positive. Among prostate cancer patients, amplification of the androgen receptor was associated with bone metastasis, while the ERG1-fusion was found less frequently in bone metastasis. Among patients with papillary thyroid cancer, chromosome-level deletion of 22q was enriched among bone metastases, while mutations in BRAF were found less frequently in bone metastases. Thus, specific tumor genetic mutations are associated with a bone metastasis phenotype. These mutations do not appear to evolve during the course of tumor progression and are likely present from an early stage during tumorigenesis.

In addition to the tumor genetic profile, the local tumor microenvironment within the bone plays a key role in metastatic colonization and growth. The bone metastasis microenvironment has been the subject of multiple recent excellent reviews and will only be discussed briefly here [22, 23]. A key finding is that the bone microenvironment supports metastasis growth through specific signaling interactions. For example, osteogenic cells secrete hepatocyte growth factor (HGF) to promote prostate cancer bone metastasis, implicating MET-HGF signaling in bone metastasis development [24]. The proteinases ADAMTS1 and MMP1 are released in a paracrine manner from the bone microenvironment to cleave Epidermal growth factor (EGF)-like growth factors and promote an osteolytic signaling cascade that promotes metastatic growth through the EGF receptor (EGFR) [25]. Both the HGF-MET and EGFR signaling pathways are therapeutically targetable.

In summary, anatomic routes of hematogenous spread, tumor genetic profile, and signaling from the bone microenvironment all contribute to the development of bone metastasis. It is notable that genetic variants associated with bone metastasis appear to be lineage-specific. Thus, genetic drivers of bone metastasis are not universal, but rather context-dependent. The successful integration of genetic biomarkers into the management of metastatic spine disease may differ based on tumor lineage and microenvironment. Signaling interactions between the tumor cells and the bone microenvironment could serve as druggable targets for systemic therapy.

Integrating Genomic Biomarkers into the Management of Metastatic Spine Tumors

Overall Prognosis and Risk Stratification

To date, the major impact of tumor genetics in the management of spine metastasis has been the improved overall survival of select molecular subgroups of patients. For example, in 2001, the addition of the HER2-targeted monoclonal antibody, trastuzumab, to chemotherapy for metastatic breast cancer patients increased 1-year overall survival from 22% to 33% [8]. In 2018, the addition of tucatinib, a HER2-targeting tyrosine kinase inhibitor (TKI), to capecitabine and trastuzumab for pretreated HER2-positive patients resulted in an improved 2-year overall survival from 27% to 45% [9]. Treatment of advanced EGFR-mutant non-small cell lung adenocarcinoma with Osimertinib, a third-generation TKI targeting EGFR, improved median overall survival from 32 to 39 months when compared to older-generation TKIs [9]. The use of combined BRAF and MEK inhibitors in BRAF-mutated metastatic melanoma has led to a 5-year overall survival rate of 34% [26]. Per the NOMS framework, patients harboring genetic mutations targetable with highly active drugs should be considered for spine interventions that maximize local tumor control.

Genetic Biomarkers of Radiosensitivity

The widespread adoption of tumor genetic profiling has allowed for the identification of tumor mutations that are associated with radiosensitivity (Table 13.1). In the era of SRS, it is now possible to deliver ablative doses that overcome intrinsic

Table 13.1 Genetic biomarkers of radiation sensitivity

Mutated gene	Class	Effect	Known function/possible mechanism
ATM [34, 35]	DNA Damage Repair	Radiosensitivity	DNA double strand break repair [31–33]
NBN [39]	DNA Damage Repair	Radioresistance (copy number gain)	DNA double strand break repair ATM signaling
RAD51 [41, 42]	DNA Damage Repair	Radiosensitivity	DNA double strand break repair ATM signaling
Ku70/Ku 80 [41, 42]	DNA Damage Repair	Radiosensitivity	DNA double strand break repair ATM signaling [43]
TP53 [47–50]	DNA Damage Repair	Radioresistance	DNA repair Altered cell senescence [51]
KEAP1 [45, 56, 57]	Oxidative Stress Response	Radioresistance	Negative regulation of NRF2 [55]
NRF2 [45, 56, 57]	Oxidative Stress Response	Radioresistance	Cellular resistance to oxidants
STK11 [58]	Oxidative Stress Response	Radioresistance	Elevated NRF2 signaling
PIK3CA [59]	Intracellular Signaling	Radioresistance	Regulation of PI3K signaling
AKT2 [44]	Intracellular Signaling	Radioresistance	Regulation of PI3K signaling
KRAS [62–65]	Intracellular Signaling	Radioresistance	Regulation of RAS signaling Regulation of DNA Repair [67, 68] Stem cell identity [69]
APC [72–74]	Intracellular Signaling	Radioresistance	Regulation of WNT signaling Stem cell identity [73] Regulation of DNA Repair [74]

radioresistance and achieve durable local tumor control, regardless of tumor histology [27]. Still, SRS is associated with treatment-related toxicities, including vertebral compression fracture, complex pain flare, and even rare but significant instances of neuropathy or myelopathy [28]. The identification of genetic markers of radiosensitivity may facilitate the de-escalation of radiotherapy dose that would reduce treatment-related morbidity.

The strongest evidence for genetic biomarkers of radiosensitivity comes from the study of the DNA damage response (DDR) pathway. Ionizing radiation primarily exerts its tumoricidal effect through DNA double-strand break, which can lead to various forms of cell death or senescence [29]. Mutations in DDR signaling inhibit or activate repair of radiation-induced DNA damage and thus alter radiosensitivity. Ataxia-telangiectasia mutated (ATM) kinase senses DNA double-stranded breaks (DSB) and subsequently promotes BRCA1 recruitment, DNA end processing, and cell cycle checkpoint regulation [30]. Human mutations in *ATM* lead to increased radiosensitivity *in vitro* [31–33]. Monoallelic and biallelic *ATM* loss-of-function mutations have been associated with 40% to 80% reductions in local failure after radiotherapy, suggesting profound radiosensitization [34, 35].

Additional molecular alterations in the ATM pathway have also been associated with altered radiosensitivity. Increased protein expression of MRE11, which activates ATM, was shown to be associated with improved disease-specific survival after chemoradiotherapy for bladder cancer [36–38]. Copy number gain of *NBN*, which is associated with MRE11 as part of the MRN complex, was shown to be associated with worse outcomes after prostate radiotherapy [39]. Decreased expression of BRCA1, BRCA2, and RAD51, proteins involved in double-strand break repair, has been associated with improved response to breast radiotherapy [40]. Specific single-nucleotide polymorphisms (SNPs) in *RAD51*, along with *Ku70* and *Ku80*, proteins that bind to DNA double-strand break ends, have been associated with increased radiosensitivity in cervical and breast cancer [41, 42]. Overexpression of *LRRC31*, which interacts with Ku70 and Ku80 and inhibits DNA repair, was shown to sensitize breast cancer cells to radiotherapy in a mouse model [43].

Beyond the ATM pathway, DDR mutations may more broadly impact tumor radiosensitivity. Tumor radiosensitivity was assessed among patients with locally advanced lung cancer who received definitive chemoradiation or postoperative radiotherapy. Patients were stratified by the presence of any mutation in a broad panel of DDR genes. Patients harboring a DDR mutation had significantly improved local-regional tumor control compared to those without a DDR pathway mutation [44, 45]. Zhao et al developed a 24-gene panel of DDR pathway mutations called Post-Operative Radiation Therapy Outcomes Score (PORTOS). Patients with a high PORTOS score who received postoperative prostate radiotherapy had a reduced rate of metastasis at 10 years compared to those with a high score who did not receive postoperative radiotherapy [46].

Mutations in *TP53*, a tumor suppressor that senses DNA damage and regulates progression through the cell cycle, have been associated with worse outcomes after radiotherapy for head and neck cancer [47]. *In vitro* studies across numerous cell types suggest that mutant *TP53* status leads to radioresistance [48–50] and may occur by inhibiting radiation-induced senescence [51]. However, other studies have found no association between *TP53* mutation status and radiosensitivity [52, 53]. A survey of radiosensitivity across 39 tumor cell lines showed substantial variability between *TP53* mutation status and radiosensitivity [54]. Therefore, the clinical impact of *TP53* mutation status on radiotherapy response may be context dependent or related to a generally more aggressive disease course.

Radiation-induced DNA damage is mediated by reactive oxygen species, which are generated through the ionization of water molecules. The KEAP1-NRF2 axis is a key regulator of the oxidative stress response. NRF2 is a transcription factor that upregulates anti-oxidant genes, while KEAP1 is an adaptor protein that regulates the stability of the NRF2 protein product [55]. Using a lung squamous cell cancer mouse model, Jeong et al. found that abrogating the KEAP1-NRF2 pathway conferred tumor cells with a radioresistant and oxidative damage-resistant phenotype [56]. The association with radioresistance has been replicated in multiple clinical cohorts [45, 56, 57]. Mutations in STK11/LKB1 have been shown to associate with increased local regional recurrence risk of inoperable non-small cell lung cancer treated with radiotherapy. The clinical observation of radioresistance was validated *in vitro* and mechanistically depended on NRF2 signaling [58].

Multiple intracellular signaling pathways have been linked to altered radiosensitivity. The Phosphoinositide 3-kinase (PI3K) signaling pathway regulates diverse cellular functions, including metabolism, growth, differentiation, and proliferation. Mutations in components of the PI3K signaling pathway, including *PIK3CA* and *AKT2*, have been associated with radioresistance in primary lung tumors [44, 59]. Inhibitors of PI3K can serve as radiosensitizing agents by suppressing DDR signaling [60]. However, PI3K inhibition did not lead to radiosensitization in head and neck squamous cell carcinoma lines, suggesting its role is context dependent [61].

The Rat Sarcoma Virus (RAS) signaling pathway, like PI3K, controls diverse cellular functions including cell growth, proliferation, differentiation, and motility. Mutations in *KRAS* have been associated with inferior local control after radiotherapy for non-small cell lung cancer [62, 63], liver metastases [64], and rectal cancer [65]. Early studies provided proof of concept data that activation of the RAS path way *in vitro*, via N-RAS or K-RAS oncogenic mutations, directly leads to radioresistance [66]. Oncogenic RAS signaling may lead to radioresistance via enhanced DDR activity [67, 68]. An alternative mechanism of RAS-mediated radioresistance is the induction of a stem-cell-like state [69]. It is unclear which RAS downstream pathway mediates the radioresistance phenotype; EGFR, PI3K-AKT, and mitogen-activated protein kinase (MAPK) pathways have all been implicated [67, 70, 71].

A recent study found that a high proportion of patients who experienced local failure after separation surgery and stereotactic body radiotherapy (SBRT) harbored mutations in the *Adenomatous polyposis coli (APC)* gene [72]. APC is a negative regulator of Wingless/integrated (WNT)-b-catenin pathway, thus implicating WNT signaling in radiosensitivity. WNT signaling has been shown to promote radioresistance via induction of a stem cell-like phenotype and by activation of the DNA repair protein DNA Ligase 4 (LIG4) [73, 74].

In summary, there are a number of genetic mutations that have been associated with altered radiosensitivity, many of which impact DDR signaling or related pathways. It appears that the impact of an individual genetic mutation may depend on disease context and cellular lineage. Whether genetic mutations or gene-expression-based radiosensitivity indexes [75, 76] can be used to guide radiotherapy dosing awaits prospective clinical validation.

Targeted Systemic Therapy for Local Spine Tumor Control

Historically, the efficacy of systemic and targeted therapies for local tumor control in bone has been limited [77–79]. An exception is the drug cabozantanib; cabozantanib is a multi-kinase inhibitor targeting VEGF, c-MET, and RET, and appears to exhibit strong activity against bone metastases. In phase II and III trials evaluating cabozantanib in the treatment of metastatic castrate resistant prostate cancer, the drug demonstrated an unprecedented 42–68% response rate on bone scan [80, 81]. The identification of genetic mutations and kinase pathways that modulate radiosensitivity opens possibilities for drug plus radiotherapy combinations. Combined modality therapy may allow dose reduction near the spinal cord while improving out-of-field tumor control in the spine. The development of such agents would require careful phase I studies to demonstrate safety and establish dosing, while ideally demonstrating pharmacokinetic properties in bone.

The Use of Circulating Tumor DNA in the Management of Spine Metastasis

CtDNA and cfDNA are fragments of genomic DNA released by tumor or normal cells, respectively, into the circulation. ctDNA and cDNA are typically released during the process of cell death [82]. They can be isolated from blood and sequenced using techniques that are optimized for the detection of low-abundance fragments. The ability to detect ctDNA can serve as a "liquid biopsy," where it is possible to detect tumor genomic DNA through a simple blood draw, rather than an interventional or surgical biopsy. There are at least five clinical applications for ctDNA, which include screening and early detection, real-time monitoring of therapy, estimating the risk of relapse, risk stratification for therapeutic intervention, and identification of actionable genetic mutations [83]. In a broad sense, each of these could be relevant to a patient with spine metastases. Here we discuss specific applications of ctDNA and cfDNA in the management of spine metastases.

1. *Identification of tumor genetic profile at the time of spine metastasis.* Since metastatic progression is a late phenomenon, biopsies obtained at the time of spine metastasis may have evolved a different mutational profile than a biopsy from

early oncogenesis. A large sequencing study that analyzed 2658 pan-cancer whole genomes identified that 40% of patients exhibit mutational spectrum changes over time [84]. Liquid biopsy, by virtue of being less invasive than surgical or interventional biopsy, can be obtained at multiple time points during a patient's cancer diagnosis and treatment; ctDNA obtained at the time of spine metastasis development may more accurately represent the current tumor mutational profile than sequencing from an earlier interventional biopsy. Tumor mutations identified through liquid biopsy could be used to predict response to radiotherapy. In the phase II ORIOLE trial that evaluated SBRT versus observation for patients with metastatic prostate cancer, ctDNA identified a set of high-risk genetic variants that were associated with reduced progression-free survival [85]. Similarly, ctDNA could be used to identify resistance mutations to systemic and targeted therapy. One limitation of liquid biopsy is that many of the genetic changes that occur during tumor progression are genome-level changes, such as copy number alterations and structural variants, which cannot be detected through ctDNA sequencing.

2. *Stratification of oligometastatic spine disease versus disseminated metastasis.* The radiotherapeutic dosing for spine metastases, in part, depends on the extent of metastatic disease. The phase III PISA trial showed that among patients with oligometastatic disease, dose escalation to 24 Gray (Gy) in a single fraction improved both local control and the risk of distant progression compared with 27 Gy in three fractions [86]. Over 50% of patients in the PISA study had disease in the spine, and over 50% of patients had a single metastatic site. Thus, patients with spine metastasis who have limited metastatic disease benefit from high-dose radiotherapy. In patients with disseminated metastatic disease, the importance of local control is overshadowed by the competing risk of distant progression. Currently, oligometastatic disease is defined radiographically by the number of discrete lesions. ctDNA has been shown to correlate well with overall tumor burden in patients with metastatic breast cancer [87], melanoma [88], and non-small cell lung cancer [89, 90]. In addition, ctDNA can identify patients at risk of relapse after definitive therapy [91, 92]. Together, these data suggest that ctDNA could be used to identify spine metastasis patients with a lower risk of systemic progression and who may benefit from oligometastasis-directed therapy [93].
3. *Determining the local treatment response of spine tumors:* Spine SRS provides high rates of local tumor control, but can be associated with treatment-related toxicity [28]. Therefore, treatment de-escalation would be preferable if excellent local control can be maintained; treatment de-escalation may be especially attractive for patients undergoing re-irradiation where the risks of normal tissue toxicity are higher. Liquid biopsy may offer an opportunity to assess treatment response during radiotherapy [94]. The half-life of ctDNA in circulation is estimated to be 35–140 minutes, based on clearance studies after surgical tumor resection [95–97]. This rapid clearance enables ctDNA to act as a biomarker of treatment response. Studies in nasopharyngeal carcinoma have shown that Epstein Barr virus (EBV) ctDNA decreases during the course of definitive radio-

therapy [98]. Interestingly, the half-life in this study was 3.8 days, which is substantially longer than observed after surgical resection and may reflect the biology of cell killing by ionizing radiation. Both the kinetics of ctDNA decline and the clearance of ctDNA by the end of radiotherapy have been shown to be prognostic for disease recurrence [99, 100]. Thus, assessment of ctDNA kinetics or clearance during spine radiotherapy may provide a marker of early treatment response that could lead to treatment de-escalation or intensification.

4. *Determining the risk of spinal cord injury from radiotherapy***.** Like tumors, healthy cells can also release DNA into the circulation under conditions of stress and cell death. For example, increased cfDNA is found after exercise overtraining [101], trauma [102], and spinal cord injury [103]. It is possible to determine the tissue of origin of cfDNA by epigenetic profiling of the DNA fragments [104, 105]. Methylation-based profiling has successfully been used to detect cfDNA from patients with inflammatory, ischemic, or traumatic brain injury [106]. This suggests a similar strategy could potentially be used to identify patients at risk for the development of myelopathy or neuropathy after spine SRS; it may be that low levels of spinal cord cfDNA will predict clinical myelopathy, just as ctDNA predicts disease recurrence. As proof of concept, methylation profiles of cfDNA were able to detect cardiac injury from DNA-damaging cancer therapy released from cardiomyocytes and were associated with subsequent cardiac dysfunction [107].

Conclusions

The development of targeted systemic agents, as well as other novel treatment strategies such as immunotherapy, has drastically improved the overall prognosis of cancer patients. As such, patients are living longer with spine metastases. For these patients, the importance of durable local control in the spine, functional preservation, and low treatment-related morbidity is critical to maintaining health-related quality of life. The development of spine SRS and minimally invasive surgical approaches has already accelerated the field of spine oncology toward this goal. DNA sequencing technologies offer further opportunity to tailor treatment based on a patient's individual tumor genomic profile. Tumor sequencing can identify actionable genetic mutations for selection of systemic therapy and may be able to guide radiotherapy dosing. Liquid biopsy is an emerging technology that is likely to revolutionize the field of precision oncology. Sequencing of ctDNA and cfDNA will potentially allow the serial detection of tumor mutations, identification of oligometastatic spine disease, treatment response after spine surgery and radiotherapy, and early detection of radiation-associated myelopathy or neuropathy. To translate into routine clinical practice, these novel concepts will require prospective clinical validation.

References

1. Van den Brande R, Cornips EM, Peeters M, Ost P, Billiet C, Van de Kelft E. Epidemiology of spinal metastases, metastatic epidural spinal cord compression and pathologic vertebral compression fractures in patients with solid tumors: a systematic review. J Bone Oncol. 2022;35:100446.
2. Wong DA, Fornasier VL, MacNab I. Spinal metastases: the obvious, the occult, and the impostors. Spine (Phila Pa 1976). 1990;15(1):1–4.
3. Cobb CA 3rd, Leavens ME, Eckles N. Indications for nonoperative treatment of spinal cord compression due to breast cancer. J Neurosurg. 1977;47(5):653–8.
4. Bach F, Larsen BH, Rohde K, Borgesen SE, Gjerris F, Boge-Rasmussen T, et al. Metastatic spinal cord compression. Occurrence, symptoms, clinical presentations and prognosis in 398 patients with spinal cord compression. Acta Neurochir (Wien). 1990;107(1–2):37–43.
5. Helweg-Larsen S, Sorensen PS. Symptoms and signs in metastatic spinal cord compression: a study of progression from first symptom until diagnosis in 153 patients. Eur J Cancer. 1994;30A(3):396–8.
6. Barzilai O, Fisher CG, Bilsky MH. State of the art treatment of spinal metastatic disease. Neurosurgery. 2018;82(6):757–69.
7. Laufer I, Rubin DG, Lis E, Cox BW, Stubblefield MD, Yamada Y, et al. The NOMS framework: approach to the treatment of spinal metastatic tumors. Oncologist. 2013;18(6):744–51.
8. Slamon DJ, Leyland-Jones B, Shak S, Fuchs H, Paton V, Bajamonde A, et al. Use of chemotherapy plus a monoclonal antibody against HER2 for metastatic breast cancer that overexpresses HER2. N Engl J Med. 2001;344(11):783–92.
9. Murthy RK, Loi S, Okines A, Paplomata E, Hamilton E, Hurvitz SA, et al. Tucatinib, trastuzumab, and capecitabine for HER2-positive metastatic breast cancer. N Engl J Med. 2020;382(7):597–609.
10. Schwartzberg L, Kim ES, Liu D, Schrag D. Precision oncology: who, how, what, when, and when not? Am Soc Clin Oncol Educ Book. 2017;37:160–9.
11. Batson OV. The function of the vertebral veins and their role in the spread of metastases. Ann Surg. 1940;112(1):138–49.
12. Saitoh H, Hida M, Shimbo T, Nakamura K, Yamagata J, Satoh T. Metastatic patterns of prostatic cancer. Correlation between sites and number of organs involved. Cancer. 1984;54(12):3078–84.
13. Paget S. The distribution of secondary growths in cancer of the breast. 1889. Cancer Metastasis Rev. 1989;8(2):98–101.
14. Zumsteg ZS, Spratt DE, Romesser PB, Pei X, Zhang Z, Kollmeier M, et al. Anatomical patterns of recurrence following biochemical relapse in the dose escalation era of external beam radiotherapy for prostate cancer. J Urol. 2015;194(6):1624–30.
15. Perez JE, Machiavelli M, Leone BA, Romero A, Rabinovich MG, Vallejo CT, et al. Bone-only versus visceral-only metastatic pattern in breast cancer: analysis of 150 patients. A GOCS study. Grupo Oncologico Cooperativo del Sur. Am J Clin Oncol. 1990;13(4):294–8.
16. Schwab JH, Boland P, Guo T, Brennan MF, Singer S, Healey JH, et al. Skeletal metastases in myxoid liposarcoma: an unusual pattern of distant spread. Ann Surg Oncol. 2007;14(4):1507–14.
17. Zehir A, Benayed R, Shah RH, Syed A, Middha S, Kim HR, et al. Mutational landscape of metastatic cancer revealed from prospective clinical sequencing of 10,000 patients. Nat Med. 2017;23(6):703–13.
18. Barzilai O, Martin A, Reiner AS, Laufer I, Schmitt A, Bilsky MH. Clinical reliability of genomic data obtained from spinal metastatic tumor samples. Neuro Oncol. 2022;24(7):1090–100.
19. Martinez-Jimenez F, Movasati A, Brunner SR, Nguyen L, Priestley P, Cuppen E, et al. Pan-cancer whole-genome comparison of primary and metastatic solid tumours. Nature. 2023;618(7964):333–41.

20. van de Haar J, Hoes LR, Roepman P, Lolkema MP, Verheul HMW, Gelderblom H, et al. Limited evolution of the actionable metastatic cancer genome under therapeutic pressure. Nat Med. 2021;27(9):1553–63.
21. Nguyen B, Fong C, Luthra A, Smith SA, DiNatale RG, Nandakumar S, et al. Genomic characterization of metastatic patterns from prospective clinical sequencing of 25,000 patients. Cell. 2022;185(3):563–75 e11.
22. Zhang W, Bado I, Wang H, Lo HC, Zhang XH. Bone metastasis: find your niche and fit in. Trends Cancer. 2019;5(2):95–110.
23. Satcher RL, Zhang XH. Evolving cancer-niche interactions and therapeutic targets during bone metastasis. Nat Rev Cancer. 2022;22(2):85–101.
24. Ono K, Kamiya S, Akatsu T, Nakamura C, Li M, Amizuka N, et al. Involvement of hepatocyte growth factor in the development of bone metastasis of a mouse mammary cancer cell line, BALB/c-MC. Bone. 2006;39(1):27–34.
25. Lu X, Wang Q, Hu G, Van Poznak C, Fleisher M, Reiss M, et al. ADAMTS1 and MMP1 proteolytically engage EGF-like ligands in an osteolytic signaling cascade for bone metastasis. Genes Dev. 2009;23(16):1882–94.
26. Robert C, Grob JJ, Stroyakovskiy D, Karaszewska B, Hauschild A, Levchenko E, et al. Five-year outcomes with dabrafenib plus trametinib in metastatic melanoma. N Engl J Med. 2019;381(7):626–36.
27. Yamada Y, Katsoulakis E, Laufer I, Lovelock M, Barzilai O, McLaughlin LA, et al. The impact of histology and delivered dose on local control of spinal metastases treated with stereotactic radiosurgery. Neurosurg Focus. 2017;42(1):E6.
28. Huo M, Sahgal A, Pryor D, Redmond K, Lo S, Foote M. Stereotactic spine radiosurgery: review of safety and efficacy with respect to dose and fractionation. Surg Neurol Int. 2017;8:30.
29. Huang RX, Zhou PK. DNA damage response signaling pathways and targets for radiotherapy sensitization in cancer. Signal Transduct Target Ther. 2020;5(1):60.
30. Goldstein M, Kastan MB. The DNA damage response: implications for tumor responses to radiation and chemotherapy. Annu Rev Med. 2015;66:129–43.
31. Cornforth MN, Bedford JS. On the nature of a defect in cells from individuals with ataxia-telangiectasia. Science. 1985;227(4694):1589–91.
32. Shiloh Y. Ataxia-telangiectasia and the Nijmegen breakage syndrome: related disorders but genes apart. Annu Rev Genet. 1997;31:635–62.
33. Taylor AM, Harnden DG, Arlett CF, Harcourt SA, Lehmann AR, Stevens S, et al. Ataxia telangiectasia: a human mutation with abnormal radiation sensitivity. Nature. 1975;258(5534):427–9.
34. Ma J, Setton J, Morris L, Albornoz PB, Barker C, Lok BH, et al. Genomic analysis of exceptional responders to radiotherapy reveals somatic mutations in ATM. Oncotarget. 2017;8(6):10312–23.
35. Pitter KL, Casey DL, Lu YC, Hannum M, Zhang Z, Song X, et al. Pathogenic ATM mutations in cancer and a genetic basis for radiotherapeutic efficacy. J Natl Cancer Inst. 2021;113(3):266–73.
36. Laurberg JR, Brems-Eskildsen AS, Nordentoft I, Fristrup N, Schepeler T, Ulhoi BP, et al. Expression of TIP60 (tat-interactive protein) and MRE11 (meiotic recombination 11 homolog) predict treatment-specific outcome of localised invasive bladder cancer. BJU Int. 2012;110(11 Pt C):E1228–36.
37. Choudhury A, Nelson LD, Teo MT, Chilka S, Bhattarai S, Johnston CF, et al. MRE11 expression is predictive of cause-specific survival following radical radiotherapy for muscle-invasive bladder cancer. Cancer Res. 2010;70(18):7017–26.
38. Soderlund K, Stal O, Skoog L, Rutqvist LE, Nordenskjold B, Askmalm MS. Intact Mre11/Rad50/Nbs1 complex predicts good response to radiotherapy in early breast cancer. Int J Radiat Oncol Biol Phys. 2007;68(1):50–8.

39. Berlin A, Lalonde E, Sykes J, Zafarana G, Chu KC, Ramnarine VR, et al. NBN gain is predictive for adverse outcome following image-guided radiotherapy for localized prostate cancer. Oncotarget. 2014;5(22):11081–90.
40. Soderlund K, Skoog L, Fornander T, Askmalm MS. The BRCA1/BRCA2/Rad51 complex is a prognostic and predictive factor in early breast cancer. Radiother Oncol. 2007;84(3):242–51.
41. Nogueira A, Catarino R, Faustino I, Nogueira-Silva C, Figueiredo T, Lombo L, et al. Role of the RAD51 G172T polymorphism in the clinical outcome of cervical cancer patients under concomitant chemoradiotherapy. Gene. 2012;504(2):279–83.
42. Willems P, Claes K, Baeyens A, Vandersickel V, Werbrouck J, De Ruyck K, et al. Polymorphisms in nonhomologous end-joining genes associated with breast cancer risk and chromosomal radiosensitivity. Genes Chromosomes Cancer. 2008;47(2):137–48.
43. Chen Y, Jiang T, Zhang H, Gou X, Han C, Wang J, et al. LRRC31 inhibits DNA repair and sensitizes breast cancer brain metastasis to radiation therapy. Nat Cell Biol. 2020;22(10):1276–85.
44. Luo LY, Samstein RM, Dick-Godfrey R, Sidiqi B, Wang C, Oro F, et al. Genomic analyses for predictors of response to chemoradiation in stage III non-small cell lung cancer. Adv Radiat Oncol. 2021;6(1):100615.
45. Shaverdian N, Shepherd AF, Li X, Offin M, Lengel HB, Gelblum DY, et al. Effects of tumor mutational burden and gene alterations associated with radiation response on outcomes of postoperative radiation therapy in non-small cell lung cancer. Int J Radiat Oncol Biol Phys. 2022;113(2):335–44.
46. Zhao SG, Chang SL, Spratt DE, Erho N, Yu M, Ashab HA, et al. Development and validation of a 24-gene predictor of response to postoperative radiotherapy in prostate cancer: a matched, retrospective analysis. Lancet Oncol. 2016;17(11):1612–20.
47. Alsner J, Sorensen SB, Overgaard J. TP53 mutation is related to poor prognosis after radiotherapy, but not surgery, in squamous cell carcinoma of the head and neck. Radiother Oncol. 2001;59(2):179–85.
48. Werbrouck C, Evangelista CCS, Lobon-Iglesias MJ, Barret E, Le Teuff G, Merlevede J, et al. TP53 pathway alterations drive radioresistance in diffuse intrinsic pontine gliomas (DIPG). Clin Cancer Res. 2019;25(22):6788–800.
49. Williams JR, Zhang Y, Russell J, Koch C, Little JB. Human tumor cells segregate into radiosensitivity groups that associate with ATM and TP53 status. Acta Oncol. 2007;46(5):628–38.
50. McIlwrath AJ, Vasey PA, Ross GM, Brown R. Cell cycle arrests and radiosensitivity of human tumor cell lines: dependence on wild-type p53 for radiosensitivity. Cancer Res. 1994;54(14):3718–22.
51. Skinner HD, Sandulache VC, Ow TJ, Meyn RE, Yordy JS, Beadle BM, et al. TP53 disruptive mutations lead to head and neck cancer treatment failure through inhibition of radiation-induced senescence. Clin Cancer Res. 2012;18(1):290–300.
52. Danielsen T, Smith-Sorensen B, Gronlund HA, Hvidsten M, Borresen-Dale AL, Rofstad EK. No association between radiosensitivity and TP53 status, G1 arrest or protein levels of p53, myc, ras or raf in human melanoma lines. Int J Radiat Biol. 1999;75(9):1149–60.
53. Brachman DG, Beckett M, Graves D, Haraf D, Vokes E, Weichselbaum RR. p53 mutation does not correlate with radiosensitivity in 24 head and neck cancer cell lines. Cancer Res. 1993;53(16):3667–9.
54. Williams JR, Zhang Y, Zhou H, Gridley DS, Koch CJ, Russell J, et al. A quantitative overview of radiosensitivity of human tumor cells across histological type and TP53 status. Int J Radiat Biol. 2008;84(4):253–64.
55. Bellezza I, Giambanco I, Minelli A, Donato R. Nrf2-Keap1 signaling in oxidative and reductive stress. Biochim Biophys Acta, Mol Cell Res. 2018;1865(5):721–33.
56. Jeong Y, Hoang NT, Lovejoy A, Stehr H, Newman AM, Gentles AJ, et al. Role of KEAP1/NRF2 and TP53 mutations in lung squamous cell carcinoma development and radiation resistance. Cancer Discov. 2017;7(1):86–101.

57. Binkley MS, Jeon YJ, Nesselbush M, Moding EJ, Nabet BY, Almanza D, et al. KEAP1/NFE2L2 mutations predict lung Cancer radiation resistance that can be targeted by glutaminase inhibition. Cancer Discov. 2020;10(12):1826–41.
58. Sitthideatphaiboon P, Galan-Cobo A, Negrao MV, Qu X, Poteete A, Zhang F, et al. STK11/LKB1 mutations in NSCLC are associated with KEAP1/NRF2-dependent radiotherapy resistance targetable by glutaminase inhibition. Clin Cancer Res. 2021;27(6):1720–33.
59. Lockney NA, Yang TJ, Barron D, Gelb E, Gelblum DY, Yorke E, et al. PIK3CA mutation is associated with increased local failure in lung stereotactic body radiation therapy (SBRT). Clin Transl Radiat Oncol. 2017;7:91–3.
60. Chang L, Graham PH, Hao J, Ni J, Bucci J, Cozzi PJ, et al. PI3K/Akt/mTOR pathway inhibitors enhance radiosensitivity in radioresistant prostate cancer cells through inducing apoptosis, reducing autophagy, suppressing NHEJ and HR repair pathways. Cell Death Dis. 2014;5(10):e1437.
61. Glorieux M, Dok R, Nuyts S. The influence of PI3K inhibition on the radiotherapy response of head and neck cancer cells. Sci Rep. 2020;10(1):16208.
62. Zhu DQ, Liu Y, Yu ZJ, Zhang RH, Li AW, Gong FY, et al. The diverse analysis identifies mutated KRAS associated with radioresistance in non-small cell lung cancer. World J Oncol. 2022;13(2):84–95.
63. Cassidy RJ, Zhang X, Patel PR, Shelton JW, Escott CE, Sica GL, et al. Next-generation sequencing and clinical outcomes of patients with lung adenocarcinoma treated with stereotactic body radiotherapy. Cancer. 2017;123(19):3681–90.
64. Hong TS, Wo JY, Borger DR, Yeap BY, McDonnell EI, Willers H, et al. Phase II study of proton-based stereotactic body radiation therapy for liver metastases: importance of tumor genotype. J Natl Cancer Inst. 2017;109(9):djx031.
65. Chatila WK, Kim JK, Walch H, Marco MR, Chen CT, Wu F, et al. Genomic and transcriptomic determinants of response to neoadjuvant therapy in rectal cancer. Nat Med. 2022;28(8):1646–55.
66. Bernhard EJ, Stanbridge EJ, Gupta S, Gupta AK, Soto D, Bakanauskas VJ, et al. Direct evidence for the contribution of activated N-ras and K-ras oncogenes to increased intrinsic radiation resistance in human tumor cell lines. Cancer Res. 2000;60(23):6597–600.
67. Minjgee M, Toulany M, Kehlbach R, Giehl K, Rodemann HP. K-RAS(V12) induces autocrine production of EGFR ligands and mediates radioresistance through EGFR-dependent Akt signaling and activation of DNA-PKcs. Int J Radiat Oncol Biol Phys. 2011;81(5):1506–14.
68. Yang L, Shen C, Estrada-Bernal A, Robb R, Chatterjee M, Sebastian N, et al. Oncogenic KRAS drives radioresistance through upregulation of NRF2-53BP1-mediated non-homologous end-joining repair. Nucleic Acids Res. 2021;49(19):11067–82.
69. Wang M, Han J, Marcar L, Black J, Liu Q, Li X, et al. Radiation resistance in KRAS-mutated lung cancer is enabled by stem-like properties mediated by an osteopontin-EGFR pathway. Cancer Res. 2017;77(8):2018–28.
70. Toulany M, Dittmann K, Kruger M, Baumann M, Rodemann HP. Radioresistance of K-Ras mutated human tumor cells is mediated through EGFR-dependent activation of PI3K-AKT pathway. Radiother Oncol. 2005;76(2):143–50.
71. Eder S, Arndt A, Lamkowski A, Daskalaki W, Rump A, Priller M, et al. Baseline MAPK signaling activity confers intrinsic radioresistance to KRAS-mutant colorectal carcinoma cells by rapid upregulation of heterogeneous nuclear ribonucleoprotein K (hnRNP K). Cancer Lett. 2017;385:160–7.
72. Chakravarthy VB, Schachner B, Amin A, Reiner AS, Yamada Y, Schmitt A, et al. Long-term clinical outcomes of patients with colorectal cancer with metastatic epidural spinal cord compression treated with hybrid therapy (surgery followed by stereotactic body radiation therapy). World Neurosurg. 2023;169:e89–95.
73. Woodward WA, Chen MS, Behbod F, Alfaro MP, Buchholz TA, Rosen JM. WNT/beta-catenin mediates radiation resistance of mouse mammary progenitor cells. Proc Natl Acad Sci USA. 2007;104(2):618–23.

74. Jun S, Jung YS, Suh HN, Wang W, Kim MJ, Oh YS, et al. LIG4 mediates Wnt signalling-induced radioresistance. Nat Commun. 2016;7:10994.
75. Scott JG, Sedor G, Ellsworth P, Scarborough JA, Ahmed KA, Oliver DE, et al. Pan-cancer prediction of radiotherapy benefit using genomic-adjusted radiation dose (GARD): a cohort-based pooled analysis. Lancet Oncol. 2021;22(9):1221–9.
76. Scott JG, Berglund A, Schell MJ, Mihaylov I, Fulp WJ, Yue B, et al. A genome-based model for adjusting radiotherapy dose (GARD): a retrospective, cohort-based study. Lancet Oncol. 2017;18(2):202–11.
77. Yu EY, Wilding G, Posadas E, Gross M, Culine S, Massard C, et al. Phase II study of dasatinib in patients with metastatic castration-resistant prostate cancer. Clin Cancer Res. 2009;15(23):7421–8.
78. Dahut WL, Scripture C, Posadas E, Jain L, Gulley JL, Arlen PM, et al. A phase II clinical trial of sorafenib in androgen-independent prostate cancer. Clin Cancer Res. 2008;14(1):209–14.
79. Yap TA, Olmos D, Brunetto AT, Tunariu N, Barriuso J, Riisnaes R, et al. Phase I trial of a selective c-MET inhibitor ARQ 197 incorporating proof of mechanism pharmacodynamic studies. J Clin Oncol. 2011;29(10):1271–9.
80. Smith M, De Bono J, Sternberg C, Le Moulec S, Oudard S, De Giorgi U, et al. Phase III study of cabozantinib in previously treated metastatic castration-resistant prostate cancer: COMET-1. J Clin Oncol. 2016;34(25):3005–13.
81. Smith DC, Smith MR, Sweeney C, Elfiky AA, Logothetis C, Corn PG, et al. Cabozantinib in patients with advanced prostate cancer: results of a phase II randomized discontinuation trial. J Clin Oncol. 2013;31(4):412–9.
82. Jahr S, Hentze H, Englisch S, Hardt D, Fackelmayer FO, Hesch RD, et al. DNA fragments in the blood plasma of cancer patients: quantitations and evidence for their origin from apoptotic and necrotic cells. Cancer Res. 2001;61(4):1659–65.
83. Alix-Panabieres C, Pantel K. Clinical applications of circulating tumor cells and circulating tumor DNA as liquid biopsy. Cancer Discov. 2016;6(5):479–91.
84. Gerstung M, Jolly C, Leshchiner I, Dentro SC, Gonzalez S, Rosebrock D, et al. The evolutionary history of 2,658 cancers. Nature. 2020;578(7793):122–8.
85. Phillips R, Shi WY, Deek M, Radwan N, Lim SJ, Antonarakis ES, et al. Outcomes of observation vs stereotactic ablative radiation for oligometastatic prostate cancer: the ORIOLE phase 2 randomized clinical trial. JAMA Oncol. 2020;6(5):650–9.
86. Zelefsky MJ, Yamada Y, Greco C, Lis E, Schoder H, Lobaugh S, et al. Phase 3 multi-center, prospective, randomized trial comparing single-dose 24 Gy radiation therapy to a 3-fraction SBRT regimen in the treatment of oligometastatic cancer. Int J Radiat Oncol Biol Phys. 2021;110(3):672–9.
87. Dawson SJ, Tsui DW, Murtaza M, Biggs H, Rueda OM, Chin SF, et al. Analysis of circulating tumor DNA to monitor metastatic breast cancer. N Engl J Med. 2013;368(13):1199–209.
88. Wong SQ, Raleigh JM, Callahan J, Vergara IA, Ftouni S, Hatzimihalis A, et al. Circulating tumor DNA analysis and functional imaging provide complementary approaches for comprehensive disease monitoring in metastatic melanoma. JCO Precis Oncol. 2017;1:1–14.
89. Winther-Larsen A, Demuth C, Fledelius J, Madsen AT, Hjorthaug K, Meldgaard P, et al. Correlation between circulating mutant DNA and metabolic tumour burden in advanced non-small cell lung cancer patients. Br J Cancer. 2017;117(5):704–9.
90. Haseltine JM, Offin M, Flynn JR, Zhang Z, Lebow ES, Aziz K, et al. Tumor volume as a predictor of cell free DNA mutation detection in advanced non-small cell lung cancer. Transl Lung Cancer Res. 2022;11(8):1578–90.
91. Tie J, Cohen JD, Wang Y, Christie M, Simons K, Lee M, et al. Circulating tumor DNA analyses as markers of recurrence risk and benefit of adjuvant therapy for stage III colon cancer. JAMA Oncol. 2019;5(12):1710–7.
92. Chaudhuri AA, Chabon JJ, Lovejoy AF, Newman AM, Stehr H, Azad TD, et al. Early detection of molecular residual disease in localized lung cancer by circulating tumor DNA profiling. Cancer Discov. 2017;7(12):1394–403.

93. Routman DM, Chera BS, Gupta GP. Circulating tumor DNA biomarkers for early detection of oligometastasis. Cancer J. 2020;26(2):116–23.
94. Sanz-Garcia E, Zhao E, Bratman SV, Siu LL. Monitoring and adapting cancer treatment using circulating tumor DNA kinetics: current research, opportunities, and challenges. Sci Adv. 2022;8(4):eabi8618.
95. Chen K, Zhao H, Shi Y, Yang F, Wang LT, Kang G, et al. Perioperative dynamic changes in circulating tumor DNA in patients with lung cancer (DYNAMIC). Clin Cancer Res. 2019;25(23):7058–67.
96. To EW, Chan KC, Leung SF, Chan LY, To KF, Chan AT, et al. Rapid clearance of plasma Epstein-Barr virus DNA after surgical treatment of nasopharyngeal carcinoma. Clin Cancer Res. 2003;9(9):3254–9.
97. Diehl F, Schmidt K, Choti MA, Romans K, Goodman S, Li M, et al. Circulating mutant DNA to assess tumor dynamics. Nat Med. 2008;14(9):985–90.
98. Lo YM, Leung SF, Chan LY, Chan AT, Lo KW, Johnson PJ, et al. Kinetics of plasma Epstein-Barr virus DNA during radiation therapy for nasopharyngeal carcinoma. Cancer Res. 2000;60(9):2351–5.
99. Han K, Leung E, Barbera L, Barnes E, Croke J, Di Grappa MA, et al. Circulating human papillomavirus DNA as a biomarker of response in patients with locally advanced cervical cancer treated with definitive chemoradiation. JCO Precis Oncol. 2018;2:1–8.
100. Chan SK, Chan SY, Choi HC, Tong CC, Lam KO, Kwong DL, et al. Prognostication of half-life clearance of plasma EBV DNA in previously untreated non-metastatic nasopharyngeal carcinoma treated with radical intensity-modulated radiation therapy. Front Oncol. 2020;10:1417.
101. Fatouros IG, Destouni A, Margonis K, Jamurtas AZ, Vrettou C, Kouretas D, et al. Cell-free plasma DNA as a novel marker of aseptic inflammation severity related to exercise overtraining. Clin Chem. 2006;52(9):1820–4.
102. Gogenur M, Burcharth J, Gogenur I. The role of total cell-free DNA in predicting outcomes among trauma patients in the intensive care unit: a systematic review. Crit Care. 2017;21(1):14.
103. Wang HC, Lin YT, Hsu SY, Tsai NW, Lai YR, Su BY, et al. Serial plasma DNA levels as predictors of outcome in patients with acute traumatic cervical spinal cord injury. J Transl Med. 2019;17(1):329.
104. Snyder MW, Kircher M, Hill AJ, Daza RM, Shendure J. Cell-free DNA comprises an in vivo nucleosome footprint that informs its tissues-of-origin. Cell. 2016;164(1–2):57–68.
105. Moss J, Magenheim J, Neiman D, Zemmour H, Loyfer N, Korach A, et al. Comprehensive human cell-type methylation atlas reveals origins of circulating cell-free DNA in health and disease. Nat Commun. 2018;9(1):5068.
106. Lehmann-Werman R, Neiman D, Zemmour H, Moss J, Magenheim J, Vaknin-Dembinsky A, et al. Identification of tissue-specific cell death using methylation patterns of circulating DNA. Proc Natl Acad Sci USA. 2016;113(13):E1826–34.
107. Yu AF, Moore ZR, Moskowitz CS, Liu JE, Dang CT, Ramanathan L, et al. Association of circulating cardiomyocyte cell-free DNA with cancer therapy-related cardiac dysfunction in patients undergoing treatment for ERBB2-positive breast cancer. JAMA Cardiol. 2023;8:697–702.

Chapter 14
Pain Management of Spine Tumors

Ingharan Siddarthan and Amitabh Gulati

Introduction

Cancer-related pain, especially back pain from metastasis, is a complex syndrome with a significant impact on the lives of patients. In this section, we describe some of the anatomic and physiologic pain generators in these patients. Then, we use this framework to describe the pharmacotherapies and interventional modalities that may be offered to improve their pain symptoms.

Epidemiology of Chronic Pain from Spine Tumors

Chronic cancer-related pain represents a significant source of morbidity for patients diagnosed with malignancy. Many pain syndromes (up to 75%) experienced by patients with cancer are caused by the disease itself [1, 2]. The remaining 25% results from either treatment of cancer (postsurgical, post radiation, or chemotherapy-related pain) or from other comorbidities of cancer such as immobility and infection. A recent meta-analysis suggests that the overall prevalence of cancer pain, especially severe cancer pain, has decreased over the last 10 years due to improved attention to cancer pain and the evolution of treatment modalities. Still, pain affects

I. Siddarthan
Department of Anesthesiology, Weill Cornell Medical College, New York, NY, USA

Department of Anesthesiology and Critical Care Medicine, Memorial Sloan Kettering Cancer Center, New York, NY, USA

A. Gulati (✉)
Department of Anesthesiology and Critical Care Medicine, Memorial Sloan Kettering Cancer Center, New York, NY, USA
e-mail: gulatia@mskcc.org

Y. Yamada et al. (eds.), *Multidisciplinary Spine Tumor Management*,
https://doi.org/10.1007/978-3-032-07519-2_14

nearly 50% of all patients with cancer [3]. Spine tumors can be especially painful; 80–95% of patients with spine metastases experience pain [4].

Mechanisms of Cancer Pain

Briefly, cancer pain can generally be subdivided into pain resulting from mechanical injury to skeletal muscle, bone or ligaments (somatic nociceptive pain), injury to organs and viscera (visceral nociceptive pain), or injury to neural tissue (neuropathic pain). Often, pain generators are multifactorial, as the chronic inflammation and injury associated with malignancy and its treatment lead to ongoing tissue damage and neural hypersensitization [5]. Postsurgical pain is most often neuropathic in nature [6]. Pain may result from either direct perioperative neural injury or, more commonly, from chronic inflammation and peripheral and central sensitization of nerves that transmit pain signals [6]. When peripheral nerves are exposed to chronic inflammation, changes in important pain receptors such as the vanilloid receptor TRPV1 and the glutamate-binding NMDA receptor lead to increased pain transmission [7–9].

Chronic malignant pain can also lead to central sensitization within the brain and spinal cord. Acutely painful stimuli become less painful with repeated exposure due to descending inhibitory pathways in the brain, such as those mediated by opioid receptors in the midbrain periaqueductal gray and alpha-2 receptors in the locus coeruleus [10].

Anatomic Origin of Pain from Tumors of the Spine and Spinal Cord

Interventional management of spine tumor pain begins with developing an understanding of what structures are causing a patient's pain. Within the spine, axial back pain may result from the anterior or posterior elements of the vertebral column and adjacent muscles, while neuropathic pain is most often a result of disease involving the spinal cord or nerve roots.

Neuroanatomy

Peripheral nerves coalesce into ventral and dorsal rami, and then into spinal nerves. Sensory neurons carrying pain signals ultimately contain cell bodies at the dorsal root ganglia (DRG). These first-order neurons traverse the intervertebral foramina and divide into dorsal roots before joining the dorsal horn of the spinal cord at each level. Here, first-order neurons synapse with several neurons at the rexed laminae, including interneurons involved in spinal reflexes and second-order sensory neurons, which then decussate to the contralateral side and ascend via the spinothalamic tract to the brain [11]. Figure 14.1 illustrates the simplified neuroanatomy representing the most important targets of pain procedures.

Several structures within this pathway are important targets of interventional procedures. Each dorsal ramus divides into medial and lateral branches. The medial branch especially provides innervation to many skeletal and muscular structures involved in axial back pain [12]. Spinal nerves form a sinuvertebral nerve (SVN) at each level, which re-enters the intervertebral foramen to provide sensory innervation to non-neural structures of the spine [13]. Finally, the sympathetic nervous system (SNS) plays an important role in sensation and pain of the vertebral column. Cadaver studies and basic science work have allowed the identification of specific nerves and branches that mediate pain from different aspects of the spine.

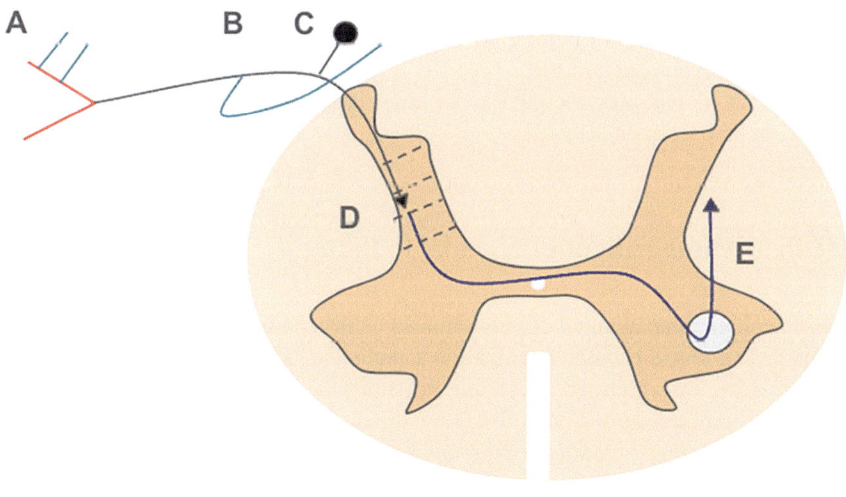

Fig. 14.1 Simplified neuroanatomy of common targets of pain procedures. (A) Dorsal and ventral rami unite to form a spinal nerve at each spinal cord level. These rami carry sensory information from peripheral nerves. The green branches represent the medial and lateral branches of the dorsal ramus, common targets of pain procedures. (B) The spinal nerves give off a sinuvertebral nerve at each level, an important sensory nerve that also receives contribution from the sympathetic trunk and carries pain from many spine structures. (C) The dorsal root ganglion (DRG) contains the cell bodies of first-order sensory neurons. (D) After the DRG, first-order neurons enter the spinal cord as dorsal root, where they synapse with second-order neurons at the rexed laminae (especially II and V). The rexed laminae are divisions of the dorsal horn. (E) Second-order neurons decussate across multiple adjacent levels and ascend to the brain, most commonly via the anterior spinothalamic tract

Posterior Elements

The posterior elements were the more classically targeted sources in treating axial back pain. These structures are primarily innervated by the medial branches of the dorsal rami and the sinuvertebral nerves. The medial branches provide innervation to the zygapophyseal joints, lamina, spinous process, and midline muscles that support the vertebral column such as the multifidus muscle [14–16]. The lateral branch of the dorsal ramus innervates the transverse process and lateral support muscles, though these have not proven to be significant targets of pain procedures except in the sacrum [17].

Anterior Elements

The anterior elements of the spine encompass the vertebral body, vertebral endplates, and intervertebral discs. The most significant contributors to their sensory innervation include the aforementioned SVNs and the sympathetic trunk. The vertebral body receives nonsegmental innervation anteriorly from the SNS, segmental innervation from the SNS laterally, and segmental innervation from the SVN posteriorly. The SVNs give off paired basivertebral nerves (BVNs) at each level, which innervate the intervertebral discs [14, 18]. The vertebral endplates are also innervated by BVNs and are emerging as an important and underrecognized source of chronic axial back pain [19, 20].

Medical Management of Oncologic Pain

Pharmacologic management of pain remains a cornerstone of the treatment of cancer pain. The World Health Organization's analgesic ladder (Fig. 14.2) provides the core structure of which agents to initiate, and when to escalate therapy [21]. In general, recommendations are to begin treatment with non-opioid medications initially, with a gradual escalation of therapy as needed to oral opioids, non-oral routes of opioid administration, and invasive/interventional therapies.

Opioid Analgesics

Opioids remain the mainstay of pain management in patients with cancer, and cancer pain remains one of the few strong indications for chronic opioid therapy. The analgesic effect of opioids is mediated by the Mu (μ)-opioid receptors, located primarily in the periaqueductal gray of the midbrain and substantia gelatinosa of the

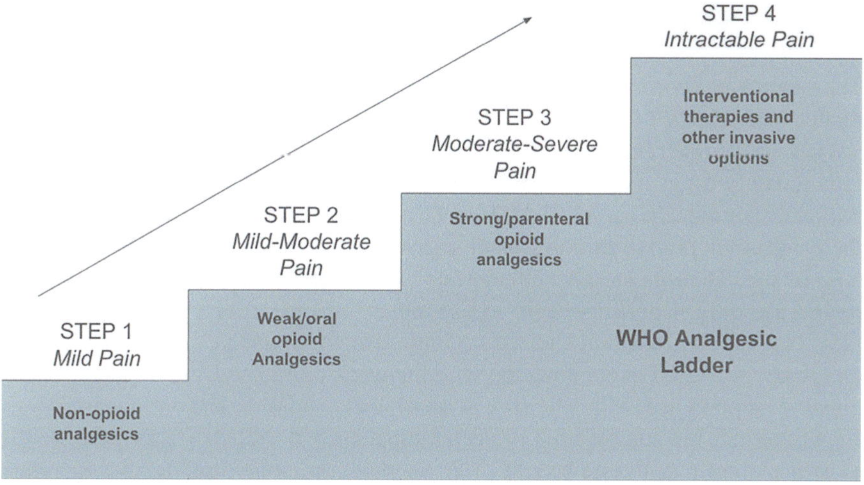

Fig. 14.2 The WHO Analgesic Ladder was initially developed in 1996 for the progression of treatment of chronic pain related to cancer. Initial therapy is aimed at multimodal management of pain with non-opioid analgesics. Refractory pain is then treated with weaker, oral opioids, followed by higher-potency opioids administered parenterally (in the inpatient setting) or via long-acting formulations. Finally, patients not responsive to pharmacologic intervention are candidates for nonpharmacologic interventional modalities, the subject of the remainder of this chapter. (Adapted from the World Health Organization [102])

spinal cord's dorsal horn. Common oral opioid regimens include full μ-receptor agonists, usually beginning with weaker agonists such as codeine, and transitioning to stronger agents such as morphine, oxycodone, extended-release oxymorphone, hydromorphone, or methadone. Partial μ-receptor agonists such as buprenorphine and atypical opioids such as tramadol and tapentadol may also be used. For patients who develop pain refractory to oral agents or intolerable side effects, alternative routes of opioid therapy can be utilized, such as a transdermal fentanyl patch. The choice of agent depends on the severity of pain and pre-existing opioid tolerance [22]. Advantages of opioid therapy include known efficacy and ease of titratability [22]. However, the literature has suggested an association between escalating opioid doses and an increase in all-cause mortality in the oncologic patient population [23]. It has been postulated that this increased mortality reflects those patients with more advanced disease and more metastatic burden, rather than a direct toxic effect of the medications [24]. Still, the concerns of increased risk of respiratory depression with escalating doses remain, and patients should be continually counseled on the risks of opioid therapy escalation.

Adjuncts to Opioid Medications

The overall goal of using non-opioid adjuncts is to reduce the degree of opioid-related side effects.

Among the most common agents used for nociceptive pain are nonsteroidal anti-inflammatory drugs (NSAIDs) and acetaminophen. Overall evidence does not support or discourage the use of NSAIDs in the management of cancer pain; considering their side effect profile, careful patient selection is crucial for considering long-term NSAID use. Their greatest benefit appears to be when given in short-term to reduce opioid use only if patients begin to experience adverse effects of opioid toxicity [25]. One randomized trial showed no improvement in analgesia when short-term diclofenac was used in combination with the weak opioid codeine [26]. The literature does support acetaminophen use as an adjunct to opioids, and one meta-analysis suggested that the combination of acetaminophen with NSAIDs may produce the most meaningful analgesic benefit [27]. Another commonly used medication class for myofascial pain includes muscle relaxants, such as tizanidine, methocarbamol, and cyclobenzaprine. These medications are useful adjuncts to opioids when patients using non-opioid adjuncts are experiencing spasticity related to upper motor neuron lesions or muscle spasm from adjacent tumors [28].

Neuropathic pain is usually not well-covered by opioid medications, and adjunct medications become especially useful in treating chronic neuropathic pain. The anticonvulsant medications gabapentin and pregabalin are commonly prescribed, and several randomized trials showed improvement in pain scores and reduction in morphine requirements when gabapentin is used for malignant neuropathic pain [29, 30]. Two antidepressant classes, specifically the serotonin-norepinephrine reuptake inhibitors (duloxetine, milnacipran) and tricyclic antidepressants using non-opioid adjuncts (especially nortriptyline), are also often used to supplement treatment and supported by evidence from randomized-controlled trials [31, 32].

Chronic opioid therapy may lead to increased pain sensitization with time, a phenomenon known as opioid-induced hyperalgesia. Evidence suggests that the NMDA receptor plays an important role in this phenomenon; therefore, medications that antagonize the NMDA receptor such as ketamine and methadone are playing an increasingly important role in chronic cancer pain management [33, 34]. Ketamine has been successfully used as a short-term infusion for treating cancer pain crises and improving response to opioids [35]. Ketamine is also being used in the outpatient setting [36], though logistic challenges may limit access to this treatment. Sodium channel blockers such as lidocaine are gaining traction for the treatment of pain sensitization syndromes, as they may disrupt pathologic signaling pathways [37]. Early evidence in cancer patients suggests improvement in pain when given as a short-term infusion and avoids some of the toxic effects of other medications [38, 39].

Cannabinoids are rapidly gaining popularity among patients with cancer due to a more tolerable side effect profile and increasing ease of access. The literature on cannabinoid effectiveness in achieving these goals is mixed; some observational data suggest a synergy with opioid medications in providing analgesia [40], though cannabinoid using non-opioid adjuncts may not actually result in opioid dose reduction [41].

Interventional Modalities for the Treatment of Chronic Pain from Spine Tumors

The basis for attempting these procedures at these authors' institutions arises from the Neurologic, Oncologic, Mechanical, and Systemic (NOMS) decision framework for patients who are candidates for some combination of radiation therapy, surgery, or stereotactic radiosurgery [42]. Interventional treatments are reserved for patients who have persistent malignant pain despite treatment of their cancer or as a result of the treatment of cancer. Interventional pain procedures are also appropriate for patients who are in too much pain to undergo treatment for cancer or whose disease may not be amenable to radiation or procedural intervention [42].

Sympathetic Plexus Blocks

The sympathetic nervous system (SNS) plays a significant role in pain transmission, and dysregulation of the SNS can lead to central sensitization. The most targeted sites include the paravertebral stellate ganglion, lumbar sympathetic ganglion, and ganglion Impar, as well as the prevertebral celiac plexus and superior hypogastric plexus. A successful diagnostic block may be followed by chemical neurolysis for sustained analgesia.

The stellate ganglion, so named for its star-like shape, is based anterior to the C7 transverse process. Stellate ganglion blocks (SGB) are most often used for ischemic pain of the cervicothoracic region, neuropathic pain that is sympathetically mediated, and for facial pain. Chronic upper extremity neuropathic pain resulting from carcinomatosis or chemotherapy may be effectively treated by the SGB, though this is not the typical first-line block for patients [43]. Blockade target is the anterior aspect of the C6 anterior tubercle (Chassaignac's tubercle), rather than C7, to reduce the risk of inadvertent vertebral artery injection. The most significant complications include hoarseness from recurrent laryngeal nerve blockade, Horner's syndrome, hematoma, inadvertent brachial plexus blockade, and pneumothorax [44].

Lumbar sympathetic blocks (LSB) may also be performed to treat chronic back pain associated with cancer [45]. As the anterior two-thirds of the vertebral body receives some sympathetic input [46], vertebrogenic pain may be effectively managed by the LSB. Radiation therapy may also result in myositis or neuritis that can be managed with sympathetic blocks, though for these patients, sympathetic blocks are not first-line. LSBs are performed by targeting the paravertebral ganglia located near L2–3 (Fig. 14.3a) [47].

The celiac plexus block does not often directly treat back pain from spine tumors but is effective in treating referred back pain from abdominal visceral malignancies such as pancreatic cancer, hepatobiliary cancer, and proximal bowel cancer [48]. The block is performed by targeting the pre-aortic celiac plexus at approximately L1 (Fig. 14.3b). Side effects primarily originate from excess parasympathetic tone and include diarrhea and hypotension [48]. Referred back pain from cancers from the distal large bowel and pelvis may be treated by blockade of the superior hypogastric plexus [49, 50]. The ganglion Impar block may be used for the treatment of referred pain resulting from perineal cancers [51] and can be useful in treating vertebrogenic pain of cancers affecting the sacrum and coccyx [52].

Procedures for Vertebrogenic Pain

The basivertebral nerves (BVNs) are primarily targeted when axial back pain is thought to occur from direct nociceptive stimuli originating in the anterior elements. Discogenic pain is especially well-targeted by BVN ablative procedures (Fig. 14.4a, b). Clinically, it can be challenging to differentiate axial back pain resulting from the anterior elements versus the posterior elements, especially zygapophyseal joint pain. Vertebrogenic pain tends to worsen with sitting and flexion while facet pain tends to worsen with extension, though this is not specific [53, 54]. Often, once vertebrogenic pain is suspected, the presence of Modic changes on MRI and failure of treatments of posterior element pain increases the likelihood of pain mediated by the BVNs [55]. Historically, the BVNs were targeted indirectly using methods such as dorsal root ganglion stimulation. More recently, evidence is emerging for direct

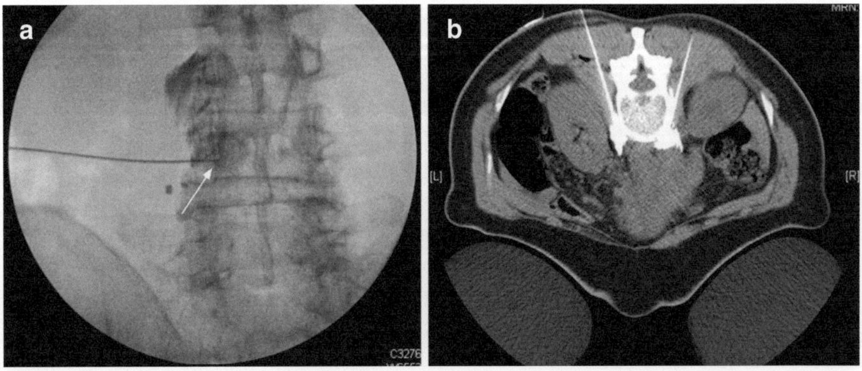

Fig. 14.3 Examples of sympathetic plexus blocks. (**a**) Lumbar sympathetic block performed under fluoroscopy. Arrow shows spread of contrast along the sympathetic chain, along the anterolateral margin of the L3 vertebral body. (**b**) Celiac plexus block performed under CT guidance, using the posterior retrocrural approach

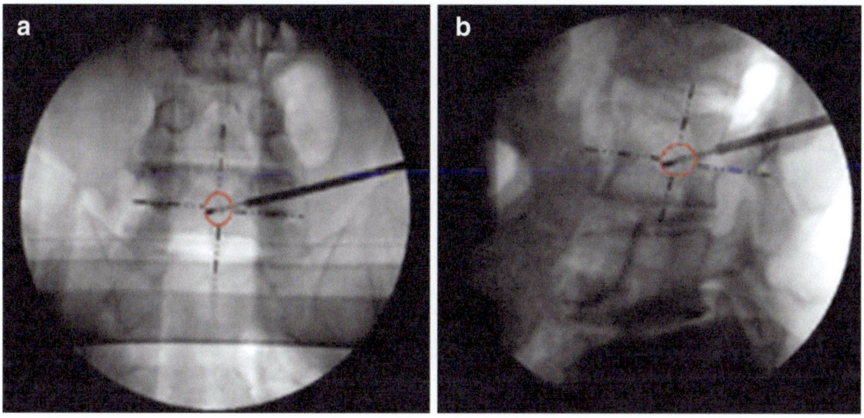

Fig. 14.4 Intradiscal basivertebral nerve (BVN) ablation performed under fluoroscopy, with anteroposterior (**a**) and lateral (**b**) views shown. This relatively new procedure offers a targeted approach to treating anterior body pain mediated by the BVNs

radiofrequency ablation of BVNs, a procedure of intraosseous thermal ablation [56]. These procedures may be most applicable to patients with anterior element pain from degenerative changes following spine surgery or radiation and are often contraindicated when pain is a result of direct tumor invasion.

Kyphoplasty

The more common method for treatment of lytic vertebral body pain is kyphoplasty. Destruction of the vertebral bodies from spine tumors results in severe nociceptive pain from vertebral body collapse [57]. The improved spine alignment and vertebral body height can significantly reduce pain in cancer patients [57, 58]. Kyphoplasty is a valuable tool in managing pain as a bridge to radiation or in patients who may not be candidates for surgical or radiation therapy.

Posterior Element Disease—Medial and Lateral Branch Blocks

The posterior elements of the spine are more often the initial targets in managing axial back pain from spine tumors. Blocks of the medial branches and lateral branches are well-tolerated by patients and associated with few side effects. Posterior element pain generally manifests with pain on lumbar extension and pain with facet loading on physical exam [59]. The medial branches are much more commonly targeted. An initial diagnostic block is performed by injecting a small volume of local anesthetic between the zygapophyseal joint and transverse process of the vertebra to target the medial branches [60–62]. After several successful diagnostic blocks, radiofrequency ablation can be performed for sustained analgesia. The lateral branches can be targeted to treat pain in tumors involving the sacrum, pelvic ilium, and sacroiliac joint [17, 63]. Because the sacroiliac joint has multiple sources of innervation, including the S1–S3 lateral branches, the superior gluteal nerve, and L4/5 dorsal rami, lateral branch blocks usually serve as a supplement to traditional intra-articular injection [17, 64]. As with BVN procedures, direct tumor invasion limits the application of these blocks in pain management.

Epidural Steroid Injections

Epidural steroid injections (ESI) have been well-established in the literature in the treatment of neuropathic pain from nonmalignant nerve root compression [65] and spinal stenosis [66], but their efficacy in malignancy is less well-studied. The most common indication for ESIs is radicular pain; this may result from cancer itself or from treatment. One retrospective study at these authors' institutions suggested that ESIs may be most effective when performed for thoracic and lumbar radicular pain [67]. Epidural steroids can be injected using a transforaminal or interlaminar approach, depending on the nature of pain and anatomy of the patient's spine (Fig. 14.5). Transforaminal approaches are preferred, when possible, as they allow for improved analgesia from focal deposition of steroid at the inflamed nerve root [67]. When this is not possible (such as if a tumor encroaches the neuroforamen), a transforaminal approach can be performed one level away, or an interlaminar approach can be performed one or two levels away.

Neuraxial-based techniques, in general, can be more challenging to perform in the oncologic population. Cancer patients may have acquired coagulopathy from

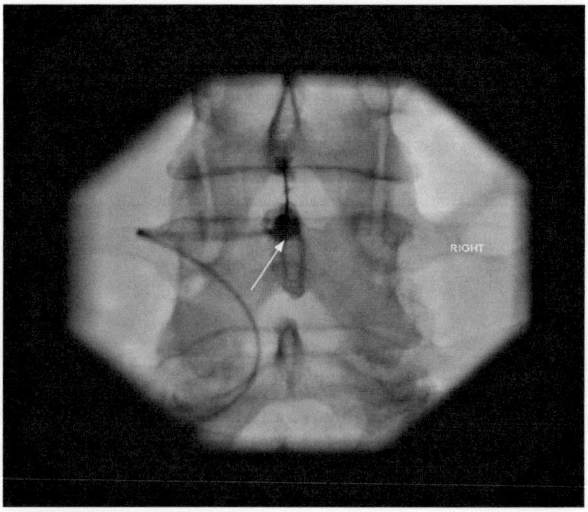

Fig. 14.5 Fluoroscopic image (AP) of an epidural steroid injection. Arrow shows correct contrast localization in the epidural space, without vascular uptake

the malignancy itself or from treatment, or may be on medications that inhibit endothelialization and increase bleeding risk, such as bevacizumab [68]. The presence of malignancy in the needle path may increase the risk of tumor seeding into the epidural or intrathecal space [69]. In these cases, a caudal epidural can be performed to deliver medication to the epidural space through the sacral hiatus and avoid tumors. Finally, treatment failure is possible, especially when neuropathic pain increases with time due to progression of the disease. Within the oncologic population, the utility of epidural injections is primarily to delineate the presence of neuropathic pain generators.

Intrathecal Drug Delivery Systems

Since their first application in 1979 [70], intrathecal drug delivery systems (IDDS) have quickly become the gold standard for management of severe, refractory cancer pain. Intrathecal therapy involves the direct delivery of medication to the cerebrospinal fluid within the subarachnoid space. A catheter is placed in the intrathecal space and is connected to an implantable or external pump that controls the rate of medication delivery (Fig. 14.6a, b). First-line medications for intrathecal pumps include morphine and ziconotide, an N-type calcium channel antagonist which reduces secretion of neurotransmitters involved in pain signaling such as calcitonin

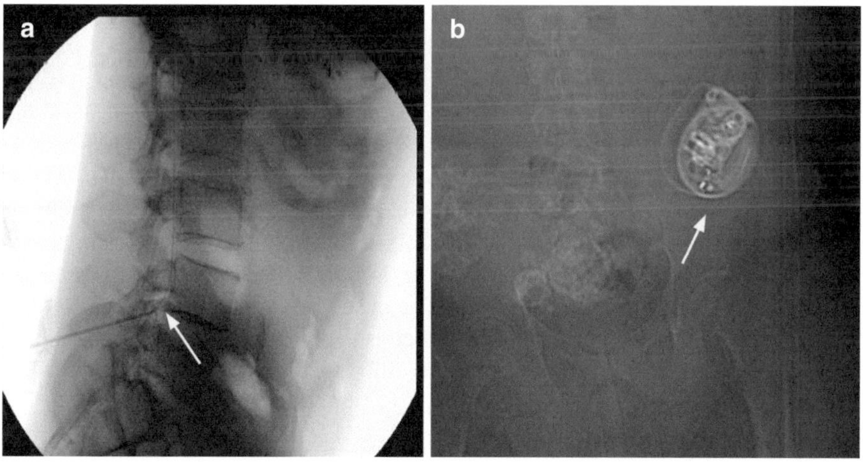

Fig. 14.6 Intrathecal drug delivery systems. (**a**) Example of intrathecal catheter placement under fluoroscopy (lateral view), with arrow indicating needle entry into thecal sac. Patients may undergo a trial of intrathecal medication before implanting a long-term catheter. (**b**) Implantable drug delivery system located in a subcutaneous pocket in the left lower quadrant of the abdomen. The catheter is connected to the pump, which then delivers the medication at a rate set by an external controller. Pumps can be refilled percutaneously, without imaging guidance, though this process can result in complications such as a pocket fill and risk of medication overdose

gene-related peptide and substance P [71, 72]. These are the only FDA-approved intrathecal medications. Other medications used by an IDDS include local anesthetics, other opioid medications such as hydromorphone, and baclofen. Dosing regimens are well-established in the literature [71, 73].

Indications for use of an IDDS include intractable pain and intolerance of side effects from oral or parenteral medication administration [74]. Retrospective data has long affirmed the improvement in pain when used in oncologic patients, especially in patients with severe pain [75]. In one randomized trial comparing intrathecal drug delivery systems (morphine) with comprehensive medical management, IDDS patients showed improvement in pain and reduction in drug toxicity [76]. There was a trend towards improved survival that was not statistically significant, potentially due to a reduction in respiratory complications of systemic opioids [76]. Another randomized trial studied ziconotide IDDS patients and demonstrated significant pain reduction, with nearly 20% of patients showing a >90% reduction in pain [77]. The polyanalgesic conference typically recommends an extensive evaluation, including a psychiatric evaluation, prior to implantation [72]. IDDS patients require extensive follow-up for pump refills and are on high doses of medication with a significant risk for withdrawal, especially those on baclofen. However, in cancer patients—especially those receiving end-of-life care, this evaluation may be foregone [78].

Complications associated with IDDS implantation can be divided into problems with the pump and problems with medication. Pump issues include lower risk complications such as superficial skin infections, catheter migration, pump motor stall or other mechanical issues, and pocket seroma or hematoma [79, 80]. More serious adverse events include serious infections such as meningitis, pocket fills of medication (where medication is inadvertently filled into the subcutaneous pocket where the pump is located), granuloma formation, and development of neurologic deficits. Granuloma formation occurs in about 1% of intrathecal catheters over 6 years, and is associated with high drug concentrations, catheter tips located in the thoracic spine, and increased distance between neuraxis entry and catheter tip location [81]. Medication adverse effects, though lower than equianalgesic doses given orally or intravenously, may persist. Despite risk of infection and neurologic deficits, intrathecal pumps are preferred over long-term epidural catheters. Continuous epidural infusions often result in treatment failure due to scarring of the epidural space [82]. Consultation with each pump manufacturer is recommended prior to obtaining MRIs for each patient, as devices have different conditions to obtain MRIs safely [83].

Spinal Cord Stimulation

Although IDDS has been the gold standard for refractory malignant pain management, neuromodulation techniques such as the use of spinal cord stimulators (SCS) are gaining popularity. Electrodes are implanted within the epidural space near the dorsal column of the spinal cord and connected to an implantable or external pulse generator (Fig. 14.7). These electrodes provide stimulatory signaling to second-order sensory neurons [84]. Different manufacturers offer different patterns of stimulation, such as tonic stimulation (where patients experience paresthesias), as well as burst or high-frequency stimulation (which often are paresthesia-free) [85]. There are several mechanisms by which pain is alleviated. One theory applies the "gate control" mechanism, where dorsal column stimulation leads to inhibitory interneuron activation, disrupting transmission of pain signals [84, 86]. Other mechanisms include an increase in GABA activity in the cord and hyperexcitation and eventual exhaustion of the wide-dynamic range neurons, which mediate central sensitization [86].

PACC guidelines recommend SCS implantation over IDDS when malignant pain is primarily neuropathic, stable with time, and not associated with progression of disease [72]. Neuromodulation may also be considered for patients with contraindications to IDDS, such as severe coagulopathy or patient refusal [87]. The literature shows significant benefits of SCS in patients with nonmalignant neuropathic pain syndromes [88, 89], but it has not been well studied in the cancer population until recently, with the advent of more MR-conditional systems [90]. Several retrospective studies have shown significant improvement in neuropathic pain in patients with radiculopathy from spine tumors [91, 92]. Even patients without pain relief showed improvement in function, such as improved mobility and successful discharge following a pain crisis [92]. Drawbacks of SCS implantation include cumulative increased risk of complications with time, such as lead migration, treatment failure, and infection [93].

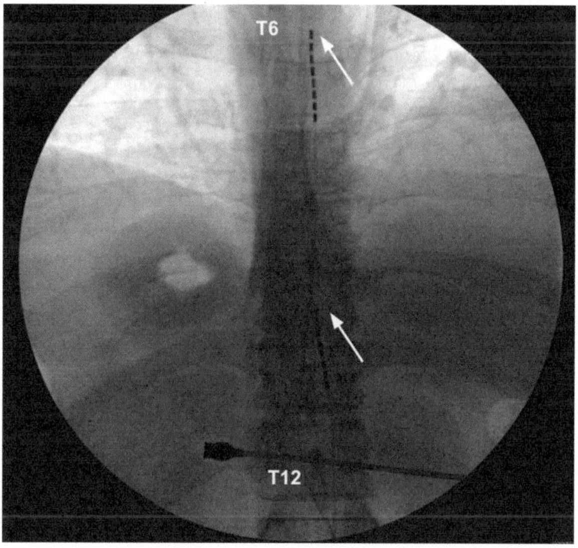

Fig. 14.7 Thoracic spinal cord stimulator implantation, with leads deployed at T6 and T10 (indicated by arrows). Leads are initially inserted percutaneously for a trial and connected to an external pulse generator. If successful, leads may be tunneled and connected to an implantable pulse generator for long-term pain management. In some cases, laminectomy may be required for placement or removal of spinal cord stimulator leads

Alternative Sites for Neuromodulation: Dorsal Root Ganglion and Peripheral Nerve Stimulation

When anatomic barriers preclude SCS placement, such as a tumor invading the posterior epidural space, alternative options for neuromodulation include dorsal root ganglion (DRG) stimulators and peripheral nerve stimulation (PNS).

DRG stimulation has several advantages over SCS. DRG may be more appropriate when specific dermatomes of neuropathic pain can be isolated, as seen in patients with CRPS and causalgia [94]. DRGs can more effectively produce analgesia without inducing paresthesias, as their dermatomal target is far more specific [95]. DRG has not yet been specifically studied for malignant pain in randomized controlled trials. A retrospective case series suggests a moderate reduction in pain scores in patients with chemotherapy-induced peripheral neuropathy, where DRG leads were implanted at two levels (L4/5 and L5/S1) [96]. Application of DRG to spine tumor pain may be limited as tumors resulting in true radiculopathy often reside near the DRGs, precluding safe lead placement.

PNS allows for management of neuropathic pain without placing a device in the neuraxis, and may become useful as a bridge to more definitive therapy or an alternative in patients who cannot receive neuraxial implants [97]. PNS first gained popularity after a randomized trial showed its efficacy in treating residual limb or phantom limb pain following amputation [98]. PNS leads are implanted percutaneously along a peripheral nerve (Fig. 14.8), connected to an external pulse generator, and remain in place for 60 days. Approximately two-thirds of patients with PNS are responders, many of whom show sustained analgesia even after the leads are

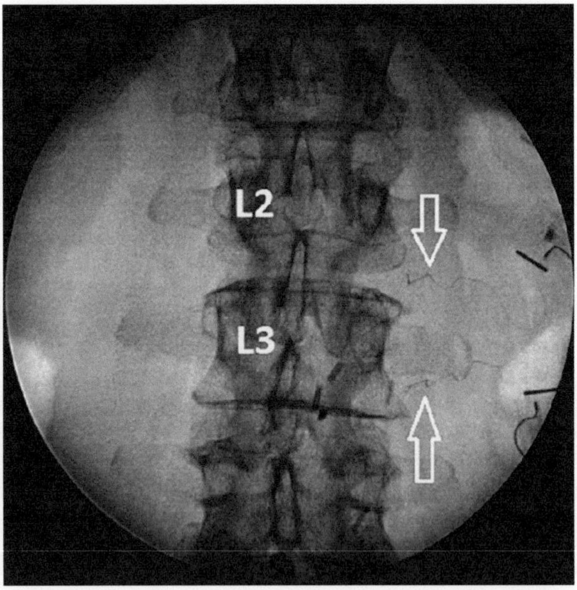

Fig. 14.8 Peripheral nerve stimulator (PNS) leads implanted to target the L2 and L3 spinal nerves, implanted using ultrasound and fluoroscopic guidance. Arrows indicate PNS leads

removed [99]. Available evidence of PNS in the oncologic population is currently limited to case reports. At these authors' institutions, a report was published on two patients who received a PNS to manage radiculopathy from metastatic cancer-causing nerve root compression [100], with lasting analgesia after 60 days. A recent case series demonstrated the potential application of PNS as a bridge to completing radiation treatment in patients with multiple myeloma whose back pain prohibited lying flat for the procedure [101]. More investigation is necessary to capture the full benefit of PNS in cancer patients, but initial evidence is promising if the technology is applied to the right patient.

Conclusion

Numerous interventional pain options exist in helping patients treat their pain resulting from spinal tumors. While there are no definite algorithms to decide how to manage pain in this population, pharmacotherapies are the mainstay of treatment choices. In many instances, local targeted blockade and denervation may be an option, while neuraxial systems may be implanted for more definitive pain therapies.

References

1. Portenoy RK. Treatment of cancer pain. Lancet. 2011;377(9784):2236–47. https://doi.org/10.1016/S0140-6736(11)60236-5. PMID: 21704873.
2. Bruera E, Kim HN. Cancer pain. JAMA. 2003;290(18):2476–9. https://doi.org/10.1001/jama.290.18.2476. PMID: 14612485.
3. Snijders RAH, Brom L, Theunissen M, van den Beuken-van Everdingen MHJ. Update on prevalence of pain in patients with cancer 2022: a systematic literature review and meta-analysis. Cancers (Basel). 2023;15(3):591. https://doi.org/10.3390/cancers15030591. PMID: 36765547; PMCID: PMC9913127.
4. Wewel JT, O'Toole JE. Epidemiology of spinal cord and column tumors. Neurooncol Pract. 2020;7(Suppl 1):i5–9. https://doi.org/10.1093/nop/npaa046. PMID: 33299568; PMCID: PMC7705531.
5. Campbell JN, Meyer RA. Mechanisms of neuropathic pain. Neuron. 2006;52(1):77–92. https://doi.org/10.1016/j.neuron.2006.09.021. PMID: 17015228; PMCID: PMC1810425.
6. Kehlet H, Jensen TS, Woolf CJ. Persistent postsurgical pain: risk factors and prevention. Lancet. 2006;367(9522):1618–25. https://doi.org/10.1016/S0140-6736(06)68700-X. PMID: 16698416.
7. Pinho-Ribeiro FA, Verri WA Jr, Chiu IM. Nociceptor sensory neuron-immune interactions in pain and inflammation. Trends Immunol. 2017;38(1):5–19. https://doi.org/10.1016/j.it.2016.10.001. Epub 2016 Oct 25. PMID: 27793571; PMCID: PMC5205568.
8. Loftis JM, Janowsky A. The N-methyl-D-aspartate receptor subunit NR2B: localization, functional properties, regulation, and clinical implications. Pharmacol Ther. 2003;97(1):55–85. https://doi.org/10.1016/s0163-7258(02)00302-9. PMID: 12493535.
9. Patapoutian A, Tate S, Woolf CJ. Transient receptor potential channels: targeting pain at the source. Nat Rev Drug Discov. 2009;8(1):55–68. https://doi.org/10.1038/nrd2757. PMID: 19116627; PMCID: PMC2755576.

10. Ossipov MH, Morimura K, Porreca F. Descending pain modulation and chronification of pain. Curr Opin Support Palliat Care. 2014;8(2):143–51. https://doi.org/10.1097/SPC.0000000000000055. PMID: 24752199; PMCID: PMC4301419.
11. Khalid S, Tubbs RS. Neuroanatomy and neuropsychology of pain. Cureus. 2017;9(10):e1754. https://doi.org/10.7759/cureus.1754. PMID: 29226044; PMCID: PMC5718877.
12. Shuang F, Hou SX, Zhu JL, Liu Y, Zhou Y, Zhang CL, Tang JG. Clinical anatomy and measurement of the medial branch of the spinal dorsal ramus. Medicine (Baltimore). 2015;94(52):e2367. https://doi.org/10.1097/MD.0000000000002367. PMID: 26717379; PMCID: PMC5291620.
13. Higuchi K, Sato T. Anatomical study of lumbar spine innervation. Folia Morphol (Warsz). 2002;61(2):71–9. PMID: 12164053.
14. Shayota B, Wong TL, Fru D, David G, Iwanaga J, Loukas M, Tubbs RS. A comprehensive review of the sinuvertebral nerve with clinical applications. Anat Cell Biol. 2019;52(2):128–33. https://doi.org/10.5115/acb.2019.52.2.128. Epub 2019 Jun 30. PMID: 31338228; PMCID: PMC6624329.
15. Bogduk N. The anatomy and pathophysiology of neck pain. Phys Med Rehabil Clin N Am. 2003;14(3):455–72, v. https://doi.org/10.1016/s1047-9651(03)00041-x. PMID: 12948338.
16. Bogduk N. The innervation of the lumbar spine. Spine (Phila Pa 1976). 1983;8(3):286–93. https://doi.org/10.1097/00007632-198304000-00009. PMID: 6226119.
17. Cohen SP, Abdi S. Lateral branch blocks as a treatment for sacroiliac joint pain: a pilot study. Reg Anesth Pain Med. 2003;28(2):113–9. https://doi.org/10.1053/rapm.2003.50029. PMID: 12677621.
18. Kim HS, Wu PH, Jang IT. Lumbar degenerative disease part 1: anatomy and pathophysiology of intervertebral discogenic pain and radiofrequency ablation of basivertebral and sinuvertebral nerve treatment for chronic discogenic back pain: a prospective case series and review of literature. Int J Mol Sci. 2020;21(4):1483. https://doi.org/10.3390/ijms21041483. PMID: 32098249; PMCID: PMC7073116.
19. Tzika M, Paraskevas GK, Piagkou M, Papatolios AK, Natsis K. Basivertebral foramina of true vertebrae: morphometry, topography and clinical considerations. Surg Radiol Anat. 2021;43(6):889–907. https://doi.org/10.1007/s00276-021-02690-0. Epub 2021 Feb 17. PMID: 33598754.
20. Sayed D, Naidu RK, Patel KV, Strand NH, Mehta P, Lam CM, Tieppo Francio V, Sheth S, Giuffrida A, Durkin B, Khatri N, Vodapally S, James CO, Westerhaus BD, Rupp A, Abdullah NM, Amirdelfan K, Petersen EA, Beall DP, Deer TR. Best practice guidelines on the diagnosis and treatment of vertebrogenic pain with basivertebral nerve ablation from the American Society of Pain and Neuroscience. J Pain Res. 2022;15:2801–19. https://doi.org/10.2147/JPR.S378544. PMID: 36128549; PMCID: PMC9482788.
21. WHO Guidelines Approved by the Guidelines Review Committee. WHO guidelines for the pharmacological and radiotherapeutic management of cancer pain in adults and adolescents. Geneva: World Health Organization; 2018. Available from: https://www.ncbi.nlm.nih.gov/books/NBK537492/.
22. Manchikanti L, Kaye AM, Knezevic NN, McAnally H, Slavin K, Trescot AM, Blank S, Pampati V, Abdi S, Grider JS, Kaye AD, Manchikanti KN, Cordner H, Gharibo CG, Harned ME, Albers SL, Atluri S, Aydin SM, Bakshi S, Barkin RL, Benyamin RM, Boswell MV, Buenaventura RM, Calodney AK, Cedeno DL, Datta S, Deer TR, Fellows B, Galan V, Grami V, Hansen H, Helm Ii S, Justiz R, Koyyalagunta D, Malla Y, Navani A, Nouri KH, Pasupuleti R, Sehgal N, Silverman SM, Simopoulos TT, Singh V, Solanki DR, Staats PS, Vallejo R, Wargo BW, Watanabe A, Hirsch JA. Responsible, safe, and effective prescription of opioids for chronic non-cancer pain: American Society of Interventional Pain Physicians (ASIPP) guidelines. Pain Physician. 2017;20(2S):S3–S92. PMID: 28226332.
23. Tölle T, Fitzcharles MA, Häuser W. Is opioid therapy for chronic non-cancer pain associated with a greater risk of all-cause mortality compared to non-opioid analgesics? A systematic

review of propensity score matched observational studies. Eur J Pain. 2021;25(6):1195–208. https://doi.org/10.1002/ejp.1742. Epub 2021 Feb 28. PMID: 33533519.
24. Amaram-Davila J, Davis M, Reddy A. Opioids and cancer mortality. Curr Treat Options in Oncol. 2020;21(3):22. https://doi.org/10.1007/s11864-020-0713-7. PMID: 32095929.
25. Derry S, Wiffen PJ, Moore RA, McNicol ED, Bell RF, Carr DB, McIntyre M, Wee B. Oral nonsteroidal anti-inflammatory drugs (NSAIDs) for cancer pain in adults. Cochrane Database Syst Rev. 2017;7(7):CD012638. https://doi.org/10.1002/14651858.CD012638.pub2. PMID: 28700091; PMCID: PMC6369931.
26. Minotti V, De Angelis V, Righetti E, Celani MG, Rossetti R, Lupatelli M, Tonato M, Pisati R, Monza G, Fumi G, Del Favero A. Double-blind evaluation of short-term analgesic efficacy of orally administered diclofenac, diclofenac plus codeine, and diclofenac plus imipramine in chronic cancer pain. Pain. 1998;74(2–3):133–7. https://doi.org/10.1016/s0304-3959(97)00157-7. PMID: 9520227.
27. Martinez V, Beloeil H, Marret E, Fletcher D, Ravaud P, Trinquart L. Non-opioid analgesics in adults after major surgery: systematic review with network meta-analysis of randomized trials. Br J Anaesth. 2017;118(1):22–31. https://doi.org/10.1093/bja/aew391. PMID: 28039239.
28. Chou R, Peterson K, Helfand M. Comparative efficacy and safety of skeletal muscle relaxants for spasticity and musculoskeletal conditions: a systematic review. J Pain Symptom Manag. 2004;28(2):140–75. https://doi.org/10.1016/j.jpainsymman.2004.05.002. PMID: 15276195.
29. Caraceni A, Zecca E, Bonezzi C, Arcuri E, Yaya Tur R, Maltoni M, Visentin M, Gorni G, Martini C, Tirelli W, Barbieri M, De Conno F. Gabapentin for neuropathic cancer pain: a randomized controlled trial from the Gabapentin Cancer Pain Study Group. J Clin Oncol. 2004;22(14):2909–17. https://doi.org/10.1200/JCO.2004.08.141. PMID: 15254060.
30. Gilron I, Bailey JM, Tu D, Holden RR, Weaver DF, Houlden RL. Morphine, gabapentin, or their combination for neuropathic pain. N Engl J Med. 2005;352(13):1324–34. https://doi.org/10.1056/NEJMoa042580. PMID: 15800228.
31. Gilron I, Tu D, Holden RR, Jackson AC, DuMerton-Shore D. Combination of morphine with nortriptyline for neuropathic pain. Pain. 2015;156(8):1440–8. https://doi.org/10.1097/j.pain.0000000000000149. PMID: 25749306.
32. Matsuoka H, Iwase S, Miyaji T, Kawaguchi T, Ariyoshi K, Oyamada S, Satomi E, Ishiki H, Hasuo H, Sakuma H, Tokoro A, Shinomiya T, Otani H, Ohtake Y, Tsukuura H, Matsumoto Y, Hasegawa Y, Kataoka Y, Otsuka M, Sakai K, Matsuda Y, Morita T, Koyama A, Yamaguchi T. Additive duloxetine for cancer-related neuropathic pain nonresponsive or intolerant to opioid-pregabalin therapy: a randomized controlled trial (JORTC-PAL08). J Pain Symptom Manag. 2019;58(4):645–53. https://doi.org/10.1016/j.jpainsymman.2019.06.020. Epub 2019 Jun 26. PMID: 31254640.
33. Bespalov AY, Zvartau EE, Beardsley PM. Opioid-NMDA receptor interactions may clarify conditioned (associative) components of opioid analgesic tolerance. Neurosci Biobehav Rev. 2001;25(4):343–53. https://doi.org/10.1016/s0149-7634(01)00018-5. PMID: 11445139.
34. Pascual D, Goicoechea C, Burgos E, Martín MI. Antinociceptive effect of three common analgesic drugs on peripheral neuropathy induced by paclitaxel in rats. Pharmacol Biochem Behav. 2010;95(3):331–7. https://doi.org/10.1016/j.pbb.2010.02.009. Epub 2010 Feb 23. PMID: 20184918.
35. Loveday BA, Sindt J. Ketamine protocol for palliative care in cancer patients with refractory pain. J Adv Pract Oncol. 2015;6(6):555–61. Epub 2015 Nov 1. PMID: 27648345; PMCID: PMC5017546.
36. Orhurhu V, Orhurhu MS, Bhatia A, Cohen SP. Ketamine infusions for chronic pain: a systematic review and meta-analysis of randomized controlled trials. Anesth Analg. 2019;129(1):241–54. https://doi.org/10.1213/ANE.0000000000004185. PMID: 31082965.
37. Hermanns H, Hollmann MW, Stevens MF, Lirk P, Brandenburger T, Piegeler T, Werdehausen R. Molecular mechanisms of action of systemic lidocaine in acute and chronic pain: a narrative review. Br J Anaesth. 2019;123(3):335–49. https://doi.org/10.1016/j.bja.2019.06.014. Epub 2019 Jul 11. PMID: 31303268.

38. Challapalli V, Tremont-Lukats IW, McNicol ED, Lau J, Carr DB. Systemic administration of local anesthetic agents to relieve neuropathic pain. Cochrane Database Syst Rev. 2005;2005(4):CD003345. https://doi.org/10.1002/14651858.CD003345.pub2. Update in: Cochrane Database Syst Rev. 2019;2019(10): PMID: 16235318; PMCID: PMC6483498.
39. Lee JT, Sanderson CR, Xuan W, Agar M. Lidocaine for cancer pain in adults: a systematic review and meta-analysis. J Palliat Med. 2019;22(3):326–34. https://doi.org/10.1089/jpm.2018.0257. Epub 2019 Jan 7. PMID: 30614748.
40. Noyes R Jr, Brunk SF, Avery DA, Canter AC. The analgesic properties of delta-9-tetrahydrocannabinol and codeine. Clin Pharmacol Ther. 1975;18(1):84–9. https://doi.org/10.1002/cpt197518184. PMID: 50159; PMCID: PMC8332526.
41. Ang SP, Sidharthan S, Lai W, Hussain N, Patel KV, Gulati A, Henry O, Kaye AD, Orhurhu V. Cannabinoids as a potential alternative to opioids in the management of various pain subtypes: benefits, limitations, and risks. Pain Ther. 2023;12(2):355–75. https://doi.org/10.1007/s40122-022-00465-y. Epub 2023 Jan 13. PMID: 36639601; PMCID: PMC10036719.
42. Laufer I, Rubin DG, Lis E, Cox BW, Stubblefield MD, Yamada Y, Bilsky MH. The NOMS framework: approach to the treatment of spinal metastatic tumors. Oncologist. 2013;18(6):744–51. https://doi.org/10.1634/theoncologist.2012-0293. Epub 2013 May 24. PMID: 23709750; PMCID: PMC4063402.
43. Menon R, Swanepoel A. Sympathetic blocks. BJA Educ. 2010;10(3):88–92. https://doi.org/10.1093/bjaceaccp/mkq012.
44. Goel V, Patwardhan AM, Ibrahim M, Howe CL, Schultz DM, Shankar H. Complications associated with stellate ganglion nerve block: a systematic review. Reg Anesth Pain Med. 2019:rapm-2018-100127. https://doi.org/10.1136/rapm-2018-100127. Epub ahead of print. PMID: 30992414; PMCID: PMC9034660.
45. Spiegel MA, Hingula L, Chen GH, Legler A, Puttanniah V, Gulati A. The use of L2 and L3 lumbar sympathetic blockade for cancer-related pain, an experience and recommendation in the oncologic population. Pain Med. 2020;21(1):176–84. https://doi.org/10.1093/pm/pnz142. PMID: 31274168; PMCID: PMC7761528.
46. Bogduk N, Tynan W, Wilson AS. The nerve supply to the human lumbar intervertebral discs. J Anat. 1981;132(Pt 1):39–56. PMID: 7275791; PMCID: PMC1233394.
47. Rocco AG, Palombi D, Raeke D. Anatomy of the lumbar sympathetic chain. Reg Anesth. 1995;20(1):13–9. PMID: 7727322.
48. Eisenberg E, Carr DB, Chalmers TC. Neurolytic celiac plexus block for treatment of cancer pain: a meta-analysis. Anesth Analg. 1995;80(2):290–5. https://doi.org/10.1097/00000539-199502000-00015. Erratum in: Anesth Analg. 1995;(81)1:213. PMID: 7818115.
49. Bosscher H. Blockade of the superior hypogastric plexus block for visceral pelvic pain. Pain Pract. 2001;1(2):162–70. https://doi.org/10.1046/j.1533-2500.2001.01017.x. PMID: 17129292.
50. Plancarte R, Amescua C, Patt RB, Aldrete JA. Superior hypogastric plexus block for pelvic cancer pain. Anesthesiology. 1990;73(2):236–9. https://doi.org/10.1097/00000542-199008000-00008. PMID: 2382849.
51. Kim CS, Jang K, Leem JG, Shin JW, Kim DH, Choi SS. Factors associated with successful responses to ganglion impar block: a retrospective study. Int J Med Sci. 2021;18(13):2957–63. https://doi.org/10.7150/ijms.60962. PMID: 34220323; PMCID: PMC8241784.
52. Gunduz OH, Sencan S, Kenis-Coskun O. Pain relief due to transsacrococcygeal ganglion impar block in chronic coccygodynia: a pilot study. Pain Med. 2015;16(7):1278–81. https://doi.org/10.1111/pme.12752. Epub 2015 Mar 20. PMID: 25801345.
53. Mok FP, Samartzis D, Karppinen J, Fong DY, Luk KD, Cheung KM. Modic changes of the lumbar spine: prevalence, risk factors, and association with disc degeneration and low back pain in a large-scale population-based cohort. Spine J. 2016;16(1):32–41. https://doi.org/10.1016/j.spinee.2015.09.060. Epub 2015 Oct 8. PMID: 26456851.

54. Tieppo Francio V, Gill B, Rupp A, Sack A, Sayed D. Interventional procedures for vertebral diseases: spinal tumor ablation, vertebral augmentation, and basivertebral nerve ablation-a scoping review. Healthcare (Basel). 2021;9(11):1554. https://doi.org/10.3390/healthcare9111554. PMID: 34828599; PMCID: PMC8624649.
55. Modic MT, Steinberg PM, Ross JS, Masaryk TJ, Carter JR. Degenerative disk disease: assessment of changes in vertebral body marrow with MR imaging. Radiology. 1988;166(1 Pt 1):193–9. https://doi.org/10.1148/radiology.166.1.3336678. PMID: 3336678.
56. Qian Z, Sun Z, Yang H, Gu Y, Chen K, Wu G. Kyphoplasty for the treatment of malignant vertebral compression fractures caused by metastases. J Clin Neurosci. 2011;18(6):763–7. https://doi.org/10.1016/j.jocn.2010.09.021. Epub 2011 Apr 19. PMID: 21507652.
57. Pflugmacher R, Taylor R, Agarwal A, Melcher I, Disch A, Haas NP, Klostermann C. Balloon kyphoplasty in the treatment of metastatic disease of the spine: a 2-year prospective evaluation. Eur Spine J. 2008;17(8):1042–8. https://doi.org/10.1007/s00586-008-0701-2. Epub 2008 Jun 17. PMID: 18560905; PMCID: PMC2518756.
58. Fischgrund JS, Rhyne A, Franke J, Sasso R, Kitchel S, Bae H, Yeung C, Truumees E, Schaufele M, Yuan P, Vajkoczy P, Depalma M, Anderson DG, Thibodeau L, Meyer B. Intraosseous basivertebral nerve ablation for the treatment of chronic low back pain: 2-year results from a prospective randomized double-blind sham-controlled multicenter study. Int J Spine Surg. 2019;13(2):110–9. https://doi.org/10.14444/6015. PMID: 31131209; PMCID: PMC6510180.
59. Yang KH, King AI. Mechanism of facet load transmission as a hypothesis for low-back pain. Spine (Phila Pa 1976). 1984;9(6):557–65. https://doi.org/10.1097/00007632-198409000-00005. PMID: 6238423.
60. Bogduk N, Long DM. Percutaneous lumbar medial branch neurotomy: a modification of facet denervation. Spine (Phila Pa 1976). 1980;5(2):193–200. https://doi.org/10.1097/00007632-198003000-00015. PMID: 6446163.
61. Cohen SP, Strassels SA, Kurihara C, Forsythe A, Buckenmaier CC 3rd, McLean B, Riedy G, Seltzer S. Randomized study assessing the accuracy of cervical facet joint nerve (medial branch) blocks using different injectate volumes. Anesthesiology. 2010;112(1):144–52. https://doi.org/10.1097/ALN.0b013e3181c38a82. PMID: 19996954.
62. Wahezi SE, Alexeev E, Georgy JS, Haramati N, Erosa SA, Shah JM, Downie S. Lumbar medial branch block volume-dependent dispersion patterns as a predictor for ablation success: a cadaveric study. PM R. 2018;10(6):616–22. https://doi.org/10.1016/j.pmrj.2017.11.011. Epub 2017 Nov 22. PMID: 29174073.
63. Hutson N, Hung JC, Puttanniah V, Lis E, Laufer I, Gulati A. Interventional pain management for sacroiliac tumors in the oncologic population: a case series and paradigm approach. Pain Med. 2017;18(5):959–68. https://doi.org/10.1093/pm/pnw211. PMID: 28339540; PMCID: PMC6279274.
64. Cox RC, Fortin JD. The anatomy of the lateral branches of the sacral dorsal rami: implications for radiofrequency ablation. Pain Physician. 2014;17(5):459–64. PMID: 25247902.
65. Chou R, Hashimoto R, Friedly J, Fu R, Bougatsos C, Dana T, Sullivan SD, Jarvik J. Epidural corticosteroid injections for radiculopathy and spinal stenosis: a systematic review and meta-analysis. Ann Intern Med. 2015;163(5):373–81. https://doi.org/10.7326/M15-0934. PMID: 26302454.
66. Liu K, Liu P, Liu R, Wu X, Cai M. Steroid for epidural injection in spinal stenosis: a systematic review and meta-analysis. Drug Des Devel Ther. 2015;9:707–16. https://doi.org/10.2147/DDDT.S78070. PMID: 25678775; PMCID: PMC4322611.
67. Oh DC, Rispoli L, Ghosh P, Gulati A. Epidural steroid injections for the management of spinal malignancy-related pain: a pragmatic review and retrospective study. Pain Pract. 2021;21(3):285–98. https://doi.org/10.1111/papr.12957. Epub 2020 Nov 1. PMID: 33025670.
68. Kazazi-Hyseni F, Beijnen JH, Schellens JH. Bevacizumab. Oncologist. 2010;15(8):819–25. https://doi.org/10.1634/theoncologist.2009-0317. Epub 2010 Aug 5. PMID: 20688807; PMCID: PMC3228024.

69. Sarma K, Kohns DJ, Berri MA, Joyce E, Smith SR. Interventional and non-interventional medical rehabilitation approaches to axial spine pain in vertebral metastatic disease. Front Pain Res (Lausanne). 2021;2:675787. https://doi.org/10.3389/fpain.2021.675787. PMID: 35295460; PMCID: PMC8915636.
70. Wang JK, Nauss LA, Thomas JE. Pain relief by intrathecally applied morphine in man. Anesthesiology. 1979;50(2):149–51. https://doi.org/10.1097/00000542-197902000-00013. PMID: 373503.
71. Deer TR, Pope JE, Hanes MC, McDowell GC. Intrathecal therapy for chronic pain: a review of morphine and ziconotide as firstline options. Pain Med. 2019;20(4):784–98. https://doi.org/10.1093/pm/pny132. PMID: 30137539; PMCID: PMC6442748.
72. Deer TR, Hayek SM, Pope JE, Lamer TJ, Hamza M, Grider JS, Rosen SM, Narouze S, Perruchoud C, Thomson S, Russo M, Grigsby E, Doleys DM, Jacobs MS, Saulino M, Christo P, Kim P, Huntoon EM, Krames E, Mekhail N. The Polyanalgesic Consensus Conference (PACC): recommendations for trialing of intrathecal drug delivery infusion therapy. Neuromodulation. 2017;20(2):133–54. https://doi.org/10.1111/ner.12543. Epub 2017 Jan 2. PMID: 28042906.
73. Malhotra VT, Root J, Kesselbrenner J, Njoku I, Cubert K, Gulati A, Puttanniah V, Bilsky M, Kaplitt M. Intrathecal pain pump infusions for intractable cancer pain: an algorithm for dosing without a neuraxial trial. Anesth Analg. 2013;116(6):1364–70. https://doi.org/10.1213/ANE.0b013e31828d670e. Epub 2013 Apr 4. PMID: 23558833; PMCID: PMC5529040.
74. Bruel BM, Burton AW. Intrathecal therapy for cancer-related pain. Pain Med. 2016;17(12):2404–21. https://doi.org/10.1093/pm/pnw060. Epub 2016 Apr 28. PMID: 28025375; PMCID: PMC5654346.
75. Sayed D, Monroe F, Orr WN, Phadnis M, Khan TW, Braun E, Manion S, Nicol A. Retrospective analysis of intrathecal drug delivery: outcomes, efficacy, and risk for cancer-related pain at a high volume academic medical center. Neuromodulation. 2018;21(7):660–3. https://doi.org/10.1111/ner.12759. Epub 2018 Feb 14. PMID: 29446171; PMCID: PMC6492925.
76. Smith TJ, Staats PS, Deer T, Stearns LJ, Rauck RL, Boortz-Marx RL, Buchser E, Català E, Bryce DA, Coyne PJ, Pool GE, Implantable Drug Delivery Systems Study Group. Randomized clinical trial of an implantable drug delivery system compared with comprehensive medical management for refractory cancer pain: impact on pain, drug-related toxicity, and survival. J Clin Oncol. 2002;20(19):4040–9. https://doi.org/10.1200/JCO.2002.02.118. PMID: 12351602.
77. Staats PS, Yearwood T, Charapata SG, Presley RW, Wallace MS, Byas-Smith M, Fisher R, Bryce DA, Mangieri EA, Luther RR, Mayo M, McGuire D, Ellis D. Intrathecal ziconotide in the treatment of refractory pain in patients with cancer or AIDS: a randomized controlled trial. JAMA. 2004;291(1):63–70. https://doi.org/10.1001/jama.291.1.63. PMID: 14709577.
78. Gulati A, Puttanniah V, Hung J, Malhotra V. Considerations for evaluating the use of intrathecal drug delivery in the oncologic patient. Curr Pain Headache Rep. 2014;18(2):391. https://doi.org/10.1007/s11916-013-0391-2. PMID: 24407749.
79. Abrecht CR, Greenberg P, Song E, Urman RD, Rathmell JP. A contemporary medicolegal analysis of implanted devices for chronic pain management. Anesth Analg. 2017;124(4):1304–10. https://doi.org/10.1213/ANE.0000000000001702. PMID: 28319551.
80. Xing F, Yong RJ, Kaye AD, Urman RD. Intrathecal drug delivery and spinal cord stimulation for the treatment of cancer pain. Curr Pain Headache Rep. 2018;22(2):11. https://doi.org/10.1007/s11916-018-0662-z. PMID: 29404792.
81. Yaksh TL, Hassenbusch S, Burchiel K, Hildebrand KR, Page LM, Coffey RJ. Inflammatory masses associated with intrathecal drug infusion: a review of preclinical evidence and human data. Pain Med. 2002;3(4):300–12. https://doi.org/10.1046/j.1526-4637.2002.02048.x. PMID: 15099235.
82. Crul BJ, Delhaas EM. Technical complications during long-term subarachnoid or epidural administration of morphine in terminally ill cancer patients: a review of 140 cases. Reg Anesth. 1991;16(4):209–13. PMID: 1911496.

83. De Andres J, Villanueva V, Palmisani S, Cerda-Olmedo G, Lopez-Alarcon MD, Monsalve V, Minguez A, Martinez-Sanjuan V. The safety of magnetic resonance imaging in patients with programmable implanted intrathecal drug delivery systems: a 3-year prospective study. Anesth Analg. 2011;112(5):1124–9. https://doi.org/10.1213/ANE.0b013e318210d017. Epub 2011 Apr 7. PMID: 21474658.
84. Smits H, van Kleef M, Holsheimer J, Joosten EA. Experimental spinal cord stimulation and neuropathic pain: mechanism of action, technical aspects, and effectiveness. Pain Pract. 2013;13(2):154–68. https://doi.org/10.1111/j.1533-2500.2012.00579.x. Epub 2012 Jul 11. PMID: 22780956.
85. Peeters JB, Raftopoulos C. Tonic, burst, high-density, and 10-kHz high-frequency spinal cord stimulation: efficiency and patients' preferences in a failed back surgery syndrome predominant population. Review of literature. World Neurosurg. 2020;144:e331–40. https://doi.org/10.1016/j.wneu.2020.08.128. Epub 2020 Sep 2. PMID: 32889188.
86. Zhang TC, Janik JJ, Grill WM. Mechanisms and models of spinal cord stimulation for the treatment of neuropathic pain. Brain Res. 2014;1569:19–31. https://doi.org/10.1016/j.brainres.2014.04.039. Epub 2014 May 4. PMID: 24802658.
87. Bulat E, Chakravarthy V, Crowther J, Rakesh N, Barzilai O, Gulati A. Exceptional cases of spinal cord stimulation for the treatment of refractory cancer-related pain. Neuromodulation. 2023;26(5):1051–8. https://doi.org/10.1016/j.neurom.2022.06.002. Epub 2022 Aug 6. PMID: 35941017.
88. de Vos CC, Meier K, Zaalberg PB, Nijhuis HJ, Duyvendak W, Vesper J, Enggaard TP, Lenders MW. Spinal cord stimulation in patients with painful diabetic neuropathy: a multicentre randomized clinical trial. Pain. 2014;155(11):2426–31. https://doi.org/10.1016/j.pain.2014.08.031. Epub 2014 Aug 29. PMID: 25180016.
89. Kemler MA, Barendse GA, van Kleef M, de Vet HC, Rijks CP, Furnée CA, van den Wildenberg FA. Spinal cord stimulation in patients with chronic reflex sympathetic dystrophy. N Engl J Med. 2000;343(9):618–24. https://doi.org/10.1056/NEJM200008313430904. PMID: 10965008.
90. Jotwani R, Mehta N, Baig E, Gupta A, Gulati A. Neuromodulation and the epidemiology of magnetic resonance utilization for lung, breast, colon, and prostate cancer. Neuromodulation. 2020;23(7):912–21. https://doi.org/10.1111/ner.13224. Epub 2020 Jul 24. PMID: 32705734.
91. Shimoji K, Hokari T, Kano T, Tomita M, Kimura R, Watanabe S, Endoh H, Fukuda S, Fujiwara N, Aida S. Management of intractable pain with percutaneous epidural spinal cord stimulation: differences in pain-relieving effects among diseases and sites of pain. Anesth Analg. 1993;77(1):110–6. https://doi.org/10.1213/00000539-199307000-00022. PMID: 8317715.
92. Crowther JE, Chen GH, Legler A, Gulati A. Spinal cord stimulation in the treatment of cancer pain: a retrospective review. Neuromodulation. 2022;25(5):693–9. https://doi.org/10.1016/j.neurom.2022.01.023. Epub 2022 Apr 9. PMID: 35410770.
93. Hayek SM, Veizi E, Hanes M. Treatment-limiting complications of percutaneous spinal cord stimulator implants: a review of eight years of experience from an academic center database. Neuromodulation. 2015;18(7):603–8; discussion 608–9. https://doi.org/10.1111/ner.12312. Epub 2015 Jun 5. PMID: 26053499.
94. Deer TR, Levy RM, Kramer J, Poree L, Amirdelfan K, Grigsby E, Staats P, Burton AW, Burgher AH, Obray J, Scowcroft J, Golovac S, Kapural L, Paicius R, Kim C, Pope J, Yearwood T, Samuel S, McRoberts WP, Cassim H, Netherton M, Miller N, Schaufele M, Tavel E, Davis T, Davis K, Johnson L, Mekhail N. Dorsal root ganglion stimulation yielded higher treatment success rate for complex regional pain syndrome and causalgia at 3 and 12 months: a randomized comparative trial. Pain. 2017;158(4):669–81. https://doi.org/10.1097/j.pain.0000000000000814. PMID: 28030470; PMCID: PMC5359787.
95. Verrills P, Mitchell B, Vivian D, Cusack W, Kramer J. Dorsal root ganglion stimulation is paresthesia-independent: a retrospective study. Neuromodulation. 2019;22(8):937–42. https://doi.org/10.1111/ner.12921. Epub 2019 Jan 30. PMID: 30701632.

96. Ege E, Briggi D, Mach S, Huh BK, Javed S. Dorsal root ganglion stimulation for chemotherapy-induced peripheral neuropathy. Pain Pract. 2023;23(7):793–9. https://doi.org/10.1111/papr.13259. Epub 2023 Jun 1. PMID: 37260046.
97. Sudek EW, Mach S, Huh B, Javed S. Use of temporary percutaneous peripheral nerve stimulation in an oncologic population: a retrospective review. Neuromodulation. 2023;S1094-7159(23):00708-0. https://doi.org/10.1016/j.neurom.2023.06.009. Epub ahead of print. PMID: 37715753.
98. Gilmore C, Ilfeld B, Rosenow J, Li S, Desai M, Hunter C, Rauck R, Kapural L, Nader A, Mak J, Cohen S, Crosby N, Boggs J. Percutaneous peripheral nerve stimulation for the treatment of chronic neuropathic postamputation pain: a multicenter, randomized, placebo-controlled trial. Reg Anesth Pain Med. 2019;44(6):637–45. https://doi.org/10.1136/rapm-2018-100109. Epub 2019 Apr 5. PMID: 30954936.
99. Naidu R, Li S, Desai MJ, Sheth S, Crosby ND, Boggs JW. 60-day PNS treatment may improve identification of delayed responders and delayed non-responders to neurostimulation for pain relief. J Pain Res. 2022;15:733–43. https://doi.org/10.2147/JPR.S349101. PMID: 35310895; PMCID: PMC8932923.
100. Mainkar O, Solla CA, Chen G, Legler A, Gulati A. Pilot study in temporary peripheral nerve stimulation in oncologic pain. Neuromodulation. 2020;23(6):819–26. https://doi.org/10.1111/ner.13139. Epub 2020 Mar 17. PMID: 32185844; PMCID: PMC7496167.
101. Mach S, Javed S, Chen GH, Huh BK. Peripheral nerve stimulation for back pain in patients with multiple myeloma as bridge therapy to radiation treatment: a case series. Neuromodulation. 2023;26(3):694–9. https://doi.org/10.1016/j.neurom.2023.01.018. Epub 2023 Mar 2. PMID: 36870933.
102. World Health Organization. Cancer pain relief and palliative care: report of WHO Expert Committee. 3rd ed. Geneva: WHO; 1996.

Chapter 15
Rehabilitation of the Spine Tumor Patient

Kristen de Vries and Lisa Marie Ruppert

Abbreviations

ADLS	Activities of daily living
AFOs	Ankle foot orthoses
ASIA	American Spinal Injury Association
CIC	Clean intermittent catheterization
CO	Cervical orthoses
CTO	Cervicothoracic orthoses
HKAFOs	Hip, knee, ankle, foot orthoses
ISNCSCI	International Standards for Neurological Classification of Spinal Cord Injury
KAFOs	Knee ankle foot orthoses
LMN	Lower motor neuron
LO	Lumbar orthoses
NOMS	Neurologic, oncologic, mechanical instability, and systemic disease
SCI	Spinal cord injury
TLO	Thoracolumbar orthoses
TLSO	Thoracolumbosacral orthoses
UMN	Upper motor neuron

K. de Vries · L. M. Ruppert (✉)
Rehabilitation Medicine Service, Department of Neurology, Memorial Sloan Kettering Cancer Center, New York, NY, USA

Department of Rehabilitation Medicine, Weill Cornell Medical Center, New York, NY, USA
e-mail: rupperl1@mskcc.org

Y. Yamada et al. (eds.), *Multidisciplinary Spine Tumor Management*,
https://doi.org/10.1007/978-3-032-07519-2_15

Introduction

Cancer patients may develop spinal column and spinal cord injury (SCI) symptoms related to primary spinal tumors or, more commonly, spinal metastases. Depending on location, spinal involvement may result in pain, weakness, sensory impairments, and autonomic dysfunction. The goals of rehabilitation interventions for patients with neoplastic spinal involvement are similar to those with traumatic injuries: relieve symptoms, prevent further complications, assess and manage medical comorbidities, enhance functional independence, and improve quality of life. In addition, they seek to educate patients and caregivers and facilitate safe discharge to the community after an acute hospitalization.

Rehabilitation in the Spine Tumor Setting

Tumors affecting the spinal column are often classified by their location as extradural, intradural-extramedullary, or intradural-intramedullary [1]. Knowing the tumor's location is vital for developing a differential diagnosis and understanding any neurologic symptoms a patient may be experiencing or be at risk of developing [2]. Patients with spinal tumors commonly present with back pain but may also have neurologic deficits at diagnosis. Physiatrists may assist the multidisciplinary spine tumor team in diagnosing these deficits, treating their associated functional impairments, and helping prevent additional related complications [3]. When establishing rehabilitation care plans, physiatrists consider an aggregate of factors, including the patient's age, type and stage of cancer, comorbid medical conditions, baseline physical fitness, and socioeconomic status.

Dr. Herbert Dietz first defined a widely accepted paradigm for cancer rehabilitation. This paradigm focuses on four categories of rehabilitation to which symptoms can be tied: restorative, supportive, preventative, and palliative rehabilitation (Fig. 15.1) [4]. Restorative rehabilitation refers to interventions aimed at returning patients to their premorbid functional status when little or no long-term impairments are anticipated. Supportive rehabilitation attempts to maximize function for permanent impairments caused by cancer and its treatment; in other words, it allows patients to circumvent their impairments. Preventive rehabilitation, more commonly known as prehabilitation, attempts to mitigate anticipated functional impairments caused by cancer and its treatment. Prehabilitation is an often underappreciated but powerful strategy, as preserving strength, flexibility, and aerobic conditioning is more manageable than restoring them once compromised. Finally, palliative rehabilitation focuses on reducing dependence in mobility and self-care activities in association with providing comfort and emotional support [4].

In the spine tumor setting, physiatrists incorporate rehabilitation paradigms and interventions into decision frameworks such as NOMS (neurologic, oncologic, mechanical instability, and systemic disease). Physiatrists may assist with clinical

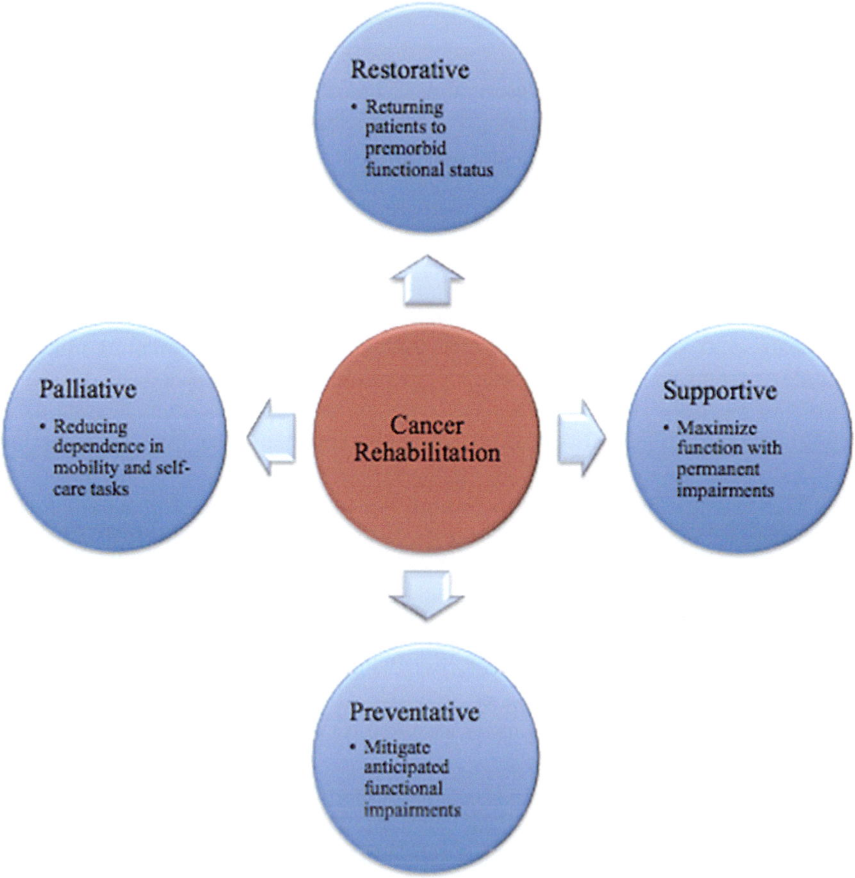

Fig. 15.1 Paradigm for cancer rehabilitation

assessment, correlating symptoms to known spinal lesions, ruling out confounding factors such as peripheral nerve and musculoskeletal injuries, distinguishing between tumor and treatment-related symptoms, improving treatment tolerance, and optimizing function.

Since cancer is a dynamic disease, reviewing the appropriateness of rehabilitation interventions and goals regularly and when disease status changes are crucial. During decision-making, physiatrists consider malignancy in distinct stages. These stages include initial diagnosis and treatment, surveillance, recurrence, temporization, and advanced disease. This approach calls attention to points along the disease trajectory that should trigger the reevaluation of anticipated deficits and redefinition of functional goals. It also ensures that shifts in prognosis and treatment requirements inform rehabilitation efforts [4].

Physiatry Evaluation

Physiatry assessments focus on presenting symptoms, neurologic impairments, and associated functional impairments [5]. These assessments help surgical, medical, and radiation oncologists understand symptom etiology and underlying diagnosis, determine appropriate oncologic treatment, and optimize function and independence for patients in their care [6]. Assessments also ensure the placement of appropriate precautions during rehabilitation interventions.

The assessment begins with a detailed history and physical examination. History questions focus on presenting symptoms, the presence of symptoms prior to cancer diagnosis, and changes in symptoms during treatment. Information obtained includes current medical comorbidities, past medical history, active medications, social history, prior and current functional status, and support system. A systematic physical examination follows the history. The examination begins with assessing posture, spinal range of motion, and palpation of spinous processes and musculature. This examination allows for the overall evaluation of known primary and metastatic disease sites with an additional focus on spine regions corresponding to presenting symptoms. During the spinal assessment, the physiatrist looks for anatomic abnormalities such as scoliosis, exaggerated kyphosis or lordosis, and pelvic obliquity. A similar examination of the appendicular skeleton follows to evaluate for bony/soft tissue abnormalities that can contribute to symptoms. Any areas of tenderness, decreased range of motion, or anatomic abnormality correlating with pain symptoms are compared to or further assessed by imaging to confirm a diagnosis and assess for potential instability.

A neurologic examination incorporating strength, tone, sensation, reflexes, proprioception, and sphincter function follows. The International Standards for Neurological Classification of Spinal Cord Injury (ISNCSCI), more commonly referred to as the American Spinal Injury Association (ASIA) examination, is recommended as a guide for use; it is essential to note that while a guide for examination, the ISNCSCI is not validated for prognostication in metastatic epidural spinal cord compression [6]. Neurological examination findings are subsequently correlated with presenting symptoms, axial and appendicular skeleton abnormalities, and imaging. The physiatry assessment also includes an assessment of cognition, blood pressure, fluid status, skin integrity, and gait mechanics (if able).

Dynamic changes from examination to examination are not uncommon. They may be related to disease progression, tumor recurrence, surgical intervention, effects of radiotherapy, or systemic effects from treatment (i.e., fatigue, neuropathy).

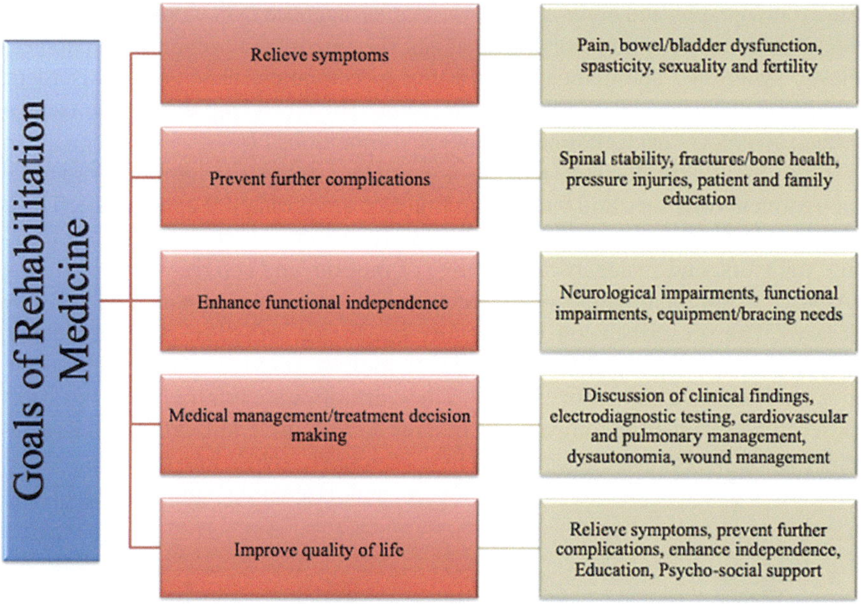

Fig. 15.2 Goals of rehabilitation in management of patients with spinal tumors

Rehabilitation Goals

Based on the rehabilitation evaluation, physiatrists will create goals and treatment plans to help optimize a patient's functional status and quality of life. When approaching patients with spinal cord dysfunction, management may encompass a variety of different aspects of patient care, including neurologic dysfunction as it relates to bowel/bladder, gait, proprioception, dysautonomia, bracing or equipment prescription, therapy prescription and precautions, pain management, sexual dysfunction, and skin care/hygiene (Fig. 15.2).

Neurologic Dysfunction and Sequelae

The physiatrist's evaluation, as mentioned above, helps determine the etiology of neurologic dysfunction. In patients suspected of having tumor-related spinal cord dysfunction, a detailed clinical assessment can help correlate symptoms to known levels of spinal involvement versus changes related to tumor-directed treatments and/or underlying comorbidities, such as peripheral neuropathies or degenerative spine changes [7].

While a detailed assessment can often narrow down the underlying diagnosis, electrodiagnosis is often a helpful extension of the physiatric physical examination.

Electromyography and nerve conduction studies diagnose radiculopathies, plexopathies, mononeuropathies, polyneuropathies (i.e., peripheral neuropathy, paraneoplastic syndrome, autoimmune neuropathies), neuromuscular junction disorders, and myopathies causing a patient's symptoms. They also help distinguish cancer-related symptoms from confounding medical conditions [7].

Once oncologic decision-making is complete, rehabilitation efforts focused on treatment tolerance and optimizing function are initiated if appropriate. These include physical and occupational therapy focusing on strength, sensory training, transfers, endurance, balance, range of motion, and activities of daily living (ADLS). Certain patients may benefit from the addition of bracing and assistive devices. The prescribed lower extremity braces, or orthotics, may supplement the desired movement, maintain range of motion, provide stability and alignment and improve gait biomechanics. These orthotics are referred to by the lower extremity joints they encompass and include AFOs (ankle foot orthoses), KAFOs (knee ankle foot orthoses), and HKAFOs (hip, knee, ankle, foot orthoses). Other supportive braces include knee orthoses and stretching splints (Fig. 15.3).

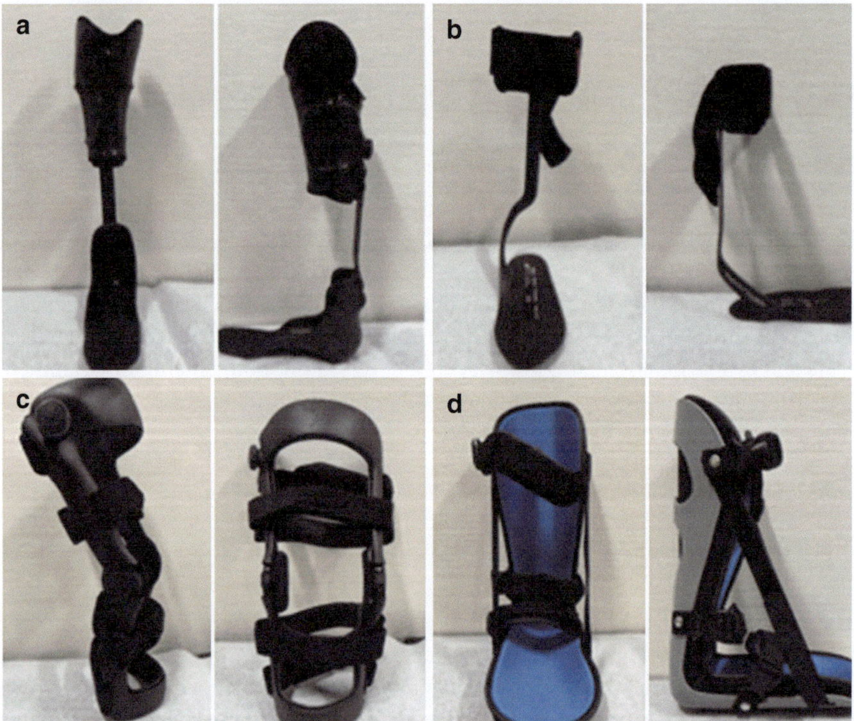

Fig. 15.3 Lower extremity orthoses. (**a**) KAFO (Knee ankle foot orthosis): Provides stability to the knee and ankle during ambulation. (**b**) AFO (Ankle foot orthosis): Provides assistance with ankle dorsiflexion during the swing and early stance phases of ambulation. (**c**) KO (Knee orthosis): Provides knee stability during stance phase of ambulation and assistance with knee extension during the swing phase. (**d**) Stretching splint: Assists in management of spasticity and ankle joint contractures

All prescribed orthoses, assistive devices, wheelchairs, and durable medical equipment must be reassessed regularly for fit and function. Rehabilitation teams educate patients and families on this and the proper maintenance of their equipment.

It is essential to recognize that, in addition to the spinal cord, any level of the central or peripheral nervous system can be impacted by cancer. For example, with central nervous system involvement, there can be a loss of supraspinal inhibitory control of spinal reflexes, resulting in spasticity [8]. Direct nerve compression, meningeal dissemination, or hematogenous or lymphatic spread can affect the peripheral nervous system. Alternatively, neuropathies can result from cancer treatment, including chemotherapy, surgery, and radiation [7]. These neurologic dysfunctions can result in pain, weakness, sensory changes, balance impairments, gait abnormalities, and autonomic dysfunction, which respond to appropriate rehabilitation interventions.

Dysautonomia

Changes to autonomic function are often seen in patients after SCI and can manifest as neurogenic shock, severe bradycardia, orthostatic hypotension, temperature dysregulation, and autonomic dysreflexia. Recognition of these consequences is of utmost importance as they can be life-threatening [9]. Physiatrists can assist in diagnosing, managing, and educating patients and staff on autonomic dysfunctions seen in this population.

Neurogenic and Spinal Shock

Neurogenic and spinal shock are separate entities and should be recognized as such. Neurogenic shock is a devastating consequence of cervical and high thoracic injuries and results from an imbalance of autonomic control related to preserved parasympathetic function from the vagus nerve and loss of sympathetic tone from the sympathetic ganglia in the thoracic spine. It manifests as severe hypotension, bradycardia, and temperature dysregulation [9].

The degree of hypotension seen is directly associated with the severity of the injury, can last up to 5 weeks, and may require vasopressor support to maintain systolic arterial blood pressure above 90 mmHg. Bradycardia may occur in up to 64–77% of patients with cervical-level injury and is also more severe within the first 5 weeks after injury [9].

Spinal shock is a muscle flaccidity and a reduction of reflexes below the level of spinal injury. The mean duration is 4–6 weeks post-injury but can vary from days to weeks. The definition of shock can vary but ends with the emergence of specific reflexes, such as the bulbocavernosus reflex [9].

Autonomic Dysreflexia

Autonomic dysreflexia (AD) is a life-threatening consequence that can occur any time after an SCI. AD generally manifests in patients with injury at or above T6 or the level of outflow to the splanchnic and renal vascular beds. The symptoms generally manifest as hypertension, piloerection, chills or shivering, pounding headache, paresthesias, flushing, diaphoresis above the lesion level, nasal congestion, anxiety, malaise, and nausea [9]. Left untreated, these can lead to severe complications, including hypertension, cerebral hemorrhage, and death [10]. These symptoms result from noxious or non-noxious stimulation below the level of injury, resulting in inappropriate activation of the nervous system. The most common trigger is urinary retention or catheter blockage, followed by bowel distension due to fecal impaction. Other noxious stimuli may include hemorrhoids, pressure injuries, ingrown toenails, fractures, menstruation, and deep vein thrombosis [9, 11].

The most crucial part of management is prevention. Patients and families must be educated on the symptoms and warning signs associated with AD. If AD does occur, the first steps in management should be non-pharmacologic. The patient should be placed upright (mitigating supine hypertension), tight or restrictive clothing loosened, and the underlying cause should be determined and removed, if possible. Pharmacologic measures should be utilized when blood pressure remains at 150 mmHg or higher, despite non-pharmacologic interventions. Nitrates and nifedipine are the most common pharmacologic interventions used [9, 11].

Orthostatic Hypotension

In addition to hypotension and bradycardia, autonomic dysregulation in these patients can manifest as orthostatic hypotension. Orthostasis can persist even after initial hypotension improves and is common in patients with cervical and high thoracic spinal cord injury levels [9]. Based on the authors' experience, all cancer patients are at a higher risk for orthostasis due to treatment-related side effects, including nausea, vomiting, and poor PO intake.

The goal of management for these patients is to prepare them for movement. Management begins with movement while in bed, followed by building tolerance to sitting upright in preparation for further mobility [12]. Initial management should be non-pharmacologic and focus on patient education, optimization of fluid status, and mechanical compression to increase vascular return. Patients are also educated on the importance of maintaining hydration and regular oral intake, increased time with transitional movements, avoiding heat, and maintaining an upright position as frequently as possible. Patients may have diurnal variations in blood pressure with lower values in the morning, limiting morning activities. Optimization of fluid status, with either oral or intravenous hydration, use of salt (in diet or tablets), and keeping the head of the bed elevated overnight can mitigate the risk of AM hypotension. Mechanical compression with abdominal and lower extremity compression, or pre-mobility exercises, can also be incorporated [13].

Pharmacologic management for orthostasis generally consists of midodrine, fludrocortisone, pyridostigmine, or droxidopa. These agents focus on vasoconstriction or volume expansion. Regardless of the agent used, pay close attention to blood pressure fluctuations, given that all carry the risk for supine hypertension [13].

Temperature Regulation

Thermodysregulation is common acutely and can persist for the lifetime of the patient. Similar to AD, patients with lesions at T6 and above are at the highest risk due to loss of descending sympathetic control in more than half of the body. Patients and families should be educated on monitoring core temperatures closely and accurately, especially if there is a concern for infection [9].

Pain

A physiatrist is vital in evaluating patients' pain and correlating symptoms with physical examination findings and spinal imaging. A physiatrist aims to improve symptoms, including pain and related functional impairments, and prevent further complications. The three classic pain patterns in patients with spine tumors are biological, mechanical, and radicular pain. Biologic pain, often worse at night, is due to periosteal stretching and inflammation from a tumor. This pain pattern is generally responsive to radiation or systemic steroids [6, 14]. Radicular pain, which often worsens with axial loading or Valsalva, is due to nerve root compression and may improve with anti-inflammatory agents, nerve stabilizers, or opioids [6]. Mechanical pain, which worsens with positional changes and increased axial loading, is related to impending or established spinal instability and generally requires stabilization [6, 14, 15].

In addition to the classic pain types seen with spine tumors, patients may experience pain from nonmalignant etiologies. This pain may be neuropathic or nociceptive. Nociceptive, or musculoskeletal pain, may be related to postural abnormalities or overuse injuries, e.g., shoulder pain using a manual wheelchair. Neuropathic pain, as noted above, may be related to spinal or nerve root involvement and other neuropathies, e.g., chemotherapy-induced and diabetes [11]. Spasticity may also play a role in pain [8].

The Joint Commission, American College of Physicians (ACP), National Comprehensive Cancer Network (NCCN), and American Society of Clinical Oncology (ASCO) guidelines support the use of pharmacologic and non-pharmacologic interventions for the management of pain [16]. Treatment recommendations target the underlying etiology. It often requires a multidisciplinary approach, which may involve pain medication, antispasmodics, radiation, interventional procedures, orthoses, physical and occupational therapy, the development of an individualized exercise program, counseling, and complementary medicine techniques [6, 8, 16].

Oral medications such as steroids, non-steroidal anti-inflammatory drugs (NSAIDs), anti-epileptic medications, and tricyclic antidepressants are options for treating pain in cancer patients [6, 16]. Baclofen and tizanidine are examples of medications used for the management of spasticity-related symptoms [8]. Opioids may be appropriate for patients with advanced cancer, but use requires caution [16]. It is imperative to understand side effect profiles of medications and potential drug interactions, particularly in cancer patients undergoing various treatments.

Interventional pain procedures for focal pain may include joint injection, muscle injection (i.e., botulinum toxin), peripheral nerve block, and ablative treatment, for patients with more complex and/or diffuse pain symptoms, spinal cord stimulation, neurolysis, or intrathecal drug delivery may be considered [6, 8, 16]. Interventional pain management may be especially beneficial in patients sensitive to potential side effects of systemic pain management or in those who do not have adequate analgesia with oral medication.

Research supports the utilization of non-pharmacologic interventions in cancer pain management. These modalities include mind-body practice, acupuncture, massage, and music therapy. Mind-body practice, including meditation and yoga, has been shown to reduce anxiety, mood and sleep disturbances and improve quality of life. Evidence also supports the use of acupuncture in musculoskeletal pain, including acute and chronic low back pain and cancer-related pain. The mechanism of action appears to be increased production of endogenous analgesic neurotransmitters and modulation of the neuronal matrix involved in pain perception [16]. While there is a lack of strong evidence to support massage therapy, studies suggest a benefit to use. Safety is paramount, and patients should receive treatment from experienced practitioners. Many randomized controlled music therapy trials have shown a significant reduction in pain, emotional distress from pain, anesthetic use, and opioid intake [16].

Bracing may offer spinal stability and pain relief in the preoperative period or for patients unable to undergo surgical fixation for spinal instability. Spinal bracing provides external support, which may improve pain, posture, and adherence to spinal precautions [15]. Similar to extremity bracing, spinal bracing is referred to by the spinal region encompassed and includes cervical orthoses (CO), cervicothoracic orthoses (CTO), thoracolumbar orthoses (TLO), thoracolumbosacral orthoses (TLSO) and lumbar orthoses (LO). The bracing prescription is determined by goals

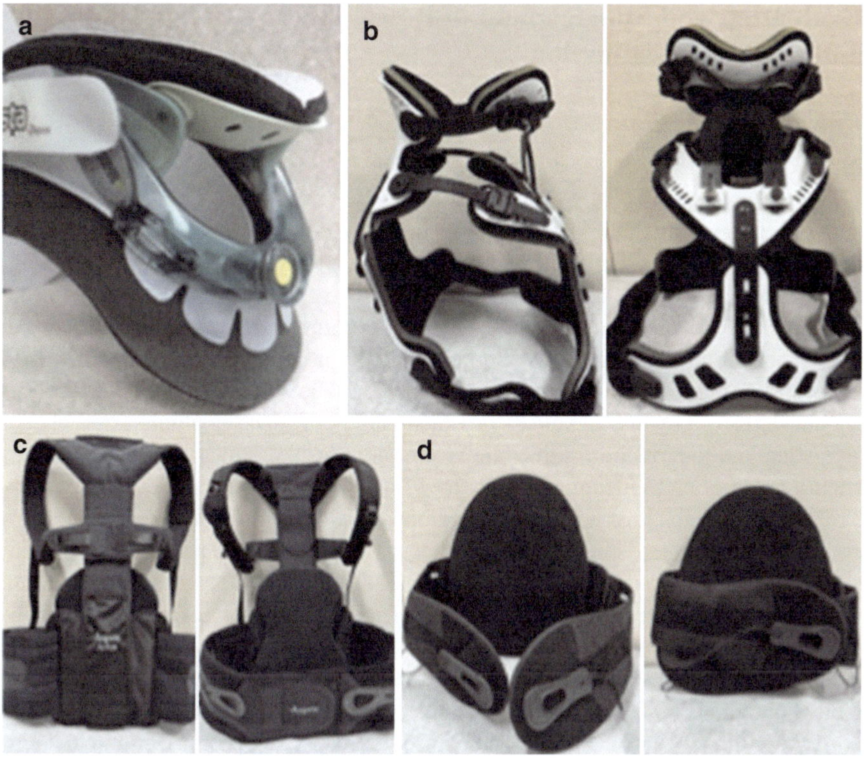

Fig. 15.4 Spinal bracing. (**a**) CO (Cervical orthosis): Provides stability and support to the cervical spine. (**b**) CTO (Cervicothoracic orthosis): Provides stability and support to the cervical and thoracic spine. (**c**) LSO (Lumbosacral orthosis): Provides support to the lumbar spine. (**d**) TLSO (Thoracolumbar orthosis): Provides support to the lumbar spine and promotes postural correction

and level of injury and in conjunction with the surgical spine team (Fig. 15.4). While there is a paucity of clinical evidence for the role of bracing, it remains a recommendation in both nursing and surgical guidelines [15].

Patients with spinal involvement may benefit from physical and occupational therapies. These therapies focus on functional mobility and self-care tasks in the preoperative and immediate postoperative period (generally within the first 2 months). After the initial healing period, the focus can shift to a core strengthening program. In all therapies, educating patients on activity restrictions and spinal precautions is vital. Spinal precautions include avoiding heavy lifting, bending, and twisting motions. These precautions should be relayed and discussed in detail with the therapy team. In addition, there should be close communication among treating and therapy team members regarding any structural or neurologic changes/concerns [17].

Evaluation and Management of Bowel and Bladder Dysfunction

Bowel Dysfunction

The level and severity of SCI can significantly impact bowel function. Injuries above the conus medullaris result in an upper motor neuron (UMN) bowel syndrome or reflexic bowel dysfunction. Patients with this type of dysfunction maintain reflex coordination and stool propulsion but lose voluntary control of the external anal sphincter [18]. Generally, these patients present with fecal retention. On the other hand, injuries at or below the conus medullaris and cauda equina result in lower motor neuron (LMN) bowel syndrome or areflexic bowel. Areflexic patterns are characterized by loss of spinal cord-mediated peristalsis, an atonic external anal sphincter, and loss of control over the levator ani muscle. This pattern leads to constipation and often to incontinence [18].

Physiatrists can assist with identifying bowel patterns through history and physical examination. Assessment begins by determining premorbid patterns and current symptoms. Bowel dysfunction symptoms include frequency, urgency, constipation, incontinence, and altered stool consistency. The Bristol Stool Form Scale is a validated tool to assess stool consistency [19]. Additional medical history, including laxative dependence, irritable bowel syndrome, lactose intolerance, diabetes, and diet, is obtained.

A thorough physical examination begins with inspecting postural alignment, spinal curvature, pelvic positioning, respiratory patterns, and shoulder symmetry. A range of motion of the spine and lower extremities and a thorough neurologic examination follow. Bowel-specific physical examination components include inspection for abdominal distension, palpation for stool and pain, abdominal percussion for air (tympanic) or stool (dull), and completion of a rectal examination to assess muscle tone, sensation, and reflexes. A formal pelvic floor evaluation with inspection for prolapse, scarring, skin irritation, hemorrhoids, fissures, and palpation for muscle tone, strength, and pain can be helpful.

Additional workup of bowel dysfunction includes abdominal plain films to assess baseline stool burden, and a CT scan if there are concerns for ileus or obstruction. Stool studies help rule out infection. Fecal occult blood studies are recommended in the setting of rectal bleeding concerns.

The findings of this assessment guide the formation of a bowel regimen (program). Bowel programs aim to ensure regular passage of stool, consistent timing of bowel evacuation, complete emptying of the rectal vault, predictable stool consistency, and completion of bowel care in a timely fashion. An effective bowel program is patient-specific, may need to be adjusted several times, and may take months to establish [20].

Regardless of the level of injury, lifestyle modifications are essential and should be the first step of a bowel program. Lifestyle modifications begin with education on adequate fluid and fiber intake for stool consistency. The Consortium for Spinal

Cord Medicine recommends that patients with SCI begin by consuming at least 15 g of fiber daily. Coarse, water-soluble fiber is preferred as it can potentially have a laxative effect and improve regularity. Physical activity and regular meals are encouraged to regulate gastric motility [20].

Bowel programs for reflexic (UMN) patterns utilize the intact anorectal reflexes to relax the sphincter via rectal stimulants (suppositories or mini enemas) or digital rectal stimulation. The ideal timing of rectal stimulation is 30 minutes after meals to maximize the gastrocolic reflex [6, 18, 20]. Of note, when using rectal stimulants, the rectal vault must first be emptied of stool so that the stimulant makes direct contact with the rectal mucosa [20]. Stool softeners and oral laxatives can be added to this program if needed.

For patients with LMN bowel dysfunction, the goal is to mitigate the risk of leakage or unplanned evacuations [20]. Manual evacuation of stool one to two times daily may be required to empty fully due to a lack of the defecation reflex. Generally, more formed stool (higher Bristol type), bulked through fiber, is preferable to maintain continence between evacuations [6, 18, 20].

Pelvic floor therapy is a conservative treatment that effectively manages fecal incontinence and constipation [21]. Aside from muscle training and myofascial release, therapy may incorporate electrostimulation and biofeedback. These treatment modalities aim to improve sphincter coordination and strength [21].

As noted above, conservative measures often successfully regulate bowel patterns. However, if these interventions fail, surgical options may be considered. These range from sacral stimulation to ostomy [11].

Bladder Dysfunction

As with the bowel, spinal involvement can significantly impact bladder function.

Patients with lesions above the sacral spinal cord (UMN) often cannot store urine due to uninhibited bladder contractions. These patients present with frequent urges to void small volumes. They can also present with detrusor-external sphincter dyssynergia, failing to relax the urinary sphincter during bladder contraction [22]. Patients with lesions at or below the level of the sacral cord (LMN) present with retention or leakage due to a highly compliant, a-contractile bladder resulting in overdistension of the bladder and inability to empty [6, 22].

It is important to note that voiding dysfunction can also result from insults to the central nervous system outside of the spinal cord and within peripheral nerves and pelvic viscera/musculature [22]. Obtaining a history of premorbid patterns, urinary tract infections, pregnancies, abdominal and pelvic surgeries, underlying neurologic conditions, and psychiatric diagnoses is crucial. Urinary symptoms, including frequency, urgency, hesitancy, poor stream, incomplete emptying, nocturia, hematuria, incontinence, and recent changes to emptying patterns, help determine the etiology of a patient's dysfunction.

A comprehensive physical examination similar to that for bowel dysfunction is necessary. A pelvic examination is critical, including, at a minimum, inspection for prolapse, tone, or scarring. Palpation of the bladder in the lower abdomen during the abdominal examination often indicates urinary retention or incomplete emptying.

Additional workup for urinary dysfunction may be indicated based on the symptoms, pattern changes, and physical examination. Post-void residuals are essential in evaluating the completeness of emptying and upon removal of an indwelling catheter. Urodynamic testing assists providers in determining a patient's filling and emptying patterns when the clinical picture is unclear. Renal ultrasound should be completed annually, especially for those with upper motor neuron patterns and high emptying pressures [6, 22].

Regardless of the emptying pattern, management should begin with patient education on behavioral modifications. These include dietary modifications and avoidance of bladder irritants like caffeine, alcohol, and carbonated beverages [23]. Education may also include information on tactile techniques (including Crede or bladder tapping), timed voiding, and bladder retraining.

For patients with UMN patterns, management aims to reduce overactive bladder symptoms and increase urethral resistance, thus improving storage. Strategies for management include behavioral modifications, pharmacologic interventions (including anticholinergic medications), pelvic floor therapy with biofeedback and electrical stimulation, neurolysis, and botulinum toxin [6, 22, 24].

Management of LMN bladder symptoms aims to improve emptying by increasing bladder contraction and reducing urethral resistance [6]. The Crede maneuver is helpful in patients with accompanying low outlet resistance. Pharmacologic interventions, including cholinergic agents, may be used [22]. Pelvic floor therapy, particularly with biofeedback, may also be of benefit [6, 24].

Circumvention of bladder dysfunction includes clean intermittent catheterization (CIC), chronic indwelling catheterization, or suprapubic catheterization [6, 22]. If hand function or support system allows, CIC is reportedly the safest to mitigate the risk of infections and urological complications [6, 11, 22]. Indwelling or suprapubic catheterization may be necessary for short- or long-term use in some patients. An example of short-term use is in patients with impaired wound healing [11].

As noted above, cancer patients' bowel or bladder dysfunction may be multifactorial [18, 22]. Use of opioids for pain control, surgical intervention, radiation therapy, hormonal deprivation therapies, chemotherapy, and premorbid bowel or bladder patterns are contributing factors to dysfunction and are to be considered when establishing appropriate management. All bowel and bladder programs must be individualized and reassessed if irregularity develops, particularly during disease progression and with treatment changes. Precautions must be considered, particularly in patients with severe thrombocytopenia, neutropenia, and post-surgical or radiation-related changes.

Skin

Pressure ulcers are a widely recognized and potentially life-threatening complication of SCI [11]. Cancer patients are at increased risk for skin breakdown and delayed wound healing due to cancer's catabolic state, treatment impacts, immobility, suboptimal nutrition, fatigue, and immunosuppression [25, 26]. Skin hygiene, especially for patients in the postoperative period, is of utmost importance to mitigate the risk of morbidity related to pressure injury, wound dehiscence, or infection.

The management of pressure injuries begins with prevention. It includes regular skin checks, avoiding pressure and shearing forces, nutritional optimization, treatment of underlying medical conditions that may contribute to skin breakdown and lifestyle/behavioral modifications. Physiatrists are well-trained in necessary pressure-relief techniques, pressure injury management, prescribing necessary equipment, including wheelchairs and cushions, and educating patients and families on management and equipment use [11].

Osteoporosis

Medical complications like osteoporosis may lead to additional complications for individuals with spinal involvement. Deterioration of skeletal microarchitecture occurs rapidly in the first 12–18 months following a SCI and can continue for several years. This bone loss places patients at increased risk for low-impact fractures [11]. Patients with cancer are at even higher risk, particularly those with malnutrition, widespread metastatic disease, and hormone deprivation therapy.

Treatment generally focuses on the reversal of bone resorption with the use of pharmacologic interventions, including bisphosphonates. Non-pharmacologic rehabilitation interventions are valuable adjuncts to bone loss prevention and management. Research supports implementing weight-bearing physical exercises with the assistance of standing devices or orthoses if necessary [11]. There should be strict adherence to spinal precautions during these activities and close attention given to other areas of metastatic disease in the skeleton. For appendicular lesions, providers should avoid passive range of motion of the involved limb, and the patients should be educated on avoiding torsional forces, which may increase the risk of fracture. In pain with functional activities, weight-bearing restrictions and offloading of the limb may be necessary until further imaging and evaluation are completed.

Sexual Function

Both SCI and cancer (or related treatment) can impair sexual function. SCI can impair libido, the ability to achieve and maintain an erection, ejaculation, and orgasm [27]. Cancer and cancer-directed treatments, including chemotherapy, hormonal therapy, radiation, and surgical interventions, can lead to fatigue, depression, body dysmorphia, weakness, skin and tissue changes (including scarring and fibrosis), and pain, significantly impacting desire, intimacy, and sexual function [28]. Addressing sexual function concerns has been shown to help improve outcomes and quality of life for these patients [27, 28].

Physiatrists and providers specializing in men's and women's health can assist with discussions and evaluating the etiology of dysfunction. They can guide patients on safe and available treatments for managing sexual and reproductive dysfunction. These may include therapeutic (both physical and psychological) and pharmacologic interventions [27, 28].

Rehabilitation Settings, Overall Outcomes, and Survival

Patients with spinal cord dysfunction related to tumors often require some degree of rehabilitation after initial management. Short- and long-term functional goals are set based on the individual's premorbid functional status, level of injury, completeness of injury, cancer-related prognosis, cancer-directed treatment plans, home environment, and social support to determine the most appropriate level of care [12]. Medical comorbidities requiring close attention are important to consider when referring for rehabilitation and may further justify the need for rehabilitation in an inpatient rehabilitation setting.

Evidence shows that patients with spinal cord dysfunction due to tumors had prolonged survival, fewer deaths from myelopathic complications, less pain, lower levels of depression, higher quality of life, and significant functional improvements, with rehabilitation, particularly in the acute rehabilitation setting [26, 29]. Other research has demonstrated that patients with this diagnosis have better outcomes when admitted to a dedicated spinal rehabilitation unit than a general rehabilitation unit. Unfortunately, despite literature support, these patients are often not considered for admission, with poor prognosis recorded as the most common reason for denial [29].

Survival rates amongst patients with nontraumatic SCI related to spinal tumors can vary widely and factor into rehabilitation planning. Patients with intramedullary tumors such as ependymomas have survival rates similar to those with traumatic SCI [29, 30]. Those with metastatic disease have the most limited survival, spending up to a third of their survival time in rehabilitation [29]. Collaborative efforts should be made to coordinate and expedite treatment scheduling to maximize rehabilitation impact and minimize length of stay for patients with poor prognosis [29, 30]. For patients with poor prognosis, rehabilitation efforts are primarily palliative, focusing on patient and family goals and training [29].

Close communication between rehabilitation and oncology teams is essential, especially during disease status and treatment changes, as patient safety and quality of life are paramount to rehabilitation interventions. The rehabilitation team pays particular attention to known areas of metastases within the axial and appendicular skeleton, blood counts, electrolytes, blood pressure, heart rate, and fall risk factors, as they may limit activities and movements.

Establishing a rehabilitation plan also requires an assessment of a patient's mental health. While the long-term psychological impacts, particularly for those with SCI related to cancer, are not well studied, there are high rates of anxiety and depression in patients with SCI and cancer, independently [31]. These can substantially impact patient participation in rehabilitation and must be addressed.

Conclusion

Spinal column or cord injury related to cancer can significantly affect an individual's function and quality of life. These injuries also have a significant risk for further medical complications, including dysautonomia, pain, and bowel/bladder dysfunction. The ultimate goal of rehabilitation interventions, particularly in the cancer population, is to maximize independence, decrease caregiver burden, and enhance the quality of life at any stage of the disease continuum [12]. The management of these patients remains multidisciplinary, and physiatry has a critical role in optimizing outcomes.

References

1. Mechtler LL, Nandigam K. Spinal cord tumors: new views and future directions. Neurol Clin. 2013;31(1):241–68.
2. Van Goethem JW, van den Hauwe L, Ozsarlak O, De Schepper AM, Parizel PM. Spinal tumors. Eur J Radiol. 2004;50(2):159–76.
3. Spratt DE, Beeler WH, de Moraes FY, Rhines LD, Gemmete JJ, Chaudhary N, et al. An integrated multidisciplinary algorithm for the management of spinal metastases: an International Spine Oncology Consortium report. Lancet Oncol. 2017;18(12):e720–30.
4. Cheville AL, Basford JR. Role of rehabilitation medicine and physical agents in the treatment of cancer-associated pain. J Clin Oncol. 2014;32(16):1691–702.
5. Ruppert LM, Cohn ED, Keegan NM, Bacharach A, Woo S, Gillis T, et al. Spine pain and metastatic prostate cancer: defining the contribution of nonmalignant etiologies. JCO Oncol Pract. 2022;18(6):e938–47.
6. Ruppert LM, Reilly J. Metastatic spine oncology: symptom-directed management. Neurooncol Pract. 2020;7(Suppl 1):i54–61.
7. Custodio CM. Electrodiagnosis in cancer rehabilitation. Phys Med Rehabil Clin N Am. 2017;28(1):193–203.

8. Billington ZJ, Henke AM, Gater DR Jr. Spasticity management after spinal cord injury: the here and now. J Pers Med. 2022;12(5):808.
9. Krassioukov AV, Karlsson AK, Wecht JM, Wuermser LA, Mathias CJ, Marino RJ, et al. Assessment of autonomic dysfunction following spinal cord injury: rationale for additions to International Standards for Neurological Assessment. J Rehabil Res Dev. 2007;44(1):103–12.
10. Hagen EM. Acute complications of spinal cord injuries. World J Orthop. 2015;6(1):17–23.
11. Sezer N, Akkus S, Ugurlu FG. Chronic complications of spinal cord injury. World J Orthop. 2015;6(1):24–33.
12. Nas K, Yazmalar L, Sah V, Aydin A, Ones K. Rehabilitation of spinal cord injuries. World J Orthop. 2015;6(1):8–16.
13. Isaacson SH, Dashtipour K, Mehdirad AA, Peltier AC. Management strategies for comorbid supine hypertension in patients with neurogenic orthostatic hypotension. Curr Neurol Neurosci Rep. 2021;21(4):18.
14. Laufer I, Rubin DG, Lis E, Cox BW, Stubblefield MD, Yamada Y, et al. The NOMS framework: approach to the treatment of spinal metastatic tumors. Oncologist. 2013;18(6):744–51.
15. Lee SH, Grant R, Kennedy C, Kilbride L. Positioning and spinal bracing for pain relief in metastatic spinal cord compression in adults. Cochrane Database Syst Rev. 2015;2015(9):CD007609.
16. Deng G. Integrative medicine therapies for pain management in cancer patients. Cancer J. 2019;25(5):343–8.
17. Guo Y, Ngo-Huang AT, Fu JB. Perspectives on spinal precautions in patients who have cancer and spinal metastasis. Phys Ther. 2020;100(3):554–63.
18. Krassioukov A, Eng JJ, Claxton G, Sakakibara BM, Shum S. Neurogenic bowel management after spinal cord injury: a systematic review of the evidence. Spinal Cord. 2010;48(10):718–33.
19. Chumpitazi BP, Self MM, Czyzewski DI, Cejka S, Swank PR, Shulman RJ. Bristol Stool Form Scale reliability and agreement decreases when determining Rome III stool form designations. Neurogastroenterol Motil. 2016;28(3):443–8.
20. Johns J, Krogh K, Rodriguez GM, Eng J, Haller E, Heinen M, et al. Management of neurogenic bowel dysfunction in adults after spinal cord injury: clinical practice guideline for health care providers. Top Spinal Cord Inj Rehabil. 2021;27(2):75–151.
21. Hite M, Curran T. Biofeedback for pelvic floor disorders. Clin Colon Rectal Surg. 2021;34(1):56–61.
22. Consortium for Spinal Cord M. Bladder management for adults with spinal cord injury: a clinical practice guideline for health-care providers. J Spinal Cord Med. 2006;29(5):527–73.
23. Wyman JF, Burgio KL, Newman DK. Practical aspects of lifestyle modifications and behavioural interventions in the treatment of overactive bladder and urgency urinary incontinence. Int J Clin Pract. 2009;63(8):1177–91.
24. Kopanska M, Torices S, Czech J, Koziara W, Toborek M, Dobrek L. Urinary incontinence in women: biofeedback as an innovative treatment method. Ther Adv Urol. 2020;12:1756287220934359.
25. Lyder CH. Assessing risk and preventing pressure ulcers in patients with cancer. Semin Oncol Nurs. 2006;22(3):178–84.
26. Ruff RL, Adamson VW, Ruff SS, Wang X. Directed rehabilitation reduces pain and depression while increasing independence and satisfaction with life for patients with paraplegia due to epidural metastatic spinal cord compression. J Rehabil Res Dev. 2007;44(1):1–10.
27. Zizzo J, Gater DR, Hough S, Ibrahim E. Sexuality, intimacy, and reproductive health after spinal cord injury. J Pers Med. 2022;12(12):1985.
28. Gleason LV. Chapter 19 – Pelvic floor dysfunction in gynecologic cancer. Elsevier; 2021.
29. New PW, Marshall R, Stubblefield MD, Scivoletto G. Rehabilitation of people with spinal cord damage due to tumor: literature review, international survey and practical recommendations for optimizing their rehabilitation. J Spinal Cord Med. 2017;40(2):213–21.

30. New PW, Eriks-Hoogland I, Scivoletto G, Reeves RK, Townson A, Marshall R, et al. Important clinical rehabilitation principles unique to people with non-traumatic spinal cord dysfunction. Top Spinal Cord Inj Rehabil. 2017;23(4):299–312.
31. Gartrell BA, Saad F. Managing bone metastases and reducing skeletal related events in prostate cancer. Nat Rev Clin Oncol. 2014;11(6):335–45.

Chapter 16
How a Multidisciplinary Spine Oncology Service Functions

Mark H. Bilsky and Yoshiya Yamada

Introduction

The concept of multidisciplinary care was credited to the Mayo brothers at the turn of the twentieth century with the Mayo Clinic model of care, which focuses on a culture of collegial multispecialty teamwork to provide quality care [3]. There is increasing awareness of the benefits of multidisciplinary medical care for patients as well as health care providers, and it is now a well-accepted practice paradigm [2]. Working as a team for optimal patient care brings together the expertise of different specialties to focus on the needs of the patient. By avoiding the "silo effect" where practitioners focus solely on the perspective of their specialty, the team approach results in better coordination between specialties and the breakdown of communication barriers between specialists.

A cohesive team approach—where no one specialist is more important than another—to complex medical problems can reduce adverse events, reduce costs, and improve patient outcomes. For example, a large retrospective study of over 18,000 breast cancer patients in Taiwan found a lower risk of breast cancer recurrence if patients received multidisciplinary care. In this retrospective study, half of the patients received multidisciplinary care, while the other half did not. Other clinical factors such as stage of disease, type of treatment, age, health status, income levels, and hospital attributes including patient volume were evenly matched. The rate of recurrence was significantly lower for the multidisciplinary care group with

M. H. Bilsky
Spinal Oncology Service, Department of Neurosurgery, Memorial Sloan Kettering Cancer Center, New York, NY, USA

Y. Yamada (✉)
Spinal Oncology Service, Department of Radiation Oncology, Memorial Sloan Kettering Cancer Center, New York, NY, USA
e-mail: yamadaj@mskcc.org

Y. Yamada et al. (eds.), *Multidisciplinary Spine Tumor Management*,
https://doi.org/10.1007/978-3-032-07519-2_16

a hazard ration of 0.87 ($p < 0.05$). Patients that experienced disease recurrence experienced a significantly higher mortality rate of 74.9% vs 16.2% for those without recurrence ($p < 0.05$), and the relative risk of mortality was also found to be significantly less for the multidisciplinary managed patients with a hazard ratio of 0.89 [13].

This paradigm also improves patient satisfaction. For example, in an outpatient one-stop multidisciplinary cancer symptom control clinic, significant improvement was noted for common cancer symptoms such as pain, nausea, depression, anxiety and well-being. Patient satisfaction was rated as excellent in 86–97% of patients. Significant improvement was observed in pain, nausea, depression, anxiety, sleep, dyspnea, and well-being. In 83 patients interviewed after the multidisciplinary clinic, satisfaction was rated as excellent (5 out of 5) in 86–97% [12].

In addition, a team working as a well-oiled machine provides greater job satisfaction for care providers and promotes greater retention of experienced personnel. The use of cohesive teams can limit adverse events, decrease the patient's length of stay in the inpatient setting, and increase patient and patient family satisfaction. It also enhances opportunities for collaborative research and innovation. Hence, effective multidisciplinary teams can provide benefits not only to patients and their families, patient care givers, and institutions and hospitals by providing better outcomes and reducing costs [4].

Multidisciplinary Spine Care

Spinal oncology is an excellent example demonstrating the benefits of multidisciplinary care. Spine tumors are often highly symptomatic, frequently requiring urgent interventions that can dramatically affect quality of life and performance status. A prime example of the need for a multidisciplinary team approach is addressing the pain generator created by spine tumors. Pain is often multifactorial, with no one solution that is best for every situation. Spine tumor pain can result from active tumor alone, i.e., biologic pain, fracture-related mechanical instability, or both. Hence, simply treating the tumor may not resolve pain if there is an additional component of mechanical instability. Ablative radiation to provide tumor control will not provide meaningful palliation for pain resulting from a mechanically unstable spine. Conversely, addressing mechanical instability alone is not sufficient to provide tumor control or the pain associated with tumoral growth. Instability resulting from a pathologic fracture often benefits from treatment with an external orthosis, percutaneous cement augmentation, such as kypho- or vertebroplasty, or open or percutaneous pedicle or lateral mass screw-rod symptoms. Physiatrists and interventional pain physicians add immeasurable value to multidisciplinary management teams, providing minimally invasive and low morbidity procedures such as C2 nerve root and greater cluneal nerve ablations to treat occipital neuralgia and sacral insufficiency fractures, respectively. The optimal care for a spine tumor patient benefits from the integration of a wide range of expertise and specialties.

The neurologic, oncologic, mechanical and systemic (NOMS) decision framework is an excellent paradigm for incorporating multidisciplinary spine tumor management [9]. In brief, NOMS is a dynamic decision framework that incorporates these four fundamental assessments to determine the role of radiation therapy, surgery, interventional radiology and or systemic therapy. The neurologic component is an assessment of the grade of spinal cord compression, myelopathy, and functional radiculopathy. The oncologic domain assesses the expected response to conventional or stereotactic radiotherapy and or systemic agents. Mechanical considerations are based upon the spine instability neurologic score (SINS) [5] and take into consideration the potential use of bracing, percutaneous cement and/or pedicle screw augmentation, or open surgery. Systemic considerations refer to the extent of systemic disease, medical comorbidities and expected overall survival.

Key Features of a Multidisciplinary Spine Program

Expertise Is Not Enough

Effective communication is a hallmark of a good multidisciplinary team [11]. Because optimal spine care requires the input of multiple specialties, poor communication can lead to confusion, misunderstandings, mistakes and poor outcomes. A systematic review of randomized trials reporting acute care multidisciplinary team-based interventions for inpatient care found that, in addition to clinical expertise, effective communication was essential for improving care. It was noted that clear communication strategies among team members can reduce emergency department readmission rates, as well as mortality, morbidity, and functional decline in patients. Hence, expertise among team members is not enough. The expertise within the team needs to be harmonized through effective communication [7]. Without good communication, multidisciplinary management may result in worse outcomes instead of better. A benefit of NOMS is that it provides a common lexicon for cross-disciplinary communication. The NOMS framework is a specialty-agnostic tool to develop treatment plans based upon a common frame of reference. The importance of multiple specialists speaking the same language cannot be overemphasized. It is crucial for effective team management that all members of the team understand each other, and NOMS provides the language to do so. Within NOMS, a radiation oncologist will understand what mechanical instability looks like and when a surgical consultation is necessary. A spine surgeon will be able to recommend radiosurgery when mechanical stabilization is not necessary. A radiation oncologist and a spine surgeon will be able to jointly recommend surgical decompression and stabilization, followed by definitive radiosurgery in the case of cord compression for oligometastatic renal cell carcinoma. Having a comprehensive treatment plan presented together by multiple specialists is can also be very reassuring to patients.

Regular Points of Contact

Regular and meaningful points of contact between team members are also a crucial component of a successful multidisciplinary team. One important reason for consistent interactions is to strengthen relationships. Respect and trust within the team are an essential part of a "well-oiled machine." Frequent interactions with the goal of building respect and trust are essential [14]. Team members must be committed to creating a culture of respect and trust, which can develop when the multidisciplinary team is focused on two fundamental priorities:

- What is best for the patient?
- What is the evidence?

Although differences of opinion are sure to arise in the discussion of complex spine tumor management, agreeing to base all decisions as a group based upon these two fundamentals as a priori guiding principles using the NOMS framework is an essential element of multidisciplinary discussions.

At Memorial Sloan Kettering Cancer Center, multidisciplinary spine care has been implemented for over 20 years. The key ways that the spine team at MSKCC has regular points of contact and function are by holding multidisciplinary weekly spine tumor boards, weekly radiosurgery contour review conferences, monthly team meetings, including research meetings, two internal spine team retreats, and an annual spine tumor symposium. One of the most effective strategies implemented early in our effort was multidisciplinary spine-tumor clinics, with the critical services being in the same physical space and coordinating up to 4 services seeing the patient in a single visit, thereby streamlining the disposition of patients to the appropriate service. The clinics also allowed us to track in real time the successes and failures of our current strategies, which allowed us to analyze and redirect our efforts as necessary. Additionally, daily email and text communications provide meaningful touchpoints particularly for issues requiring urgent or emergent decisions. The other critical component improving delivery of care for referring physicians is a single institutional spine-tumor number, which provides a mechanism to initiate a consult without having to decide whether to send to a spine surgeon, radiation oncologist or interventional radiologist.

The weekly spine tumor board is consistently attended by radiation oncologists, neurosurgeons, orthopedic surgeons, interventional radiologists, interventional anesthesiologists, pain and palliative medicine specialists, and physiatrists. Medical oncologists often attend when they have patients to present to the tumor board. Complex and difficult spine cases are presented to the tumor board for review and expert consensus multidisciplinary panel evaluation. Thus, surgeons, radiation oncologists, medical oncologists, neuroradiologists, physiatrists, and pain management specialists can add their expertise to find solutions for such cases. For example, when managing a patient with significant positional pain and instability due to a spinal metastasis but not medically cleared for surgery, bracing may be a viable alternative with nerve blocks, optimizing medical pain management and definitive radiosurgery may be a viable alternative to surgical stabilization and radiation. Although scheduling a time that is ideal for all involved can be very challenging, stakeholders need to commit to regular attendance at this meeting. As an academic center, this tumor board is particularly helpful in the training of residents and fellows of different specialties, who can see firsthand the multidisciplinary process at work. Attendees can learn and appreciate which factors are important for each specialty to consider in developing a treatment plan. All discussions are couched in the NOMS framework. Currently, the meeting is held virtually on a teleconference platform to ease the burden of attendance.

Stereotactic Spine Radiotherapy Contour Conference is a weekly meeting attended by neurosurgeons and radiation oncologists. All stereotactic body radiation therapy (SBRT) target contours are presented for peer review prior to treatment. This meeting is an important quality control tool to make sure that all patients undergoing spine SBRT will get the same treatment, independent of the geographic location of treatment administration and the treating physician. Because the actual treatment planning of spine SBRT cases is completed automatically using expedited constrained hierarchical optimization [15], the only human input for radiation treatment planning are the target and normal tissue contours. By controlling the quality of the target and normal tissue contours, ECHO will provide consistently excellent radiotherapy treatment plans regardless of other factors such as potential variation from individual practitioners. Other factors such as the dose and fractionation of radiotherapy for a given patient are also discussed in a multidisciplinary fashion.

Monthly spine tumor meetings can be operational or research-oriented. During these meetings, discussions about workflow and practical problems with patient care such as scheduling or other operational concerns can be undertaken. Treatment policies and practices can be discussed and agreed upon as a multidisciplinary group. Multidisciplinary input regarding outcomes can be an important item for discussion. For example, since the same group of neuroradiologists read spine MRIs, they have brought up patterns of toxicity such as paraspinal myositis or vertebral body fractures that individual practitioners had not recognized. These meetings provide important avenues for communication so that the right hand knows what the left hand is doing.

At an academic institution, research and innovation are an important part of the output of the multidisciplinary spine oncology service. Innovations such as intraoperative dural plaque brachytherapy [6] and temporary organ displacement through the placement of catheters to introduce a saline bolus to displace bowel and kidneys away from radiation fields [10] were ideas spawned from multidisciplinary discussions of vexing clinical problems.

The integration of dynamic contrast-enhanced MRI imaging of the spine for assessment of treatment response to spine radiosurgery in routine clinical practice is another example of multidisciplinary translational collaboration. Preclinical models have suggested that endothelial vascular collapse by activating the acid sphyngomylienase pathway in the cell membrane of tumor endothelial cells is a unique and important mechanism of response to stereotactic radiosurgery [1], an effect that can be demonstrated with dynamic contrast-enhanced (DCE) MRI. Hence, significant effort was undertaken to use DCE MRI to assess the effect of radiosurgery on spinal tumors. In our hands, this technique has high specificity and sensitivity [8] for tumor response, and it has now been routinely incorporated into the clinic. Research protocols can be reviewed in these meetings to ensure that there are no elements of a protocol that could adversely affect the function of any given specialty, and feedback from team members can be given to improve the workflow of the study that the study author may not have fully appreciated. Authorship of peer-reviewed papers should represent the multidisciplinary nature of the work. It has been our experience that working as a team has promoted and accelerated academic productivity. In 2023, the MSKCC spine team has contributed 18 original peer-reviewed papers in the field of spine oncology.

Semiannual spine tumor service retreats are also an important tool to maintain multidisciplinary team cohesiveness. These meetings generally run for an afternoon and can serve several functions. Generally, all participating specialties are represented on the agenda. Discussions can focus on proposals for changes in practice, review of complications, or refreshers for different aspects of care. For example, a review of contour guidelines for radiation treatment can be helpful for the entire group. A more comprehensive understanding of how radiation target volumes are generated can help surgeons plan surgery when postoperative radiation is also planned. Physiatrists can better appreciate how to diagnose late radiation reactions when they have a clear understanding of how the radiation is given. Neuroradiologists can better appreciate where to expect radiation effects in normal tissues when reading MRI scans. Each discipline has an opportunity to introduce new ideas, technologies, and workflows to enhance the care of patients related to their specialty in a multidisciplinary environment to discuss the pros and cons. Ultimately a group consensus is required for changes related to spine care.

The MSKCC Spine Service also runs an annual Spine Oncology Symposium. Although the theme and emphasis of the meeting may differ from year to year, the primary goal is to promote education and training. These symposia provide vehicles to present and discuss cutting-edge technologies, emerging potentially practice-changing clinical data, and inform current practices and procedures. These meetings also serve as a way to promote dialogue between centers of excellence, remaining a constant year to year by inviting faculty with expertise from other institutions and allowing the MSKCC Spine Service to stay current and on the cutting edge of all aspects of spine oncology treatment and management.

Summary

The multidisciplinary spine oncology service at MSKCC is fundamentally successful because team members have individual expertise and skills that are brought to bear for the optimal care of a spine oncology patient in a collaborative, cohesive environment. Communication is facilitated by the NOMS framework and mutual trust, and understanding is fostered by multiple and regular meaningful points of contact within the group. In essence, team members are committed to the concept of multidisciplinary care to optimize patient care. In the end, having the right people makes it work.

References

1. Bodo S, Campagne C, Thin TH, Higginson DS, Vargas HA, Hua G, Fuller JD, Ackerstaff E, Russell J, Zhang Z, Klingler S, Cho H, Kaag MG, Mazaheri Y, Rimner A, Manova-Todorova K, Epel B, Zatcky J, Cleary CR, et al. Single-dose radiotherapy disables tumor cell homologous recombination via ischemia/reperfusion injury. J Clin Invest. 2019;129(2):786–801. https://doi.org/10.1172/JCI97631.
2. Choi BC, Pak AW. Multidisciplinarity, interdisciplinarity, and transdisciplinarity in health research, services, education and policy: 2. Promotors, barriers, and strategies of enhancement. Clin Invest Med. 2007;30(6):E224–32. https://doi.org/10.25011/cim.v30i6.2950.
3. Clapesattle H. The Doctors Mayo. The University of Minnesota Press; 1941.
4. Epstein NE. Multidisciplinary in-hospital teams improve patient outcomes: a review. Surg Neurol Int. 2014;5(Suppl 7):S295–303. https://doi.org/10.4103/2152-7806.139612.
5. Fisher CG, DiPaola CP, Ryken TC, Bilsky MH, Shaffrey CI, Berven SH, Harrop JS, Fehlings MG, Boriani S, Chou D, Schmidt MH, Polly DW, Biagini R, Burch S, Dekutoski MB, Ganju A, Gerszten PC, Gokaslan ZL, Groff MW, et al. A novel classification system for spinal instability in neoplastic disease: an evidence-based approach and expert consensus from the Spine Oncology Study Group. Spine (Phila Pa 1976). 2010;35(22):E1221–9. https://doi.org/10.1097/BRS.0b013e3181e16ae2.
6. Folkert MR, Bilsky MH, Cohen GN, Voros L, Oh JH, Zaider M, Laufer I, Yamada Y. Local recurrence outcomes using the (3)(2)P intraoperative brachytherapy plaque in the management of malignant lesions of the spine involving the dura. Brachytherapy. 2015;14(2):202–8. https://doi.org/10.1016/j.brachy.2014.10.007.
7. Hickman LD, Phillips JL, Newton PJ, Halcomb EJ, Al Abed N, Davidson PM. Multidisciplinary team interventions to optimise health outcomes for older people in acute care settings: a systematic review. Arch Gerontol Geriatr. 2015;61(3):322–9. https://doi.org/10.1016/j.archger.2015.06.021.
8. Kumar KA, Peck KK, Karimi S, Lis E, Holodny AI, Bilsky MH, Yamada Y. A pilot study evaluating the use of dynamic contrast-enhanced perfusion MRI to predict local recurrence after radiosurgery on spinal metastases. Technol Cancer Res Treat. 2017;16(6):857–65. https://doi.org/10.1177/1533034617705715.
9. Laufer I, Rubin DG, Lis E, Cox BW, Stubblefield MD, Yamada Y, Bilsky MH. The NOMS framework: approach to the treatment of spinal metastatic tumors. Oncologist. 2013;18(6):744–51. https://doi.org/10.1634/theoncologist.2012-0293.
10. Maybody M, Soliman MM, Yamada Y, Tahour D, Hsu M, Moskowitz CS, Katsoulakis E, Solomon SB. Temporary organ displacement to escalate radiation dose to retroperitoneal

tumors and decrease toxicity to organs at risk. J Vasc Interv Radiol. 2020;31(10):1578–86. https://doi.org/10.1016/j.jvir.2020.01.011.

11. Penson RT, Kyriakou H, Zuckerman D, Chabner BA, Lynch TJ Jr. Teams: communication in multidisciplinary care. Oncologist. 2006;11(5):520–6. https://doi.org/10.1634/theoncologist.11-5-520.
12. Strasser F, Sweeney C, Willey J, Benisch-Tolley S, Palmer JL, Bruera E. Impact of a half-day multidisciplinary symptom control and palliative care outpatient clinic in a comprehensive cancer center on recommendations, symptom intensity, and patient satisfaction: a retrospective descriptive study. J Pain Symptom Manag. 2004;27(6):481–91. https://doi.org/10.1016/j.jpainsymman.2003.10.011.
13. Tsai CH, Hsieh HF, Lai TW, Kung PT, Kuo WY, Tsai WC. Effect of multidisciplinary team care on the risk of recurrence in breast cancer patients: a national matched cohort study. Breast. 2020;53:68–76. https://doi.org/10.1016/j.breast.2020.07.001.
14. van Baalen S, Carusi A. Implicit trust in clinical decision-making by multidisciplinary teams. Synthese. 2019;196:4469–92. https://doi.org/10.1007/s11229-017-1475-z.
15. Zarepisheh M, Hong L, Zhou Y, Oh JH, Mechalakos JG, Hunt MA, Mageras GS, Deasy JO. Automated intensity modulated treatment planning: the expedited constrained hierarchical optimization (ECHO) system. Med Phys. 2019;46(7):2944–54. https://doi.org/10.1002/mp.13572.

Index

A
Ablative SRS, 126
Acetaminophen, 218
Actinomycin, 185
Acute onset of myelopathy, 12
Aggressive hemangiomas, 102–103, 112
Aneurysmal bone cysts, 46, 104, 112
Anterior elements, 216
Antibody-drug conjugates, 191
Anti-PD-1/anti-PD-L1, 190, 191
Anti-RANKL (receptor-activator of nuclear kappa B ligand) antibody, 78
Arc therapy, 146, 147
Automated ECHO plans, 162
Automated planning, 150, 152
  using MSK-ECHO
    ECHO, 155, 156, 159–161
    new disease site/new prescription, 158, 159
    step constrained hierarchical optimization, 157
    technical challenges, 157, 159
Autonomic dysreflexia (AD), 242

B
Back pain (fracture pain), 18
Basivertebral nerves (BVNs), 216, 220
Bevacizumab, 170, 187, 188
Bilateral pediculectomy, 14
Bilateral transpedicular approach, 22, 23
Biologic effective dose (BED), 123
Bone Fillers, 24
Bowel dysfunction, 246–247
Bracing, 244
BRAF inhibitors, 189
Bragg peak effect, 42

C
Cancer pain, 213, 214, 216, 218, 223, 244
  mechanisms of, 214
Cancer Patient Fracture Evaluation (CAFE) study, 18
Cannabinoids, 218
Carbon-fiber reinforced polyetheretherketone (CFRP) pedicle screw, 67
Celiac plexus block, 220
Cell free DNA (cfDNA), 198, 204
Cement augmentation, 56–59
Chondrosarcoma, 39
Chordomas, 5, 10, 39–44, 46, 47, 111
  clinical background, 89
  follow-up, 91
  outcomes, 90, 91
  treatment, 89, 90
  workup, 89
Chronic cancer-related pain, 213
Chronic opioid therapy, 218
Chronic pain, 213–214, 217, 219–227
  from spine tumors, 213–214
Circulating tumor DNA (ctDNA), 198, 204–206
Cohesive team approach, 255
Collapsed vertebral body, 17, 34
Colorectal carcinoma, 10

Y. Yamada et al. (eds.), *Multidisciplinary Spine Tumor Management*,
https://doi.org/10.1007/978-3-032-07519-2

Conventional external beam radiation therapy (cEBRT), 3, 4, 6–9, 12, 52, 58
vs. surgical decompression, 52
Corticosteroids, 170
CT/MRI fusion, 144–145
CT myelogram, 144–145
CT scanning protocol, 144
Cytotoxic chemotherapy, 183, 184

D
Deep venous thrombosis (DVT), 12
De novo spine, 150, 168, 169, 176, 179
neurologic tissues, MSK dosimetric guidelines for, 169
Dermatitis, 189
Disseminated metastasis, 205
DNA damage response (DDR), 202
DNA double stranded breaks (DSB), 202
Dorsal epidural tumor, 54
Dorsal root ganglion, 226–227
Doxorubicin, 184
Dysautonomia, 240–243

E
EGFR inhibitors, 188
EGFR-targeted therapy, 10
Electromyographic (EMG), 178
En bloc excision, 40, 43, 47
En bloc spondylectomy, 10, 40
En bloc surgical excision, 39
En bloc techniques, 41
En *bloc* wide excision, 40
Endoscopic spine surgery, 69
Enneking appropriate (EA), 41, 46
Enneking classification, 39, 40
Enneking surgical staging system, 76
Enneking-appropriate (EA) resection, 76, 77
Enneking-inappropriate (EI) resection, 76
Ependymoma, 96–97, 112
Epidermal growth factor receptor (EGFR), 46
Epidural or foraminal venous plexus, 26
Epidural spinal cord compression (ESCC), 4, 6–10, 14, 65, 68
Epidural steroid injection (ESI), 20, 222, 223
Epidural tumor, 14
Epstein Barr virus (EBV) ctDNA, 205
Erector spinae paraspinal injections, 20
Esophageal displacement, 46
Esophageal toxicity, 175, 176
management of, 177
minimizing risk of, 176
Evoked potentials testing, 178
Ewing's sarcoma (EWS), 95, 96, 111
Expedited constrained hierarchical optimization (ECHO)
benefits, 161
performance, 159–161
workflow, 155, 156

F
5-Fluorouracil, 185
Flattening-filter-free (FFF) photon beams, 147
Frailty, 12
Free vascularized fibula (FVF) strut grafts, 82

G
Gemcitabine, 185, 186
Giant cell tumor, 39, 46, 105, 112
Giant cell tumor of bone (GCTB), 78
Gluteus maximus advancement flaps, 83

H
Hemangioblastomas (HB), 106, 112
Hematologic tumor, 17
HER2-amplification negative, 199
High-dose radiation, 135
Hormone receptor (HR) positive, 199
Hybrid therapy, 5, 7–10, 55, 58, 59, 65

I
Image-guided intensity modulated radiation therapy, 42
Immune checkpoint inhibitors (ICI), 189
Immunotherapy, 189, 190, 198
Inflated bone tamps, 22, 25
Intensity modulated radiation therapy (IMRT), 146–148
Intracompartmental chordoma, 43
Intradural-extramedullary tumors, 69
Intrathecal pumps, 223
Irinotecan, 186

K
KEAP1, 203
Ketamine, 218
Knowledge-based planning (KBP), 152
Kyphoplasty, 17–19, 21, 22, 26–36, 56, 57, 66
trocars, 22, 26, 32, 33, 35

L

Laser interstitial thermal therapy (LITT), 69
Liquid biopsy, 206
L2 kyphoplasty, 34
Lumbar sympathetic blocks (LSB), 219
Lytic disease, 13

M

Mammalian target of rapamycin (mTOR), 46
Mechanical instability, 11, 14
Mechanical stability, 65
Meningiomas, 100–102, 112
Metastatic epidural disease, 52
Metastatic epidural spinal cord compression (MESCC), 52, 53, 58, 59
Metastatic sacral tumors, 83, 84
Metastatic Stage IV papillary thyroid carcinoma, 13
Metastatic thoracolumbar compression fractures, 67
Minimally invasive spine surgery (MISS)
- application of, 65
- endoscopic spine surgery, 69
- laser interstitial thermal therapy, 69
- limitations, 70
- metastatic thoracolumbar compression fractures, 67
- navigation, 68
- NOMS framework, 65
- robotics, 69
- in spinal tumor management, 65
- in spine oncology
  - PPSI, 66
  - spinal cord or nerve root decompression with tumor resection, 68
  - surgical stabilization, 66–68
  - vertebral cement augmentation, 66
- stabilization, 65
- *vs.* traditional open spine surgery, 64

Minimally invasive surgical approaches, 198
Mobile spine chordoma, 47
Mobile spine tumors, 44
MSK-IMPACT, 199
MSK vertebral ablation, 35
Multidisciplinary care, 255
Multidisciplinary management
- metastatic sacral tumors, 83, 84
- primary sacral tumors, 76–83
  - complications, 79, 80
  - emerging medical therapies, 78
  - Enneking-appropriate resection, 76
  - Enneking-inappropriate resection, 76
  - outcomes, 78–79
  - reconstruction, 81–83
  - sacral anatomy and biomechanics, 80–81
  - salvage options, 77, 78
  - tumor ablation, 76

Multidisciplinary spine care, 256–257
Multidisciplinary spine oncology service functions, 255, 256
- program, features of, 257
- regular points of contact, 258–260

Multi-disciplinary spine tumor care, 1
Multiple criteria optimization (MCO), 152
Multiple robotic systems, 69
Myelopathy, 126, 168
- management of, 170
- minimizing risk, 169, 170

Myokymic discharge, 178
Myositis, 173–175

N

Neuraxial-based techniques, 222
Neuroanatomy, 214–215
Neurologic dysfunction and sequelae, 239–240
Neurologic, oncologic, mechanical, systemic (NOMS) framework, 198, 257
Neurologic status, 65
Neurologic tissues, 168, 169
- MSK dosimetric guidelines for, 169

Neuromodulation, 224–227
- alternative sites for, 226–227

Neuropathic pain, 218
Neuropathy, 126
New England Spinal Metastases Score, 12
Nifedipine, 242
Nitrates, 242
NOMS decision framework, 65, 126
- assessment, 14
- case study, 13
- mechanical instability, 11
- neurologic consideration, 6
- oncologic consideration, 6–7
- radiosensitive tumors, 7
  - ESCC 0 to 1c, SSRS, 8
  - ESCC 2 without myelopathy, 9
  - ESCC 2-3 with or without myelopathy, 9, 10
- systemic assessment, 11–14
- unknown tumor with myelopathy, 10

Non-steroidal anti-inflammatory drugs (NSAIDs), 218
NRF2, 203

O
Oligometastatic disease, 35, 205
Oligometastatic spine disease, 205
Oncologic pain
  medical management of, 216–219
    opioid analgesics, 216
Oncologic status, 65
Opioid analgesics, 216
Opioids, 244
Orthostatic hypotension, 242–243
Osteogenic sarcoma, 46
Osteoporosis, 249

P
Pain, 243–245
Pain flare, 167, 168
  management of, 168
  minimizing risk of, 168
Pain management, 1
  intrathecal drug delivery systems, 223, 224
  spinal cord stimulation, 224–227
  spine tumors, 213
    adjuncts to opioid medications, 218
    anterior elements, 216, 217
    cancer pain, mechanisms of, 214
    epidural steroid injections, 222, 223
    interventional modalities, 219
    kyphoplasty, 221
    neuroanatomy, 214, 215
    opioid analgesics, 216
    posterior element disease, 221, 222
    posterior elements, 216
    sympathetic nervous system, 219, 220
    vertebrogenic pain, procedures for, 220, 221
Paragangliomas, 107, 112
Patient immobilization, 142, 143
Patient setup, 154, 155
Pedicled VRAM pull-through flap, 83
Percutaneous instrumentation, 59
Percutaneous kyphoplasty (PKP), 17, 19, 21, 32
Percutaneous pedicle screw instrumentation (PPSI), 66
Percutaneous vertebroplasty (PVP), 17, 21
Peripheral nerve stimulation, 226–227
Photon-based stereotactic radiosurgery, 42
PI3K, 203
Plan check tool (PCT), 154
Planning risk volume (PRV), 145
Platelet-derived growth factor receptor (PEGFR), 46
Plexopathy, 177, 178
  management of, 179
  minimizing risk of, 178
Pneumonitis, 185
Polymethyl methacrylate (PMMA), 17, 18, 24–26, 29–33, 35, 55
  bone cement augmentation, 68
Posterior element disease, 221–222
Posterior elements, 216
Post-Operative Radiation Therapy Outcomes Score (PORTOS), 202
Post radiation paraspinal myositis, 28
Post-surgical cardiopulmonary complications, 14
Precision oncology, 206
Pressure ulcers, 249
Primary bone tumors, 46
Primary sacral tumors, 76–83
  complications, 79, 80
  emerging medical therapies, 78
  Enneking-appropriate resection, 76
  Enneking-inappropriate resection, 76
  outcomes, 78–79
  reconstruction, 81–83
  sacral anatomy and biomechanics, 80–81
  salvage options, 77, 78
  tumor ablation, 76
Primary sarcomas of the spine, 93–95, 111
  background, 93
  follow-up, 95
  outcomes, 94
  treatment, 94
  workup, 94
Proton-beam and carbon ion radiation techniques, 42
Proton beam radiation, 42

Q
Quality assurance (QA), 153

R
Radiation-induced DNA damage, 203
Radiation-induced plexopathy (RIP), 177
Radiation myositis, 173
Radiation recall reactions, 176
Radiation therapy, 17, 29
Radiation toxicity, 42
Radiobiology, 125
Radioresistance, 203
Radioresistant solid tumor histologies, 126
Radiosensitive tumors, 7

ESCC 0 to 1c, SSRS, 8
ESCC 2 without myelopathy, 9
ESCC 2-3 with or without myelopathy, 9, 10
Radiosensitivity, 10, 201–204
genetic biomarkers of, 201–204
Radiotherapy (RT), 183
actinomycin, 185
antibody-drug conjugates, 191
anti-PD-1/anti-PD-L1, 190, 191
bevacizumab, 187, 188
BRAF inhibitors, 189
cytotoxic chemotherapy, 183, 184
doxorubicin, 184
EGFR inhibitors, 188
5-fluorouracil, 185
gemcitabine, 185, 186
immunotherapy, 189, 190
irinotecan, 186
systemic therapies, 192
targeted therapies, 187
taxanes, 187
T-DM1, 191
Rat sarcoma virus (RAS) signaling pathway, 203
Rectal injury, 79
Rehabilitation
medicine, 1
in spine tumor
autonomic dysreflexia, 242
bladder dysfunction, 247, 248
bowel dysfunction, 246, 247
dysautonomia, 240, 242
goals, 239
neurologic dysfunction and sequelae, 239, 240
orthostatic hypotension, 242, 243
osteoporosis, 249
outcomes and survival, 250, 251
pain, 243–245
physiatry evaluation, 238
setting, 236, 237
sexual function, 250
skin, 249
Re-irradiation spine, 168, 169, 177, 179
neurologic tissues, MSK dosimetric guidelines for, 169
Relative biological effectiveness (RBE), 42, 43
Robotics, 69
Rotational VRAM pull-through flap, 83

S
SABR-COMET trial, 12
Sacral chordoma, 75–77
Sacral neuropathy, 43
Sacral tumors
metastases, 83, 84
primary
complications, 79, 80
emerging medical therapies, 78
Enneking-appropriate resection, 76
Enneking-inappropriate resection, 76
outcomes, 78–79
reconstruction, 81–83
sacral anatomy and biomechanics, 80–81
salvage options, 77, 78
tumor ablation, 76
Schwannoma, 100, 112
Segmental instrumentation, 52
Semiannual spine tumor service, 260
Separation surgery, 65
historical evolution, 52–54
hybrid therapy, 58
minimally invasive trends, 58–59
surgical technique, 54–57, 60
Sexual function, 250
Single nucleotide polymorphisms (SNPs), 202
SINS criteria, 11, 14
Skin, 249
Small intercompartmental tumors, 40
SMARCB1, 46
Solitary plasmacytomas, 113
Solitary plasmacytomas of bone (SBP), 109, 111
SORG nomogram, 12
Spinal cord, 214–216
astrocytomas, 98–100, 112
decompression, 10, 55, 56, 59
delineation
with CT myelogram or CT/MRI fusion, 144, 145
Spinal cord injury (SCI), 136, 236
Spinal cord stimulation, 224–225
Spinal instability neoplastic score (SINS) system, 65, 66, 172
Spinal navigation, 68
Spinal oncology, 256
Spine metastases, 197
biology of, 198–200
genomic biomarkers
local spine tumor control, targeted systemic therapy for, 204
overall prognosis and risk stratification, 200
radiosensitivity, 201–204
management of, 198
management, circulating tumor DNA in, 204–206

Spine metastases (*cont.*)
stereotactic radiosurgery and stereotactic body radiation therapy, 124
high-dose stereotactic radiosurgery, 125, 126
radiobiology, 125
reirradiation, 136, 137
re-irradiation with spine SBRT, 127–129
stereotactic body radiation therapy, 126, 135
surgery and SRS/SBRT, 135, 136
stereotactic radiotherapy for, 124
Spine radiation toxicity and management
esophageal toxicity, 175, 176
management of, 177
minimizing risk of, 176
myelopathy, 168
management of, 170
minimizing risk, 169, 170
myositis, 173–175
pain flare, 167, 168
management of, 168
minimizing risk of, 168
plexopathy, 177, 178
management of, 179
minimizing risk of, 178
vertebral compression fracture, 171
management of, 172
minimizing risk of, 171
Spine SBRT, 111, 112, 126, 127, 131, 135, 136, 138, 141–163, 167–169, 171, 173–176, 178, 180, 189, 259
algorithm, surgical evaluation prior to, 173
Spine stereotactic radiosurgery (sSRS), 3–10, 52, 53, 126, 130
Spine tumor, 256
pain management of, 213
adjuncts to opioid medications, 218, 219
anterior elements, 216, 217
cancer pain, mechanisms of, 214
epidural steroid injections, 222, 223
interventional modalities, 219
intrathecal drug delivery systems, 223, 224
kyphoplasty, 221
neuroanatomy, 214, 215
opioid analgesics, 216
posterior element disease, 221, 222
posterior elements, 216
spinal cord stimulation, 224–227
sympathetic nervous system, 219, 220
vertebrogenic pain, procedures for, 220, 221
rehabilitation in
autonomic dysreflexia, 242
bladder dysfunction, 247, 248
bowel dysfunction, 246, 247
dysautonomia, 240, 242
goals, 239
neurologic dysfunction and sequelae, 239, 240
orthostatic hypotension, 242, 243
osteoporosis, 249
outcomes and survival, 250, 251
pain, 243–245
physiatry evaluation, 238
sexual function, 250
skin, 249
thermodysregulation, 243
setting
rehabilitation in, 236, 237
Spinopelvic skeletal reconstruction, 83
Stellate ganglion blocks (SGB), 219
Stereotactic body radiation therapy (SBRT), 40, 42, 43, 45–47, 65, 68, 69, 123, 135–136, 141
automated planning using MSK-ECHO
ECHO benefits, 161
ECHO performance, 159–161
ECHO workflow, 155, 156
new disease site/new prescription, 158, 159
step constrained hierarchical optimization, 157
technical challenges, 157, 159
imaging, simulation, and immobilization, 142
CT scanning protocol, 144
patient immobilization, 142, 143
spinal cord delineation with CT myelogram or CT/MRI fusion, 144, 145
target delineation, 146
imaging techniques, 141
implemention, 141
patient setup and treatment delivery, 154, 155
planning techniques, clinical criteria, plan evaluation
automated planning, 150, 152
clinical criteria, 148, 149
IMRT and arc therapy, 146, 147
MSKCC, dosimetric guidelines, 150, 151
quality assurance, 153
Stereotactic radiosurgery (SRS), 124, 135–136, 198

Stereotactic radiotherapy
  for spine metastases, 124
  and stereotactic body radiation therapy, 124
    high-dose stereotactic radiosurgery, 125, 126
    radiobiology, 125
    reirradiation, 136, 137
    re-irradiation with spine SBRT, 127–129
    stereotactic body radiation therapy, 126, 135
    surgery and SRS/SBRT, 135, 136
Stereotactic Spine Radiotherapy Contour Conference, 259
Surgery, 135–136
Systemic status, 65
Systemic therapies, 192

T
Target delineation, 146
Targeted systemic therapies, 198
Targeted therapies, 187
Taxanes, 187
Temperature regulation, 243
T6 laminectomy, 14
Total sacrectomy, 78, 81–83
TP53, 202
Transformative pillars, 198
Transpedicular approach, 22–24
Trastuzumab-emtansine (T-DM1), 191
Tumor ablation, 76
Tumor radiosensitivity, 10

V
Vascular endothelial growth factor receptor (VEGFR), 46
Vertebral body fractures, 135
Vertebral cement augmentation (VCA), 66
  cancer treatments, 17
  end of life care, 36
  final AP and lateral X-rays, 26
  fluoroscopy, 34, 35
  fracture progression, 19, 26–34
  kyphoplasty, effects of, 26–29
  MRI, 21, 22
  patient selection, 18–20
  persistent or recurrent pain post kyphoplasty—post-kyphoplasty fracture progression, 28–31
  PMMA, 17, 24–26
  primary goal or indication, 19–21
  RF ablation, 35
  technical aspects, 21, 22
Vertebral compression fracture (VCF), 171
  management of, 172
  minimizing risk of, 171
Vertebroplasty, 57, 66
Vertebroplasty effect, 32
Vertical rectus abdominis musculocutaneous (VRAM) pull-through flap, 83
Visual Analogue Scale (VAS) pain score, 19, 21
Volumetric arc therapy, 42
Volumetric modulated arc therapy (VMAT), 147

MIX
Papier aus verantwortungsvollen Quellen
Paper from responsible sources
FSC® C105338

If you have any concerns about our products,
you can contact us on
ProductSafety@springernature.com

In case Publisher is established outside the EU,
the EU authorized representative is:
Springer Nature Customer Service Center GmbH
Europaplatz 3, 69115 Heidelberg, Germany

Printed by Libri Plureos GmbH
in Hamburg, Germany